Clinical Assessment and Treatment of HIV
Rehabilitation of a Chronic Illness

Edited by
Mary Lou Galantino, MS, PT
Assistant Professor, Division of Physical Therapy
Stockton State College
Pomona, NJ, USA

Private Practice, L.I.F.E. Physical Therapy

SLACK Incorporated, 6900 Grove Road, Thorofare, NJ 08086-9447.

Cover design by Bob Hochgertel

Printed in the United States of America

Library of Congress Catalog Card Number: 90-53246

ISBN: 1-55642-181-8

Published by: SLACK Incorporated
               6900 Grove Road
               Thorofare, NJ 08086-9447

       Last digit is print number: 10   9   8   7   6   5   4   3   2

DEDICATION

You are with one who is dying in the same way you are with yourself. Open, honest, and caring. You are simply there, listening with a heart that is willing to hold the joy or pain of another with equal compassion, with a mind that does not separate life from death, that does not live in concepts and shadows but in the direct experience of the unfolding.

The pages of this book unfold through people living with HIV and those no longer with us, whose spirits reside throughout my work. I dedicate this book to my patients who have taught me how to explore treatment approaches when the AIDS epidemic first presented itself in the early 1980s. They have supported me in continuing in the adventures of this field.

It is they who inspire me to continue to write and lecture.

Contents

Foreword

"Immunoagility:" can it be achieved? We are caught up in a race between ecodestruction and viral besiegement. Viruses are using our lack of consideration for Mother Earth as an ally in their assault upon the living. As our environment qualitatively deteriorates, our natural ability to resist entities such as viruses is reduced.

Viruses are opportunists and, as such, constantly search for the Achilles heel so that they can make entry into host cells and alter the nucleic acid proteins therein. Viruses are extremely adept at mutational change. The life span of a virus can be measured in hours. The virus is a protein bag of nucleic acids (both DNA and RNA) that requires penetration of a host cell in order to reproduce. In so doing, it changes the nucleic acids in the host cell to suit its own purpose and enhance its replicating abilities. Even though the life span of a virus can be measured in hours, it is capable of causing significant host cell and self mutation during that time. We all want to survive. Perhaps even the virus, somewhere in its genetic makeup, has a survival gene and instinct that acts at the expense of the life of its host.

In the case of HIV, it is most difficult to find a magic potion that will be effective against the invading virus because the virus establishes itself inside the host cell. Thus, the medicinal molecule must enter the host cell and not be as toxic to the host as it is to the virus. Second, as the new generations of viruses are born, they seem able to mutate in order to resist and successfully adapt to the new drug. We must continue to pursue this allopathic avenue of treatment, keeping in mind the extreme adaptive ability of the virus and the fact that we could kill the host as well as the virus.

Another avenue of approach to the problem of HIV invasion is the enhancement of host resistance, and what I call "immunoagility." Quite simply, the healthier the host and the better the immune system function, the better the host's ability to improvise effective defenses against viral invasions.

How do we improve the health of humankind? We improve the environment and the living conditions for all, not just for select societal segments. To reduce the strength of HIV invasion, we must reduce the number of vulnerable hosts. It would seem that the HIV virus may be demonstrating to all of us that there can be no health or biologic isolationism. People need to live in healthy, clean places with good nutritious food on a daily basis. People need to live where there is clean air to breath; clean water to drink; nontoxic and fertile land in which to grow food; and clean oceans, seas and lakes for aquatic life. HIV will not let us forget our responsibilities in this area--to ourselves and to others.

We must also recognize that good physical health cannot exist without motion. Bodies, tissues, cells and their membranes, fluids and molecules all have to move. Stasis is the precursor of death. All therapies that establish motion must work together to enhance health. Exercise, the multitude of manipulative techniques, massage therapy, fluid-moving therapies, craniosacral therapy, myofascial release therapy, energy therapies and all the others must be eclectically used without prejudice to establish the optimal physical mobility possible. Health care professionals must transcend political and/or therapeutic differences in attempts to facilitate movement in our patients.

The immunity against HIV can be enhanced by the use of immunostimulant vaccines. This virus seems a little more difficult to understand than some of the others against which vaccines have been so successful (ie. smallpox, measles, polio). One report stated that 20 variants of HIV were identified in a single host from one tissue sample. If this is true, the implications are incredible! They strongly suggest that we will do better by enhancing host resistance and "immunoagility" than we will by trying to kill a virus as resourceful as this one or by trying to "outguess it" with a vaccine.

HIV, as a chronic illness, mandates a collective work effort. Ego and power politics can retard this effort. HIV is reminding humankind that we must clean up, respect and love Mother Earth.

I believe we all bear the responsibility and can work in cooperation toward a solution to this problem. No single discipline or therapeutic approach has the answer. Can we extract something positive from the HIV epidemic? Can we more equally share the gifts of Mother Earth and life with each other? Can we learn to appreciate and not exploit our environment? Time will tell. Perhaps sooner than we would like to admit.

—John E. Upledger, DO, FAAO

Preface

Greek mythology tells us that in his second Labour, Hercules son of Zeus, was called upon to confront the nine-headed Hydra of Lerna. The Hydra proved to be the most formidable of foes for several reasons. Legend has it that the middle head of the Hydra was immortal. As Hercules would smote and sever one of the mortal heads, two more, equally as venomous, grew back only to make his efforts that much more difficult. The prototype for all great warriors, Hercules not only overpowered but was able to outwit his adversaries as well. He fought to immobilize the immortal head and sequentially reduce the power of the beast by conflagration of the mortal heads. When the beast was most vulnerable, he impaled the immortal head with poisonous arrows. Ironically, the arrows were also dipped in the blood of the Hydra so that no antidote could be formulated.

The ravages of HIV have been understated, overstated and misstated in the past ten years. Miscommunication has led to mistrust and ultimately to dispositions based on myths rather than facts. Just as Franklin Delano Roosevelt cautioned his fellow Americans that their fear was more of fear itself rather than Nazi Germany, the providers of health care should perhaps take note of successful responses to crises throughout history.

A notable example of such a response was America's effort during World War II. First, as Roosevelt so vividly discerned, negative energy spent on fear had to be rerouted in a positive direction. The ideology was unselfishness and the methodology was hard work. So as fear (in this case the immortal head) was immobilized, the power of the mortal heads was reduced in the battles fought in the various campaigns worldwide.

Victory for many was not altogether sweet. For some, victory meant survival and a chance to rebuild. In the name of victory, many died or were scarred for life. Family units were disrupted and childhoods shortened. Yet, the aftermath of war brought a period of reconstruction unparalleled in history. Out of destruction and devastation came construction and innovation.

Now we are at war with a virus and a disease that is reminiscent of past wars. Epidemiology, immunology and medical research are attempting to immobilize the immortal head of the Hydra by containing the fear surrounding HIV. With the advent of life-sustaining drugs, the allied health professions must coordinate their efforts to enhance the quality of life. Lawmakers must be firm and fair regarding the legislation affecting providership of care. Adequate knowledge of the scope and capabilities of other disciplines provides the clinician with the ability to deliver care focally. The clinician can then fight one head of the Hydra and be confident that the other heads are equally confronted by his allies. The creative aspects of interchange among clinicians and patients offer insights into another domain of function and quality of life. Ultimately, this will prevent engulfment of the patient as well as the clinician by the ravages of the Hydra.

The road to victory in this battle is a long and arduous one. Hercules would advise us to 1) carefully but quickly discern the enemy's strengths and weaknesses, 2) engage the adversary with an organized plan of action, and 3) contest the foe vigorously but retreat when indicated. With knowledge, the fear of this monster will not loom so ominously over humankind. With a unified effort by patients, health care providers, care givers, and business and government, the physical, personal, social, moral, legal, ethical and emotional problems can be diminished and eventually eliminated. The valiant efforts of people during crises throughout history should serve as the template for successfully overcoming the ravages of this disease. As with the Lernaed Hydra, HIV will fall not to poison arrows but rather to intelligence, strength, perseverance and courage.

—Rick Dellagatta, MEd, PT

Acknowledgments

As the list of contributors shows, many individuals have demonstrated their expertise in the formulation of this book. Throughout the 1980s, I have been honored to be associated with many professionals, several of whom have become close friends.

I am grateful to the staff at Rehabilitation Data Systems and Maple Leaf Physical Therapy, particularly Steve Ranere, assistant CEO, for his "brainstorm ideas" in manuscript preparation and entire technical layout of this project; and to my support staff at Rice Village Physical Therapy—Maria McGinnis, Savitry Ramsaran and my associate Osie Steinberg—for their commitment and dedication to my work.

To Arthur Slaughter, who maintained my pursuit of writing through the memories of Gary. To David Turner and Terri Segal for their creative illustrations and bringing forth many concepts. To Grace Ann Bertram, PT and Kelly Sacky, PTA who provided technical assistance. To Marti Brewer, who bravely explored a clinical affiliation with me at a hospice setting as a premedical student, only to discover her role in writing.

To my family, who has come to understand my professional commitment to the HIV population. To Michael Pizzi, who continues to live in the enthusiasm of this work through our writing and lectures. To Ricky Dellagatta, who essentially became my coeditor and truly exemplified the meaning of the word "partnership" on many levels.

And ultimately, to people living with HIV, who spent endless hours in their own "soul-searching" as they wrote their innermost thoughts to share with the reader.

Thank you.

Introduction

The continuum of time is often symbolized by the purifying and seemingly endless journey of a river. As the tributaries merge to form the river's body, old and new models of health care coalesce to create new direction for health care providers' thoughts. This theme echoes throughout the HIV epidemic. In recent years, the concepts of health and illness, along with methods of health care delivery, have been critically evaluated. The belief that medicine, grounded in the natural sciences, provides the only means for disease intervention is being questioned. Sufficient notoriety now exists to warrant the investigation of complementary therapies of health care that are both noninvasive and noniatrogenic.

Looking at the possible models of available health care, we can view three distinct arenas. The first is a direct intervention model by one primary health care professional. In the second model, more than one health care professional can evaluate and manage by their own model within the realm of their specialty. The third arena is an interactive model of multifocal intervention with function of the individual as the ultimate goal. The intent of this book is twofold: first, to provide a treatise on the various modes of intervention in HIV disease and second, to promote harmonious interaction among these disciplines for the purpose of improving quality of life.

Through my experience with persons with HIV disease, I have borne witness to the behaviors that result from resistance to changes in one's model of life. For instance, imagine that an illness has severely and cruelly depleted your body's energy stores, and you cannot participate in the world in the ways you have become accustomed. Imagine, also, the erosion of your personal and professional stability and consider its potentially devastating consequences. Denial and resistance to change imposed by this illness are caused by one's desire for things to be other than they are. As the jaws of the vise close tighter, the model of life as you have known it is no longer viable. How painful it is when you can no longer fulfill your imagined reality. You wonder to yourself: "Who am I?" "Who is dying?" "Who is living?"

You don't know quite who you are because you can't carry out your specialty any longer. As your role and identity in the world is greatly threatened, you are embattled from within yourself. The grace and serenity of moving on are violently restrained by adherence to the arbitrary values of a time past.

Can we go beyond this already existing model? Against a background of fear and uncertainty, persons with HIV disease develop major concerns while navigating their way through the complex health care system and relating to the people responsible for their care. As patients strive to go beyond known models and roles, health care professionals also have the opportunity to expand the traditional boundaries of medicine. The established foundations of medicine in conjunction with holistic health may more completely address the spiritual, environmental and physical domains of our lives. The merger of these ideologies transcends the boundaries of health care recipient or provider.

A holistic approach to rehabilitation may necessitate a shift in our perception of current practices. Emphasis can be placed on sharing decision making and establishing goals for both patient and therapist. A central factor in holistic rehabilitation depends equally on what one does with a patient and how one does it. It is essential to focus on the interdependence between client and practitioner as well as between disciplines. Sharing power, exchanging views and interpreting actively, engage the patient in his or her own recovery. Emphasis is placed on the whole rather than on the symptom.

As a chronic illness, HIV disease further depicts this concept of comprehensive rehabilitation. Just like other diseases requiring long-term care, the HIV spectrum of disorders is deserving of rehabilitation services. Health is regarded as unique to each individual, depending on his or her lifestyle and including not only the absence of symptoms but a complete state of physical and mental well-being.

My hope is that the reader will challenge existing models, assimilate the knowledge presented in this book, search for new dimensions of care for humans and above all, allow for self-exploration in the journey; for it enhances the adventure along the way.

—Mary Lou Galantino, MS, PT

About the Editor

Mary Lou Galantino, MS, PT, has made her professional commitment to the transformation of rehabilitation through continued research and clinical application in the arenas of chronic pain, oncology and HIV disease. She graduated from University of Pittsburgh in 1982 and acquired her Advanced Master's Degree in Physical Therapy at Texas Women's University in 1989.

She has published numerous articles and presented workshops in Europe and the United States on holistic rehabilitation for these patients. Formerly Director of Physical Therapy for the Institute for Immunological Disorders in Houston, Texas, Mary Lou is the founder of Living In Full Expression (LIFE) Physical Therapy, a private practice, and is presently an Assistant Professor at Stockton State College in New Jersey. She is a consultant in HIV, hospice and chronic illness.

Contributing Authors

Michael H. Antoni, PhD
Department of Psychology
University of Miami
Coral Gables, Florida

Rick Dellagatta, MEd, PT
CEO of Rehabilitation Data Systems
Assistant Professor of Stockton State College
Private Practice: Maple Leaf Physical Therapy
Hammonton, New Jersey

Byron St. Dizier, PhD
Associate Professor of Communication Studies
University of Alabama
Birmingham, Alabama

Richard C. Elbein, MS, RD, LD
Director of Dietary Services
Belle Park Hospital
Houston, Texas

Robert L. Falletti, MS
Project Director
AIDS Regional Education and Training Center for
Texas and Oklahoma Health Professionals
Houston, Texas

Mary Ann Fletcher, MD
Department of Medicine
University of Miami School of Medicine
Miami, Florida

Paul R. Gustafson, MD, FACP
Internal Medicine and Oncology
Houston, Texas

Mary Hilliard, RN, MS, LPC
Unity Total Health Program
Creative Psychotherapy
Houston, Texas

Arthur LaPerriere, PhD
Center for Biopsychosocial Studies of AIDS
Department of Psychiatry
University of Miami School of Medicine
Miami, Florida

Joel K. Levy
Baylor College of Medicine
Department of Psychiatry
Houston, Texas

Peter W.A. Mansell, MS, MB, BCh, FRCS
Medical Consultant
President of Physicians Association for AIDS Care
Houston, Texas

Grace Moffat Minerbo, MD, PhD
Visiting Associate Professor
Texas Woman's University
Houston, Texas

Guy McCormack, MS, OT
Associate Professor
San Jose State University
San Jose, California

Deirdre McDowell, PT
Texas Medical Center
Houston, Texas

Ann Giffin Monson, MS, PT
Director of Rehabilitation Services
University of Tennessee Medical Center at Knoxville
Knoxville, Tennessee

Eugenie A.M.T. Obbens, MD, PhD
Clinical Associate Professor of Neurology
University of Arizona Health Sciences Center
Tucson, Arizona

Michael W. O'Dell, MD
Physical Medicine and Rehabilitation
The Graduate Hospital
Philadelphia, Pennsylvania

Michael Pizzi, MS, OTR/L
Private Practice
Occupational Therapist
Wellness Consultant
Silver Spring, Maryland

Neil Schneiderman, PhD
Department of Psychology
University of Miami
Coral Gables, Florida

William A. Scott, CSW
President of N.G.L.H.S.
Private Practice:
New Counseling Center
Houston, Texas

Donald Skipwith, Attorney at Law
Houston, Texas

Tina Sweezey, MS, PT
Department of Physical Therapy
Mediplex Rehabilitation-Camden
Camden, New Jersey

People living with HIV (Chapter 19)
Christine, Michael, Brad: Houston, Texas
Stuart: Ten Mile Lake, Minnesota
Byron: Birmingham, Alabama

1

An Introduction to the Medical Management of HIV Infection

Peter W. A. Mansell, MA, MB, BCh, FRCS

Living is not only living good, but living well. The wise man, therefore, lives as long as he should, not as long as he can. He will think of life in terms of quality not quantity.

—Lucius Annaeus Seneca

INTRODUCTION

As the natural history of HIV continually unfolds, improved methods of treating the opportunistic infections of the disease become available. This chapter is an introduction to the medical management of the human immunodeficiency virus (HIV) infection and an overview of some of the drug therapies in current use.

The acquired immunodeficiency syndrome (AIDS) is caused by infection with HIV, which was originally discovered in 1983 at the Pasteur Institute in Paris. A retrovirus, HIV is transmitted either sexually, perinatally or by means of contaminated blood or blood products. The infection is chronic with a mathematically projected AIDS-free median time of 11 years after seroconversion (Phuir et al., 1989; Luis et al., 1988).

The virus infects cells in the immune system preferentially and also targets epithelial cells and cells in the central nervous system (CNS). Large quantities of the virus are found in body fluids such as semen, blood and vaginal secretions and has been isolated in small quantities in other fluids such as saliva. HIV infection is a relentless condition resulting in autoimmune dysfunction, with resultant death due to secondary infections.

Although treatment methods have improved, the long-term prognosis remains poor.

COURSE OF THE DISEASE

The course of HIV is progressive and the various stages can be categorized by signs, symptoms and cell count. The Centers for Disease Control (CDC) classifies HIV infections into four groups according to signs and symptoms. The Walter Reed Staging System correlates events of the disease progression with the quantity of T-helper cells within six stages (see Appendix A) (Centers for Disease Control, 1986; Redfield et al., 1986). For discussion purposes, the CDC Classification System will be used to depict the progression and management of HIV.

Group I—Acute Infection

Frequently after initial infection, there is a brief febrile illness that may be accompanied by a generalized rash and a mononucleosis. This condition often clears within two weeks, leaving the patient well and usually unaware of what has happened.

Group II—Asymptomatic Infection

A period of asymptomatic infection then follows during which the patient feels well, can work and can pass the infection on to others. This period may last for several years. People in this stage of the disease are theoretically in the most advantageous period for treatment with an antiviral agent. Unfortunately patients are seldom, if ever, identified at this early stage because the flu-like symptoms are so mild. Aseptic meningitis may or may not be present during this phase. Patients may be classified on the basis of complete blood count (CBC), platelet count and T4 and T8 counts.

Group III—Persistent Generalized Lymphadenopathy

The next easily recognizable point in the spectrum of infection is that of lymphadenopathy. At this stage, a painless enlargement of lymph nodes usually appears at two or more extrainguinal sites. In some cases, the nodes can get very large and sometimes tender. This seems to be an indication of an immune response at the cellular level. Subclassifications in this group may be made by laboratory analysis as in group II.

Group IV—Other Diseases

The next stage of the disease may occur with or without lymph node swelling. This stage is defined by five separate but not necessarily distinct subgroups from A to E. The groups consist of constitutional, neurologic, secondary infectious diseases; secondary cancers; and other diseases.

Subgroup A, constitutional diseases, formerly termed AIDS related complex (ARC) or wasting syndrome is defined as a collection of symptoms that include the following:

1. fever lasting more than one month
2. weight loss of greater than 10 percent
3. night sweats and diarrhea lasting more than one month

Patients can be extremely ill or die in subgroup A without the manifestations of the other subgroups.

Subgroup B (neurologic disease) may include the presence of dementia, myelopathy and peripheral neuropathy, which may be observed singly or in combination. Acute and subacute myelopathies include transverse myelitis due to varicella zoster virus or herpes zoster virus (HZV), spinal epidural or intradural lymphoma, and polyradiculopathy secondary to cytomegalovirus (CMV) (Devinsky et al., 1987; Miller et al., 1989; Tucker et al., 1985). Some subacute as well as chronic progressive myelopathies appear to be far more common than the acute myelopathies. Slow progressive vacuolar myelopathies are usually seen with dementia and are conventionally referred to as AIDS dementia complex (Navia et al., 1986; Petito et al., 1985). Myelopathy in the HIV-1 infected individual may be caused by coinfection of a second retrovirus, human lymphotrophic virus type I (HTLV-I) (Brew et al., 1989; Rosenblum et al., 1989).

Peripheral neuropathies occurring in the latter phases of HIV-1 infection are most commonly those caused by herpes zoster virus and CMV (Eidelberg et al., 1986) as well as distal sensory axonal neuropathies (Snider et al., 1988). Toxic axonal neuropathies caused by antiviral and autonomic neuropathies have been noted in this subcategory (Price et al., 1990; Yarchoan et al., 1989; Craddock et al., 1987; Lin-Greenberg & Taneja-Uppal, 1987).

Subgroup C is further subdivided into category C-1 (secondary infectious diseases). Opportunistic infections such as *Pneumocystis carinii* pneumonia (PCP), toxoplasmosis and CMV infection are representative but not all inclusive of this grouping. Other specified secondary infectious diseases such as oral hairy leukoplakia, multidermatomal herpes zoster, oral candidiasis and tuberculosis comprise some of the listings of category C-2.

Subgroup D, the secondary cancers, includes Kaposi's sarcoma (KS), non-Hodgkin's lymphoma and primary lymphoma of the brain. Most noteworthy is Kaposi's sarcoma, which was first described in 1872 by Moritz Kaposi, a Hungarian dermatologist. In its classic form, this rare lesion was a multicentric, pigmented sarcoma usually appearing on the legs, predominantly in older men of Jewish and Eastern European origin (Ziegler & Dorfman, 1988).

Through the decades, four types of KS have been identified: 1) modular, 2) florid, 3) infiltrative, and 4) lymphodemopathic. In 1980, the first cases of AIDS were heralded by an unexplained appearance of KS in homosexual men. In the early years of the epidemic, KS accounted for over 40 percent of AIDS; Since 1986, the proportion of KS in AIDS patients has gradually dropped below 20 percent (Ziegler, 1990).

Typical treatment regimens include a host of antineoplastic drugs including vincristine, vinblastine, bleomycin and local low-dose radiation treatments. These treatments may have various side effects, including chemotherapy-induced peripheral neuropathy pain and overall decreased functional ambulation secondary to lesion enhancement in the lower extremities.

KS may also appear on the mucous membrane of the oral cavity, particularly on the hard palate. When this occurs, adequate nutritional intake may be prohibited because eating and swallowing may be painful. Additional sources of pain may be referred from the viscera with extensive KS lesions, leading to further painful syndromes (see Chapter 10). A rehabilitative approach to therapy attempts to facilitate adequate nutrition and promote and maintain functional ambulation. Pain management is often necessary to facilitate other functional goal achievement. The HIV-infected patient may show a marked deficiency in cell-mediated immunity.

Subgroup E (other conditions) is comprised of diseases not classifiable in the former subgroups and may yet be attributable to HIV infection or indicative of a defect of cell-mediated immunity. Chronic lymphoid interstitial pneumonitis, along with signs and symptoms, could be attributed to HIV infection or to a coexisting disease not classified elsewhere. Examples include constitutional symptoms not listed in subgroup IV-A, infectious diseases not listed in IV-C, and neoplasms not listed in IV-D (Centers for Disease Control, 1986).

TREATMENT OF HIV

The treatment of HIV infection and its complications depends on the stage of the disease and the particular manifestations at the time. Azidothymidine (AZT) was approved by the Food and Drug Administration (FDA) for the treatment of the viral infection in 1987, after a relatively limited trial in patients who had experienced one episode of PCP (Fischl, 1990). A statistically significant improvement was noted in survival for the treated group. In 1989, another trial with the same drug has shown that patients with less than 500 CD4+ cells also benefit from taking the drug. Although evidence suggests that other antiviral drugs also benefit the patient, several drugs have not yet been approved and are still under investigation (Table 1-1). There is no general agreement on whether asymptomatic patients should be treated with AZT unless their CD4+ cell count is less than 500. Serious problems associated with long-term use of the drug include severe and painful myopathy and bone marrow depression, often leading to symptomatic anemia that requires transfusion. Because other drugs may not be available, managing the patient, in whom the disease has progressed, but who can no longer take AZT, either due to toxicity or to the development of resistant strains, becomes difficult. Although DDI looks promising, the drug has at least two serious side effects: pancreatitis and severe, painful peripheral neuropathies. It seems clear that both of these drugs are useful but must be administered in combinations to reduce their toxicities. The combination should probably include a biologic response modifier (BRM) to boost or restore the immune system, as neither drug shows evidence of restoring the immune system to normal by itself simply by reducing the viral load. A number of other drugs that have been investigated but not approved are suramin, foscarnate, dideoxyadenosine, ampligen, AL 721, dextran sulphate and compound Q, either due to lack of effect or unacceptable toxicity (Table 1-1).

Once the patient becomes symptomatic, the use of an antiviral drug is more easily justified. In a patient with simple lymphadenopathy, treatment should be guided by the level of immune dysfunction and whatever symptomatic treatment is needed. When group III-related symptoms are evident, grave therapeutic problems arise. At this stage, the CD4+ count will almost certainly be low enough to justify

the use of AZT, or another antiviral, if available. The management of the group III-related symptoms is often difficult due to nonspecific fever, diarrhea, weight loss, fatigue and night sweats. Explicit care in history taking and physical examination is necessary. Fever can often be controlled with small doses of steroids, which can be given safely without further compromising an already damaged immune system. Steroids do have undesirable side effects unless carefully monitored; therefore, therapy should be administered only under close supervision. Diarrhea can often be controlled using agents such as Lomotil, activated charcoal or deodorized tincture of opium. Weight loss, a serious problem for the HIV-infected patient at all stages of the disease, should be anticipated and treated with early nutritional intervention, as later efforts may not be effective. Weight loss appears best managed by a dietitian who understands the unique problems of the HIV disease process. Weight loss can result from an inability to eat because of pain or infection in the upper digestive tract; loss of appetite because of infection, fever, loss of taste or smell; or an inability to pay for palatable or well-balanced meals. Proper nutritional counseling and appropriate enteral and parenteral nutrition are critical components in the overall schema of management (see Chapter 6).

Fatigue is often a function of weight loss and poor nutrition, sleeplessness and depression. Interventions, such as a supervised exercise program and a proper eating regimen, are often beneficial to the patient with chronic fatigue. The rehabilitation specialist may elect to use an HIV Evaluation Form (Appendix C) to further assess overall function. If depression is a major factor, psychosocial intervention and medication can be incorporated. Although many drugs are useful in the management of group III infections, side effects caused by drug interaction must be considered. The therapist may be consulted to treat a patient who is actually overdosed with narcotics, hypnotics or even steroids. Many patients self-medicate, and the drugs, many of which may be categorized as alternative medicines, have side effects and interactions of their own. Physical and occupational therapists often develop in-depth communication with their patients and may actually know about these alternative medications before the attending physician or nurse practitioner.

When group IV stage of HIV is reached, the therapeutic picture changes. At this stage there is a defined illness to treat whether it be an opportunistic infection or a malignancy (the problem is slightly different if the diagnosis is dementia). Presently, each opportunistic infection or malignancy has standardized treatment regimens (as in the case of PCP). Investigational protocols continue to observe side effects and efficacy of new drugs for opportunistic infections. In the gamut of HIV infection, the patient who has

Table 1-1
AGENTS FOR THE TREATMENT OF HIV INFECTION ANTIVIRALS

AGENT	PURPOSE	EFFECT
AL721	-alters outer envelope of HIV -inhibits infectivity of HIV by preventing attachment of virus	-little objective evidence has supported this agents use -available over the counter
Azidothmidine (AZT) Zidovudine (zdv) Retrovir	-antiviral -thymidine nucleoside analog -inhibits HIV replication	-toxicity: bone marrow -blood transfusions may be needed for anemias
Axidouridine (AzdU)	-similar to AZT	-In Phase I Study -less toxic than AZT

Dideoxycytidine (DdC)	-cytidine nucleoside analog	-inhibits reverse transcriptase
		-toxicity:
		  peripheral neuropathy
		  rash
		  stomatitis
		  fever

Dideoxyinosine
Videx
(DdI)
	-dideoxynucleoside agent	-inhibits reverse transcriptase
		-toxicity:
		  peripheral neuropathy
		  acute pancreatitis

Dextran Sulfate	-treatment for hyperlipidemia -interferes with the ability of HIV infected cells to form "giant" cells	-anticoagulant -questionable antiviral activity, still under study
Peptide T	-mimics the HIV envelope protein, gp120 -little toxicity	-blocks CD4 receptor on T helper cells
Ribavirin	-antiviral	-under investigation
Alpha-interferon	-antiviral -anti neoplastic -immunomodulator -treatment of HIV and KS	-inhibits transcription of viral messenger RNA and protein synthesis
Ampligen	-antiviral -still under investigation	-mismatched double stranded RNA that has viral activity against HIV
Beta-interferon	-antiviral -anti neoplastic -immunomodulator -protein produced with recombinant technology	

continued . . .

access to a program of investigational treatment is at a distinct advantage. Costly medications are more readily available and treatment regimens are often more sophisticated. Such programs usually are found at academic institutions, although community research is currently being developed.

Antibiotics, chemotherapy, radiation and the various supportive regimens have side effects, many of which include weakness, myopathy, neuropathy and arthralgia. Therapists may frequently treat the sequelae of drug therapy as well as problems directly related to HIV. Rehabilitation, as part of a complete plan of management, can promote, maintain or remediate function as well as alleviate pain. Rehabilitation may be initiated in a hospital setting and later delivered at home or in an outpatient setting as part of the overall plan of continuing care.

Table 1-1 (continued)
AGENTS FOR THE TREATMENT OF HIV INFECTION

AGENT	PURPOSE	EFFECT
CD4	-soluble CD4 binds to the gp120 receptor of HIV -blocks the ability to infect or destroy T-4 helper cells	-synthetic mimic of the CD4 molecule -studies at San Francisco General (SFG) & National Cancer Institute (NCI)
Erythropoietin (EPO)	-stimulates bone narrow to produce viable erythroid precursors and RBCs	-efficacious for the patient with anemia (Hct<30)
Imuthiol (DTC)	-immune stimulator -increases CD4 cells -still under investigation	-induces the liver to produce a substance, hepatosin, which is a thymic hormone -antabuse properties
Interleukin-2 (IL-2)	-glycoprotein by stimulated T-helper lymphocytes	-undergoing trials with antiviral agents
IMREG-1	-enhances production of IL-2 and gamma interferon	-under investigation
Isoprinosine	-synthetic immuno modulator	-under investigation
Lentinan	-stimulate production of lymphokines -enhances cell-mediated immunity	-may be synergistic with AZT -under study at San Francisco General Hospital
Trichosanthin (Compound Q)	-selected inhibitory activity against HIV	-isolated from the Chinese cucumber root -under investigation
Alpha-interferon Adriamycin Bleomycin VP16 Vincristine Vinblastine	-treatment of Kaposi's sarcoma	-cytopenia -peripheral neuropathies -immunosuppression
Adriamycin Cytoxan Methotrexate Prednisone Vincristine VP16	-treatment of B-cell lymphoma	-granulocytopenia

COST

Health care consumes about 11 percent of the gross national product and is estimated to rise steadily as the population ages. HIV infection is one of the contributors to the soaring cost of health care delivery. The medical cost of HIV alone in 1991 reached approximately $16 billion and the lifetime costs of caring for an HIV patient vary between $40,000 and $150,000, depending on the length of illness and the area of the country (Centers for Disease Control, 1988). One way, indeed the main way, of reducing cost is to change HIV infection from a disease treated predominantly in the hospital to one treated at home or in an outpatient clinic. The responsibility for the delivery of cost-effective quality health care is a triple constraint function borne by the patient (consumer), the provider and the third-party guarantors. HIV-seropositive individuals may benefit from careful and frugal procurement of the health care services they require. The cost of similar services may vary significantly from one provider to another. Third-party payors must monitor and report overcharging and fraud.

One particularly costly item on many bills is the use of the intensive care unit (ICU). During the life of the Institute for Immunological Disorders, a comprehensive center exclusively for the HIV client in Houston, Texas, 350 patients were admitted over 14 months with an average in-hospital stay of nine days. No patient was admitted to the ICU. Indeed, a small number of patients should or must be admitted to the ICU, but they are perhaps the exception rather than the rule. Many conditions for which patients are readily admitted to the ICU may be managed comparably in the ward with skillful nursing and the use of physical and respiratory therapists.

COMPLEMENTARY THERAPIES

HIV infection, like cancer, is a chronic disease that is difficult to treat successfully. Individuals suffering from chronic illness or life-threatening diseases are susceptible to the philosophies of alternative or complementary therapies. Many of these approaches are referred to as *holistic* and may include Chinese medicine, yoga, biomedicine, vitamin therapy (see Chapter 6), acupuncture, touch/massage therapy and metaphysical approaches. Many patients are drawn to these therapies because of a sense of hopelessness. The *holistic* approach gives the patient some control and a sense of hope. Unfortunately, just as conventional therapies can be abused, alternative therapies may be associated with many misconceptions.

A significant disadvantage of some therapies is the effect on the patient's overall health. Various approaches may be attempted to restore the immune system, including detoxifying the body, restoring proper nutrition and providing enormous amounts of different vitamins or other substances that may not contribute to the individual's health. Alternative therapies may also place guilt on the patient, conveying the idea that "this would not have happened if you had a better lifestyle." This message can profoundly compound the psychological problems that the patient may already be facing. Finally, complementary medicine may be very expensive and is often not paid for by third-party payors. Despite these disadvantages, however, complementary alternatives, if integrated with traditional therapies, may be beneficial. Integration may help the patient find the right balance to deal with anger and uncertainty, take responsibility for his or her condition and give the proper sense of hopefulness (Steinberg, 1990). When a patient is considering using some form of complementary therapy, the health care professional must be able to provide objective information. Items to consider include the following:

1. Inquire about the projected therapeutic intervention and its origin.
2. Listen to the client carefully.
3. Watch for biased judgment regarding complementary therapies.
4. Be careful not to quickly interpret various comments.
5. Help the patient turn personal insights about motivation into a method for dealing with health-related anxieties.

It is also important to inform the entire health care team about participation in complementary therapies so the therapies can be monitored properly for side effects and interactions.

Patients are often advised to take certain medications or try certain therapies as prophylaxis, especially to prevent infection. Long-term use of antibiotics has not always been effective, except in the prevention of respiratory infections (see Chapter 8), and may result in serious side effects and the development of resistant organisms. Nevertheless, the use of aerosolized pentamidine for the prevention of PCP has been proven effective as has the continued use of some other agents to prevent the recurrence of infections such as toxoplasmosis, CMV retinitis and cryptococcal meningitis.

COMPLICATIONS

It is important to realize that infection by HIV causes an immune dysfunction; all the other manifestations, such as opportunistic infections and malignancies, are complications of this dysfunction. Some direct effects of HIV are also recognized, such as dementia and the wasting syndrome, which are probably caused by specific damage to target cells caused by the virus itself. In general, treatment should have two objectives: 1) to eliminate the virus and restore the immune system to normal, neither of which have been achieved so far and 2) to treat the complications as they arise, whether they are diagnosed as group III or group IV. Since the bone marrow is affected, the treatment of many of the complications is much more difficult than in an immunologically competent host. The treatment of lymphoma in HIV is much more difficult than anticipated because the side effects of chemotherapy are generally much more severe in the HIV-infected patient. In addition, some of the methods used to restore the immune system (ie. bone marrow transplantation) have made little progress since the probability of eliminating the virus is low. Much of the early work with immune modulators, such as IL-2, requires further study to determine their ability to control the viral cause of the immune dysfunction.

Infection with HIV poses a great challenge to humankind, not only scientifically and medically but also politically, economically, morally, legally and theologically. Both the luster and tarnish of humankind is often brought forth in the face of adversity. In *A Christmas Carol* Scrooge is symbolized as *Hate* and *Fear* hiding beneath the skirts of *Igno-rance*. He is forewarned that ignorance is the greatest enemy of humankind. Dickens' theme appears as true today as it was in the 19th century and nowhere more than in societal attitudes toward HIV. HIV infection is not an exclusively homosexual disease, although many persist in regarding it as such. The greatest threats to public health probably now lie in the intravenous drug-using population, young sexually active heterosexuals and relatively poorly educated ethnic minorities (Centers for Disease Control, 1990). For this reason, pediatric HIV infection is a formidable problem, particularly in large urban areas. Sexual habits and addictive behavior may be considered social mores and are difficult to discuss, even within the veil of patient confidentiality.

The magnitude and presence of HIV is worldwide. The infection has been reported from almost every country in the world and WHO statistics further note that there is tremendous under-reporting (World Health Organization, 1989). The estimates of 250,000 cases in early 1990 are quite conservative as are the estimates of the total number of infected people. For some countries, such as Uganda and Zaire, the economic disaster is frightening. With up to 30 percent of the population infected, the future is bleak, especially since there are few prospects for controlling the situation in the foreseeable future. The tragedy and travesty of HIV abounds because young people who carry so much of the hope for the future in such countries are infected in greater numbers each year. In Brazil, there is an uncontrolled increase in HIV, particularly among the poor urban populations of Rio de Janeiro and Sao Paulo. In Bangkok, Seoul and Hong Kong thousands of people engage in solicited and unsafe sexual practices each week. HIV is not aware of color or creed nor can it be contained by territorial boundaries or prison bars. Ironically, the infection is quite preventable. No vaccine appears on the immediate horizon and for now, education is the means of reducing the threat.

While some behavioral patterns of civilization's sub-cultures may appear comparable to those described by Gibbons, the disease remains one whose means of travel is due more to ignorance than to lasciviousness. Clearly, a change of behavior patterns, continued education and intense laboratory and clinical research are humankind's aegis in the battle against this apocalyptic disease.

SUMMARY

This chapter presented a general overview of the medical course of HIV disease. The Centers for Disease Control classification was described and the Walter Reed Classification referred to in Appendix A. A number of drug interven-

tions were noted (Table 1-1). Rehabilitation specialists can play a major role in managing the entire continuum of symptoms associated with chronic HIV disease.

Acknowledgment

The author would like to acknowledge Rick Dellagatta, MEd, PT and Grace Ann Bertram, PT, for assistance in manuscript additions to this opening chapter.

References

Brew, B.J., Hardy, W., Zuckerman, E., et al. (1989). AIDS-related vacuolar myelopathy is not associated with co-infection by HTLV-1. *Annals of Neurology*. 26:679.

Brew, B.J., Cooper, D.A., Perdices, M.J., et al. (in press). The neurological complications of HIV infection in the absence of significant immunodeficiency. *Australian & New Zealand Journal of Medicine*.

Centers for Disease Control. (1986). Classification for Human T-lymphotrophic Virus Type III / Lymphadeno-pathy-associated virus infections. *Morbidity and Mortality Weekly Report*. 38:334.

Centers for Disease Control. (1988, February). HIV/AIDS Surveillance Report. 36. Centers For Disease Control. (1989, February). HIV/AIDS Surveillance Report. 37 and 38.

Centers for Disease Control. (1990, February). HIV/AIDS Surveillance Report. 1-18.

Craddock, C., Pasvol, G., Bull, R., et al. (1987). Cardiorespiratory arrest and autonomic neuropathy in AIDS. *Lancet*. 2:16.

Devinsky, O., Cho, E.S., Petito, C.K., et al. (1987). Herpes zoster myelitis (abstract). *Neurology*. 37:319.

Eidelberg, D., Sotrel, A., Vogel, H., et al. (1986). Progressive polyradiculopathy in acquired immune deficiency syndrome. *Neurology*. 36:912.

Fischl, M. (1990). Treatment of HIV infection. In Sande M.A. and Volberding, P.A. (Eds.): *The Medical Management of AIDS*. (pp 3-113) Philadelphia: W.B. Saunders.

Gibbons, E. (1955). The Decline and Fall of the Roman Empire. In Great Books of the Western World. *Encyclopedia Britannica*. 40.

Lin-Greenberg, A., and Taneja-Uppal, N. (1987). Dysautonomia and infection with the human immunodeficiency virus. *Annual Internal Medicine*. 106:167.

Luis, K.J., Darrow, W.W., and Rutherford, G.W. (1988). A model basis estimate of the mean incubation period for AIDS in homosexual men. *Science*. 240:1335.

Miller, R.G., Storey, J., and Greco, C. (1989). Successful treatment of progressive polyradiculopathy in AIDS patients (abstract). *Neurology*. 39:271.

Navia, B.A., Cho, E.S., Petito, C.K., et al. (1986). The AIDS dementia complex II. Neuropathology. *Annals of Neurology.* 19:525.

Petito, C.K., Navia, B.A., Cho, E.S., et al. (1985). Vacuolar myelopathy pathologically resembling subacute combined degeneration in patients with acquired immunodeficiency syndrome (AIDS). *New England Journal of Medicine.* 312:874.

Phuir, J.P., Munoz, A., Kengsley, L., et al. (1989). Incidence of AIDS in homosexual men developing HIV-1 specific antibody. Presented at the 5th International Conference on AIDS, Montreal, Canada.

Price, R.W., Brew, B.J., and Rosenblum, M. (1990). The AIDS dementia complex and HIV-1 brain infection: A pathogenetic model of virus-immune interaction. In Waksman (Ed.): *Immunologic Mechanisms in Neurologic and Psychiatric Disease.* New York: Raven Press.

Redfield, R.R., Wright D.C., and Tremont E.C. (1986). The Walter Reed Staging Classification for HTLV-III/LAV Infection. *New England Journal of Medicine.* 314:131.

Rosenblum, M.R., Brew, B.J., Avdhow, H.A., et al. (1989, June 5-9). Clinical pathological features of HTLV-1 associated myelopathy (H & M) in AIDS (abstract).

Presented at the 5th International Conference on AIDS, Montreal, Canada.

Snider, W.D., Sipson, D.M., Nielsen, S., et al. (1988). Neurological complications of acquired immune deficiency syndrome: Analysis of 50 patients. *Annals of Neurology.* 14:403.

Steinberg, C.I. (1990). Integrating traditional medicine with other therapies in the treatment of HIV-infected individuals. *Maryland Medical Journal.* 39(2):183.

Tucker, T., Dix, R.D., Datzen, C., et al. (1985). Cytomegalovirus and herpes simplex virus ascending myelitis in a patient with acquired immune deficiency syndrome. *Annals of Neurology.* 18:74.

World Health Organization. (1989). Acquired immunodeficiency syndrome (AIDS): Global projections of HIV/AIDS. *Weekly Epidemiologic Record.* 64:229.

Yarchoan, R., Mitsuya, H., Thomas, R.V., et al. (1989). In vivo activity against HIV and favorable toxicity profile of 2', 3' dideoxyinosine. *Science.* 245:412.

Ziegler, J.L., and Dorfman, R.E. (1988). *Kaposi's Sarcoma.* New York: Marcel Dekker.

Ziegler, J.L. (1990). *Journal of Acquired Immune Deficiency Syndromes.* 3:S3.

2

The Epidemiology of HIV Infection and AIDS

Robert L. Falletti, MS

It was only when Ivan realized the total meaninglessness of his life that he was overwhelmed by the pain of his cancer. As long as there seemed to him to be a valid meaning to his existence, he could resist it and retain control and dignity.

—Fyodor Dostoyevsky

INTRODUCTION

Epidemiology is the study of the distribution of disease in human populations. Like any investigator, an epidemiologist asks the important questions, who, what, when and where, in order to identify, analyze and help prevent disease. The first step in identifying an epidemic is to determine that a cluster of unusual events with some common characteristics has occurred. These characteristics or risks are then evaluated for their potential role in causing or transmitting disease. This evaluation can lead to identifying multiple causes, a single biologic agent or a combination of many cofactors. Ultimately, all this information is used to establish a strategy for preventing further cases by directing public health policy and targeting interventions.

Epidemics are not new to human history. In this century alone, there were two before AIDS: the influenza epidemic of 1918-1919 and the polio epidemic of the 1950s. AIDS has taken its place in history as both the last epidemic of the 20th century and the first epidemic of the 21st century.

The AIDS nomenclature was first established in mid-1981 (Centers for Disease Control, 1981) with identification amongst five homosexual men, aged 29 to 36 years, in Los Angeles, California. They had been diagnosed with PCP, which is associated with severely immunocompromised individuals. More cases, all associated with high mortality,

followed in both New York and California (Centers for Disease Control, 1981). By the end of 1981, well over 100 diagnosed cases had been described since 1978. The list of illnesses and conditions associated with this syndrome began to grow: Kaposi's sarcoma (a rare form of cancer in older men); Burkitt's lymphoma (endemic in parts of Africa); and fungal, viral and protozoan infections. In conjunction with these infections and cancers was a reduced immune function—specifically low numbers of thymus-dependent helper lymphocytes (T4 cells, CD4 cells).

RISKS

By mid-1982 the United States (U.S.) Public Health Service, through the Centers for Disease Control, had established the term acquired immunodeficiency syndrome (AIDS), a working case definition and reporting format for local and state health departments, physicians and hospitals, and had recorded nearly 600 cases. From this information, certain characteristics, only hints in the first few cases, began to emerge as significant. Although the overwhelming majority of cases were in homosexual or bisexual men, by the end of 1982 there were cases among intravenous (IV) drug users, Haitians, hemophiliacs, blood transfusion recipients, female sexual partners of infected men and infants born to IV-drug-using women.

BEHAVIORS AND TRANSMISSION

Although there has been a great deal of concern about the mode of transmission of the virus, there has been little if any change in the way HIV has been acquired since the early 1980s. Today the emphasis is not so much on risk groups, but on the behaviors that put people at risk for the disease. These risky behaviors fit into the following transmission categories:
- male homosexual/bisexual contact
- IV drug use (female and heterosexual male)
- male homosexual/bisexual contact and IV drug use
- hemophilia treatment
- heterosexual contact (male or female)
- transfusion/blood component recipient
- being born to a parent with/at risk for AIDS

From these behaviors, three modes of transmission have been identified:
1. sexual contact with an infected person
   * homosexual and/or heterosexual
2. exposure to blood or blood products
   * needle sharing among IV drug users
   * transfusions/blood products from 1977 to mid-1985
   * occupational exposure in the health care setting
3. transmission from an infected woman to her fetus or infant.

Intensive study has centered around identifying new modes of transmission. Some of these investigations include repeated household studies, health care worker studies, mosquito smashing studies and institutional living studies. The results only serve to reinforce the three established ways that HIV is transmitted and to further dispel the fear of casual contact transmission.

It is now clear that the HIV epidemic is really a combination of many subepidemics, in which there are different rates of transmission, infection and diagnosis of HIV/AIDS. The risk for acquiring HIV infection for gay males, IV drug users, female sexual partners, and blood product recipients differs because behaviors vary. Enmeshed within these subepidemics are the timing and varying effects of education and prevention programs on those individuals at risk. For example, gay males and IV drug users in the late 1970s and early 1980s had no warning of this virus, whereas those engaging in high-risk behaviors during the mid to late 1980s may have received the benefit of prevention messages. Unfortunately, because the time from infection to onset of symptoms averages seven years,

the benefits of these prevention programs may not materialize until the early 1990s.

ETHNIC GROUPS

Increases in the rate of AIDS among black and Hispanic IV drug users, their heterosexual partners, and newborns have continued; but the rate seems to be declining among white gay males (Centers for Disease Control, 1990). Morbidity and mortality will continue to be high among young and middle-aged black and Hispanic minorities in which the use of IV drugs is higher than in the general population. In time, drug-related AIDS will have a significant impact in urban centers across the nation, not just along the eastern seaboard. Also of continued concern is the large number of black and hispanic men who acquire their infection from male-to-male sexual contact; 45 percent of the black men and 47 percent of the Hispanic men reported with AIDS were exposed to HIV due to sexual contact with other men (Centers for Disease Control, 1990). For minority women, the behaviors at highest risk are IV drug use and sexual contact with male partners who use IV drugs. This subepidemic among urban minorities involved with IV drug use, needle sharing, and sex-for-drugs is complicated by the fact that it involves a drug-addicted population. Ultimately, this cycle leads to another subepidemic of HIV-infected newborns.

PEDIATRIC AIDS

Reported AIDS cases among persons diagnosed at less than 13 years of age increased 17 percent from 1988 to 1989 (Centers for Disease Control, 1990). Approximately 83 percent of the pediatric cases were attributed to the HIV-infected mother. Ten percent of cases were due to transfusions with blood components and five percent were due to the treatment of hemophilia. Among the HIV-seropositive mothers, most were IV drug users or became infected through sexual contact with a male partner who used IV drugs.

THE VIRUS

In 1983, a retrovirus was identified as the causative agent for AIDS. It was originally named lymphadenopathy-associated virus (LAV) in France (Barre-Sinoussi et al., 1983) and human T-cell lymphotropic virus, type III (HTLV-III) in the United States (Gallo et al., 1983). In 1986, an international committee on taxonomy of viruses renamed it human immunodeficiency virus (HIV) to reflect a new human pathogen (Coffin et al., 1986).

PAST AND PRESENT NAMES FOR THE AIDS VIRUS

LAV	Lymphadenopathy-associated virus; 1983, Montagnier, France
HTLV-III	Human T-cell lymphotropic virus type 3; 1983, Gallo, United States
ARV	AIDS related virus; 1984, Levy, United States
HIV-1	Human immunodeficiency virus type 1; 1986, International Committee
HIV-2	Human immunodeficiency virus type 2; 1987, West Africa

HIV-2 is related to HIV-1 in its structure and it also causes AIDS. However, it differs in geographic distribution from HIV-1. First isolated in West Africa (Clavel et al., 1987) it was identified only in persons from West Africa in the United States in 1987 (Centers for Disease Control, 1988). It is believed to be transmitted in the same manner as HIV-1. Its existence suggests that HIV-1 and HIV-2 share a common viral ancestor, perhaps the simian immunodeficiency virus (SIV), which infects the macaque monkey. HIV-2, like HIV-1, has spread rapidly in Central Africa and in Europe, and additional blood screening programs are needed to detect it along with HIV-1, especially for blood banking purposes.

ANTIBODY TEST

In mid-1985, a test to detect antibodies for the AIDS virus was licensed. The HIV antibody test was first used to screen the donor blood supply and then to clinically test persons wishing to know their HIV status. The test can detect only antibodies to the AIDS virus and not the virus itself. Thus, if a person is exposed to HIV and antibodies have not yet developed, they would test negative yet still be infected. On average it may take three to six months for antibodies to develop. However, there are reports of individuals being infected with HIV and not producing antibodies for a year or more.

The procedure for antibody detection is an enzyme-linked immunosorbent assay (ELISA) test followed by a supplemental test called a Western Blot (WB). Both of these tests must be performed to confirm the presence of antibodies to HIV. Persons are notified and counseled only with confirmed results.

CENTRAL AFRICA

With the advent of HIV serologic testing, other nations, including those in central Africa, began testing current and past blood samples and their populations. HIV infection was widespread in Africa and transmitted in a different pattern than that in the United States. It is estimated that 10 to 20 percent of all infants born in central Africa are born to mothers infected with HIV (Fauci, 1987). Surveys of prostitutes indicate that up to 88 percent are infected, as compared with a 10 to 18 percent HIV infection rate in the general population. This rate is in sharp contrast to the estimated U.S. rate of 0.03 percent for the general population. Such high infection rates allow the virus to be spread evenly between males and females through sexual contact. This results in a male/female ratio of 1:1 in central Africa as compared to the U.S. ratio of 14:1.

The striking differences between central Africa and the United States represent a specific example of the global diversity of the epidemiology of HIV infection. Dr. Jonathan Mann (1988) of the World Health Organization (WHO) has delineated three patterns of HIV infection based on transmission trends and the length cf time the virus has spread within a country. These patterns are described in Table 2-1 and Figure 2-1.

HEALTH CARE WORKERS

Because health care workers were in contact with persons with AIDS and HIV infection early on, there was concern that they might be infected through occupational exposure. After extensive investigations of many health care workers exposed to HIV by needle sticks, splashes, bites, punctures and aerosols of blood, only 0.47 percent showed transmission of HIV (Centers for Disease Control, 1989). This rate is in complete contrast to hepatitis B with a 25 percent transmission rate. Therefore, universal precautions and guidelines have been developed by the CDC to prevent hepatitis B and HIV exposure in the health care setting (see Appendix B, Chapter 4). These guidelines have been adopted by the U.S. Department of Labor, the National Institute for Occupational Safety and

Table 2-1
PATTERNS OF HIV-1 INFECTION IN THE WORLD

PATTERN 1	PATTERN 2	PATTERN 3
Homosexual/bisexual men and IV drug users are the major affected groups.	Heterosexuals are the main population group affected.	More recent introduction with spread among persons with multiple sex partners.
Introduced: Mid-1970s or early 1980s.	Introduction: Early to late 1970s.	Introduction: Early to mid 1980s
Sexual Transmission: Predominantly homosexual. Limited heterosexual transmission, but expected to increase.	Sexual Transmission: Predominantly heterosexual. Up to 25% of the 20-40 year age group in some urban areas infected, and up to 90% of female prostitutes. Homosexual transmission not a major factor.	Sexual Transmission: Both homosexual and heterosexual transmission just being documented. Very low prevalence of HIV infection even in persons with multiple partners, ie. prostitutes.
Parenteral Transmission: IV drug use accounts for the next largest proportion, even in Europe. Transmission via blood or blood products not a continuing problem, yet tens of thousands infected before 1985.	Parenteral Transmission: Transfusion of HIV-infected blood is a major factor. Nonsterile needles and syringes as well.	Parenteral Transmission: Not a significant problem at present. Some infections in recipients of imported and non-imported or blood products (ie. Rumanian children).
Perinatal Transmission: Mainly female IV drug users, sex partners of IV drug users, and women from HIV-1 endemic areas.	Perinatal Transmissions: Significant problem in areas where 5% to 15% of women are HIV-1 antibody positive.	Perinatal Transmission: Currently not a problem.
Distribution: Western Europe, North America, some area of South America, Australia, New Zealand.	Distribution: Africa, Caribbean, some areas of South America.	Distribution: Asia, the Pacific Region (except Australia and New Zealand), the Middle East, Eastern Europe, some rural areas of South America.

Developed by Robert L. Falletti, MS.

Health (NIOSH) and the Occupational Safety and Health Association (OSHA).

HIV INFECTION

With the advent of the HIV antibody test, the full spectrum of the disease became apparent. Stages of infection from initial exposure to preliminary symptoms to diagnosed AIDS could be identified, assessed and treated. It also became possible to estimate from stored blood samples the length of the incubation period (exposure to symptoms), which may extend up to 10 or even 14 years. Unfortunately, because the time from symptomatic infection to advancement of HIV disease may average seven years, the majority of the persons infected in the early 1980s have not yet been counted as AIDS cases and most likely will not be symptomatic until the mid-1990s. According to estimates by the Centers for Disease Control, approximately 1 to 1.5 million people in the United States are infected with HIV. To determine trends and transmission pattern years before diagnosis, a number of HIV testing programs and seroprevalence surveys are underway in the United States. HIV antibody testing data are being collected from sexually transmitted disease, tuberculosis and IV drug clinic clients; selected hospital patients; military entrants; job corp applicants; women of reproductive age; prisoners; college students; migrant workers; and blood donors (Tables 2-2, 2-3 and 2-4).

Because HIV infection varies among different populations and different geographic regions, the overall percentage infected with HIV in the United States cannot be determined from these surveys. Instead, results show

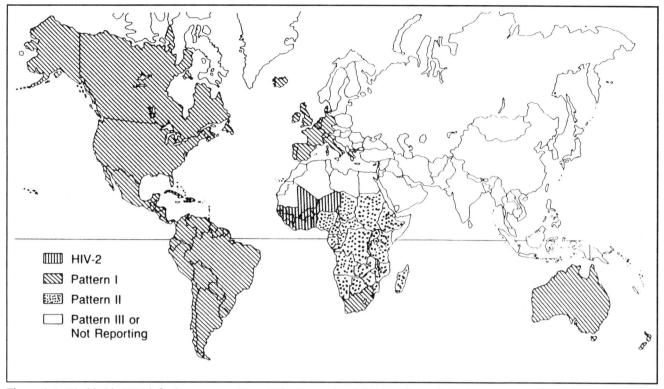

Figure 2-1. Worldwide HIV infection patterns. From "The International Epidemiology of AIDS," Mann, et al. *Used with permission. Copyright 1988 by Scientific American, Inc. All rights reserved.*

that the various subepidemics are spreading through specific groups and communities.

TRENDS

- AIDS cases have been reported from all states, the District of Columbia, and four U.S. territories; yet the geographic distribution has shifted from the Mid-Atlantic region to other U.S. regions and from urban to rural areas.
- Approximately 90 percent of AIDS cases since 1982 are adult males, yet the percentage of adult cases in women has increased from 7 percent in 1984 to 10 percent in 1989.
- Nationally, blacks are 3.2 times and Hispanics are 2.8 times more likely than whites to have AIDS.
- IV drug use as a risk behavior for AIDS has increased from 17 percent in 1985 to 31 percent in 1989.
- Nationally, in 1987, AIDS was the leading cause of death in men aged 25 to 44 years old.
- The U.S. Public Health Service projects that 365,000 AIDS cases and 263,000 deaths will occur by the end of 1992 (Figure 2-2).
- The Harvard Institute of International Development (Mann et al., 1988) estimates that by 1995 the annual loss due to AIDS deaths in Zaire will be $350 million or eight percent of that country's gross national product.
- In the United States, the 1991 estimated mortality cost of AIDS, based on lifetime earnings, ranges between $28.6 and $36.3 billion (Scitovsky & Rice, 1987).
- The cumulative medical costs (varying due to length of stay and inpatient hospital costs) of caring for AIDS patients in the United States by 1991 will range from $6.3 to $45.5 billion (Bloom & Carliner, 1988).

SUMMARY

AIDS and HIV infection will most certainly challenge the current public health and health care systems in both the developed and developing world. The WHO estimates that between six and eight million persons are infected with HIV and that there are over 600,000 estimated cases of AIDS worldwide (Nakajima, 1990). The potential economic im-

Table 2-2
HIV IN DRUG USERS
RESULTS OF STUDIES AVAILABLE IN 1988

STATE	CITY	SETTING	PERCENT POSITIVE	NUMBER TESTED
New York	New York City	Methadone maintenance	57	731
		Drug treatment	49	487
New Jersey	Asbury Park	Methadone maintenance	43	60
	Trenton	Methadone maintence	12	57
Michigan	Detroit	Non-AIDS hospitalization	30	76
		Non-AIDS hospitalization	19	31
		Non-AIDS hospitalization	12	96
District of Columbia	Washington	Non-AIDS hospitalization	28	47
Massachusetts	Worcester	Jail	16	189
		Drug treatment	14	311
Wisconsin	Milwaukee	STD clinic	8	24
California	Los Angeles	Methadone maintenance	3	205
Ohio	9 cities	Methadone maintenance	1	509
Texas	San Antonio	STD clinic	1	149

Source: HIV/AIDS division, Centers for Disease Control, Atlanta, Georgia.

Table 2-3
HIV IN REPRODUCTIVE-AGED WOMEN
RESULTS OF STUDIES AVAILABLE IN 1988

STATE	CITY	SETTING	PERCENT POSITIVE	NUMBER TESTED
New Jersey	Newark	Delivery	4.3	604
Florida	Miami	Delivery	3.6	2061
New York	New York City	Delivery	3.1	223
		MIC clinic	1.5	1497
		Abortion clinic	1.4	1491
		Delivery	1.3	1934
		Family planning	0.8	2112
	Upstate	Family planning	0.2	2413
Massachusetts	Boston	Delivery	1.7	1000
Maryland	Baltimore	Prenatal	1.3	1245
California	San Francisco	Prenatal	1.0	207
	San Diego	Prenatal	0.6	532
Pennsylvania	Philadelphia	Delivery	0.0	384

Source: HIV/AIDS division, Centers for Disease Control, Atlanta, Georgia.

Table 2-4
HIV INFECTION IN CHILDBEARING WOMEN
NEONATAL SURVEYS

STATE	MONTHS OF SURVEY	POSITIVE PERCENT	NUMBER OF SPECIMENS TESTED
New York	December 1987 – November 1988	0.66	276,609
Florida	July – December 1988	0.49	60,133
New Jersey	July – September 1988	0.49	29,309
Massachusetts	December 1986 – June 1987	0.21	30,708
	January – December 1988	0.25	88,924
Texas	April – July 1988	0.09	86,180
California	July 1988	0.08	43,301
Michigan	July – December 1988	0.06	71,758
Colorado	February – December 1988	0.04	41,269
New Mexico	October 1987 – December 1988	0.02	24,880

Source: HIV/AIDS division, Centers for Disease Control, Atlanta, Georgia.

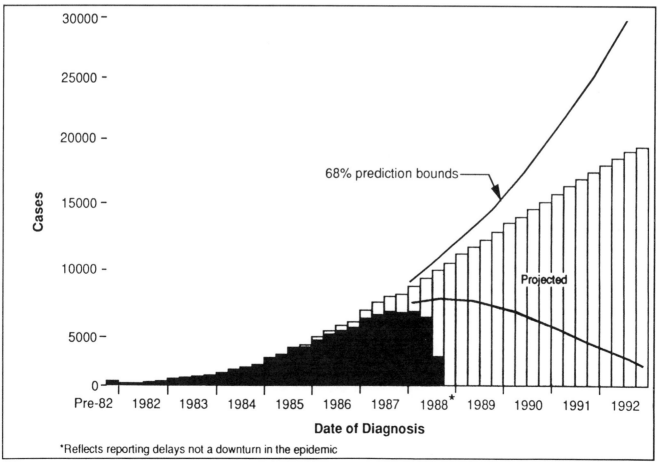

Figure 2-2. Incidence of AIDS in the United States, 1982 -1992. *Source: HIV/AIDS Division, Centers for Disease Control, Atlanta, Georgia.*

pact of AIDS on developing countries that already have health care delivery problems is staggering. In the developed world, especially in the United States, morbidity and mortality will continue to increase in the next few years. Most affected will be young and middle-aged men in the white, black and Hispanic communities. Although the major modes of transmission are known, more information is needed about the occurrence of HIV infection in local areas to help target, implement and evaluate prevention programs. To that end, the role of epidemiology in the HIV epidemic is best stated by James W. Curran (1988), Director, HIV/AIDS Division, Centers for Disease Control:

Epidemiologic principles should provide the basis for directing the considerable resources needed to prevent sexual, perinatal, and IV drug abuse transmission of HIV. Progress in prevention efforts and control of HIV infection will require a long-term commitment of both science and society.

References

Barre-Sinoussi, F., Chermann, J.C., Rey, F., et al. (1983). Isolation of a T-lymphotropic retrovirus for a patient at risk for acquired immunodeficiency syndrome. *Science.* 220:868.

Bloom, D.E., and Carliner, G. (1988). The economic impact of AIDS in the United States. *Science.* 239:604.

Centers for Disease Control. (1981, June). Pneumocystis pneumonia—Los Angeles. *Morbidity and Mortality Weekly Report.* 30:250.

Centers for Disease Control. (1981, July). Kaposi's sarcoma and Pneumocystis pneumonia among homosexual men—New York City and California. *Morbidity and Mortality Weekly Report.* 30:305.

Centers for Disease Control. (1988, January). AIDS due to HIV-2 infection—New Jersey. *Morbidity and Mortality Weekly Report.* 37:33.

Centers for Disease Control and National Institute for Occupational Safety and Health. (1989, February). *Guidelines for Prevention of Transmission of Human Immunodeficiency Virus and Hepatitis B virus to Health-care and Public-safety Workers.* Atlanta:Author.

Centers for Disease Control. (1990, February). Update: Acquired immunodeficiency syndrome—United States, 1989. *Morbidity and Mortality Weekly Report.* 39:81.

Centers for Disease Control. (1990, March). *HIV/AIDS Surveillance Report,.* 1-22.

Clavel, F., Mansinho, K., Chamaret, S., et al. (1987). Human immunodeficiency virus type 2 infection associated with AIDS in West Africa. *New England Journal of Medicine.* 316:1180.

Coffin, J., Haase, A., Levy, J.A., et al. (1986). International Committee on Taxonomy of Viruses. What to call the AIDS virus? *Nature.* 321:10.

Curran, J.W., Jaffe, H.W., Hardy, A.M., et al. (1988). Epidemiology of AIDS and HIV infection in the United States. *Science.* 239:610.

Fauci, A.S. (1987). AIDS: Pathogenic mechanisms and research strategies. *American Society for Microbiology News.* 53:264.

Gallo, R.C., Sarin, P.S., Gelman, E.P., et al. (1983). Isolation of human T-cell leukemia virus in acquired immune deficiency syndrome (AIDS). *Science.* 220:865.

Mann, J.M., Chin, J., Piot, P., and Quinn, T. (1988). The international epidemiology of AIDS. *Scientific American.* 259:82.

Nakajima, H. (1990). Opening speech at World Health Organization's AIDS Program Management Committee. *United Press International.*

Scitovsky, A.A., and Rice, D.P. (1987). Estimates of the direct and indirect costs of acquired immunodeficiency syndrome in the United States: 1985, 1986, and 1991. *Public Health Reports.* 102:5.

3

Immunologic Aspects in HIV

Grace Moffat Minerbo, MD, PhD

Nothing in life is to be feared. It is only to be understood.

—Marie Curie

INTRODUCTION

From the time of Metchnikoff, there has been debate as to whether cells or soluble substances are responsible for immunity. In the 19th century, greater emphasis was placed on the humoral response. It was known that serum factors could transfer immunity to the host from the donor, but immunity was not conferred by all microorganisms. For example, immunity to TB cannot be transferred by serum factors but only by mononuclear cells (lymphocytes, polys, macrophages) since the tubercle bacillus is an intracellular organism. It thus became apparent that an antigenic stimulus resulted in predominantly one kind of response: either the cell-mediated or humoral response. Examples of cell-mediated responses are allograft rejection, immunity to obligative intracellular organisms such as TB and fungi and tumor immunity. Examples of humoral immune responses are antitoxins (diphtheria and cholera), agglutinating or opsonizing antibodies to bacteria (antibody synthesis and release) and virus neutralizing antibody. Antigenic factors that determine the type of immune response are route of entry, type and size of microorganisms, and biologic activity.

HUMORAL AND CELLULAR IMMUNITY

The immune response (cell-mediated or humoral response) is lymphocyte dependent. Gowans et al. (1962) found that body types of immune responses, both cellular and humoral, were mediated by the same cell, the lympho-cyte. One of the primary immune organs is the thymus, a bursa-like lining (similar to the bursa of Fabricius found in birds where stem cells differentiate into T- and B-cells, respectively). With the removal of the bursa of Fabricius from birds, the humoral response is lost or severely reduced, whereas the cell-mediated immune response remains intact. With the removal of the thymus before the third day of life, cell-mediated immunity is lost, decreasing the patient's ability to tolerate skin grafts, whereas antibody production, although intact, is reduced.

Bone marrow provides the stem cell precursors of lymphocytes. These stem cells migrate into the bursa or thymus, where they differentiate into bursa cells (B-cells or B lymphocytes) and thymus cells (T-cells or T lymphocytes), respectively. From the thymus and the bursa (primary immune organs), the lymphocytes enter the lymphatic-blood circulation where they migrate to the secondary lymphoid organs, and T-cells migrate to the paracortical areas of the lymph nodes and periarterial areas of the spleen. Normally, 60 to 70 percent of the small lymphocytes in serum are T-cells and 30 to 40 percent are B-cells.

RETICULOENDOTHELIAL SYSTEMS AND PHAGOCYTOSIS

The reticuloendothelial system is the anatomic basis of the immune system. Phagocytosis is the primary process by which immunity is achieved. The reticuloendothelial system consists of reticular fibers with fixed cells. Phagocytic cells may be either fixed or circulating. Examples of the fixed population of phagocytic cells are Kupffer cells (liver), reticular cells (lymph nodes and spleen) and alveolar cells (dust cells in the lungs). Examples of circulating phagocytic cells are the polymorphonuclear leukocytes (polys) and monocytes.

Phagocytosis involves a series of steps. First, the particle is enveloped in pseudopods, which leads to their enclosure in a cytoplasmic vacuole or phagosome. Then, lysosomes fuse with the phagosome, emptying their enzymatic contents into the *digestive vacuole*. The enzymes are acid hydrolysis and lysosomes that enzymatically digest the foreign matter, causing the degradation and elimination of the digested bacteria and other foreign substances. If the foreign matter is not digestible, as with silica or sand particles, it may also be toxic to the macrophages, contributing to inhalation lung disease.

The phagocytic cells collaborate with the cells of the immune system. In response to most foreign substances, a preparative step is usually required whereby the phagocyte interacts with the antigen and prepares it for presentation to the immune system. By definition, antigens (Ag) are recognized by cells and antibodies of the immune system as foreign. Antibodies (Ab) are protein molecules produced by the immune system after antigenic stimulation. Antibodies are synonymous with immunoglobulins. When not aided by antibody or complement, the activities of the phagocytic system differ from the immune system in several ways. The phagocytic system is characterized by being relatively non-specific: Phagocytes cannot distinguish between one foreign substance and another. Phagocytosis proceeds in an all-or-none manner. Phagocytes lack memory and are incapable of learning. Having ingested a given substance at one time, they do not ingest a similar particle encountered later with any greater speed or efficiency. The ability to distinguish between self and non-self substances, however, is characteristic of phagocytes.

LYMPHOCYTE CIRCULATION

The pathway of the lymphocyte involves the blood vascular circulation and the lymphatic circulation. During the 1960s, Gowans et al. (1962) in England found that lymphocytes follow a given pathway in the body whereby afferent lymphatic vessels lead to the lymph nodes where the lymph is filtered. The lymph is carried away from the lymph nodes through the efferent lymph ducts to the blood system via the thoracic lymph duct. The secondary immune organs are the lymph nodes and the spleen.

The arteries of the circulation system deliver the lymphocytes to the spleen and tissue fluid of the body in the capillary networks of tissue. The lymphocytes may return to the circulation via the vessels or migrate from the capillaries into the tissues as a response to inflammation. From the tissues, lymphocytes may return to the lymphatic system via the afferent lymphatics draining the tissue to the proximal lymph nodes. Lymph nodes filter tissue fluid (lymph) while the spleen filters blood. Both the spleen and lymph nodes can process antigens.

STRUCTURE AND FUNCTION OF IMMUNOCOMPETENT CELLS

T-cells and B-cells cannot be morphologically distinguished from each other with the light microscope. Therefore, *markers* are needed to distinguish B- and T-cell lymphocytes. Human thymus cells (T-cells) bind sheep red blood cells to their cell membrane, thereby forming cell clusters or rosettes. B-cells do not bind sheep red blood cells; however, they can be identified by making an antibody against human immunoglobulins, tagging the antibody with fluorescein and reacting the tagged antibody with lymphocytes. B-cells stain for surface immunoglobulins (Igs) but T-cells do not. The immunoglobulins on the B-cell surface thus act as B-cell markers. Fluorescent B-cells are seen by dark-field microscopy.

Physiologic differences between T- and B-cells can be observed. T-cells synthesize lymphokines after interacting with antigens; B-cells synthesize antibodies after interacting with antigens. Lymphokines are proteins that have the ability to influence the movement and activities of macrophages. Therefore, T-cells produce lymphokines that serve to regulate control cell-mediated immunity. B-cells produce antibodies that control humoral immunity.

The advent of the development of blood serum electrophoresis placed immunology on the forefront of medical research by the 1960s. Electrophoretic investigation demonstrated that antibodies migrate primarily with the protein class immunoglobulins. The antibodies, although of different types, all migrated in electrophoresis as a single class of globulins. It was not until the 1960s that a large quantity of a single type of immunoglobulin could be obtained from multiple myeloma patients. These patients have cancer of usually one class of plasma cells, thereby producing only one class of immunoglobulins in large quantities.

The molecular structure of the antibody molecule was determined shortly thereafter (Hood, L.E. et al., 1984). It was found that all antibody molecules are proteins that consist of two pairs of polypeptide chains of amino acids linked by disulfide bonds. The large inner chains are called heavy chains, and the smaller outer chains are called light chains (H or L chains). At the amino terminal portion is the antigen-combining site, which consists of both light and heavy chains. The binding of antigen at these sites does not involve chemical reactions such as covalent bonding but rather physical forces of protein-protein interactions, whereby the antigen molecule fits into the groove of the antibody as a key fits into a lock.

There are five classes of immunoglobulins, categorized by the heavy chains: IgM, IgG, IgA, IgE or IgD. The class of Ab determines to a large extent the distribution of the immunoglobulins in the tissue and blood of the patient (Table 3-1). The fraction/centrifuge (Fc) portion of the Ab molecule confers two other important biologic functions to the Ig classes. First, it confers the ability to react with another protein system known as the complement system. Second, it confers the ability to interact with phagocytes (macrophages) and mast cells. In addition to allowing the Ig molecule to activate complement, the Fc portion also makes possible the interaction of the Ig molecule with other cells. The Fc portion of the Ig molecule promotes interaction of antigen-antibody complexes between the monocyte and macrophage. The monocyte is a circulating macrophage; it is called a macrophage when it leaves the blood and goes into the tissue. The monocytes and macrophages possess a receptor for the cell-fixing portion of the IgG molecule, the Fc receptor.

The importance of the IgG Fc receptor site on macrophages is well known. If the bacteria are coated with specific IgG antibody, the interaction of the Ab-coated bacteria with the Fc portion of the monocyte-macrophage receptor leads to enhanced phagocytosis and killing of the bacteria known as opsonization. The monocyte also has a cell surface receptor for an activated component of complement (C3B receptor). If, in addition to specific Ab, complement is now added to the system, the complement-coated antibody is phagocytized and killed at an even faster rate. Thus, the Fc portion of the Ig molecule allows for interaction not only with the complement system but also with receptors on various cells. Neutrophils have recently been shown to possess receptor sites for IgG and IgA molecules. Mast cells and basophils possess Fc receptor sites for IgE molecules. Interaction of IgE antibody antigen (allergen) complexes with mast cells leads to the liberation of a variety of vasoactive substances, such as histamine and slow-reacting substances, which play a role in asthma and the anaphylactic phenomena.

If a specific antigen interacts with the surface immunoglobulins of a clone of B-cells specific for that antigen (eg. B-3), B-3 clones proliferate. After a number of cell divisions, B-cells differentiate to form a larger cell that produces a single, specific antibody. This antibody-producing cell, known as the plasma cell, is the end-product cell of B-cell differentiation. It is metabolically geared to produce as many as 2,000 antibody molecules per second. It should be reemphasized that the plasma cell produces antibody that is similar in antigen specificity to the surface immunoglobulins present on the precursor B-cell. The expanded clone of precursor B-cells is the basis of immunologic memory. On a subsequent encounter with antigen 3, a large number of cells can respond to the stimulus for cell division and

Table 3-1
FIVE CLASSES OF IMMUNOGLOBULINS

IMMUNOGLOBULIN	STRUCTURE AND LOCATION	TOTAL SERUM
IgM	This is a large molecule consisting of five linked Ig molecules (pentameter). It is found intravascularly only. The large structure of the molecule does not allow it to cross the placenta.	10%
IgG	Consists of one small immunoglobulin molecule. It is found extravascularly surrounding body cells in tissue fluid. Only IgG crosses the placenta. It is responsible for the protection of the newborn during the first six months of life.	75%
IgA	Found in body secretions (salvia, tears, mucus, vaginal and prostatic secretions). It is the chief source of defense of the respiratory tract.	15%
IgE	Found in body secretions in response to allergies or parasites. It comprises only 0.04 percent of the total serum immunoglobulins but binds with very high affinity to mast cells via its Fc region.	0.04%
IgD	Found only in newborns; its function is unknown.	-0-

Table 3-2
SUMMARY OF ANTIGEN-ANTIBODY EVENTS (HUMORAL) IN THE IMMUNE RESPONSE

INFLAMMATION SITE

When a specific antigen gains access to tissues, an inflammatory focus develops. Phagocytic cells enter the site of inflammation and begin to digest and process the antigen.

LYMPH NODES (B-CELL CLONES)

The drainage of antigens of phagocytic cells containing antigen into the afferent lymphatics from the inflammatory site leads to the encounter between antigen and a specific clone of B-cells in germinal centers of the regional lymph nodes.

PLASMA CELL DIFFERENTIATION AND MEMORY B-CELL FORMATION

Presentation of the antigen to a clone of B-cells within the germinal centers leads to the proliferation of B-cells which results in an increased number of antibody-producing plasma cells and an increased number of specific memory B-cells.

RELEASE OF MEMORY B-CELLS AND SPECIFIC ANTIBODIES FROM LYMPH NODES

Plasma cells usually remain in the lymph nodes. Memory B-cells and antibody, however, leave by way of the efferent lymphatics to ultimately gain access to the blood and other lymph nodes.

Ab AT INFLAMMATORY SITE

Antibody reaches the original inflammatory site from the circulation. Under optimal circumstances, antibody with the aid of phagocytic cells and complement will effectively eliminate the antigen.

---

antibody production. A latent period, which varies from days to weeks, follows antigenic interaction with B-cells before the antibody appears. During this time, there is proliferation of the B-cell clone (memory cells) and the production of plasma cells.

Initially, the plasma cells produce primarily IgM. The IgM response may last from several days to weeks, after which IgM has a greater affinity than the IgM for the original antigen. After the IgM response, high rates of IgG production may last for several weeks, after which there is a general decrease in the serum-Ab levels, which corresponds to the elimination of the antigen. The switch from IgM to IgG production is known as the primary immune response and is not fully understood. If the same person is exposed to the same antigen at a later date, months or even years later, a secondary immune response occurs. The secondary immune response consists of a shorter latency period before the appearance of IgM. The duration of IgM response is shorter, and the switch to the more efficient IgG production occurs earlier. The net effect of the secondary response is to produce a higher level of IgG antibodies, which persists for a longer time, thereby decreasing the latency period. This result is due to the creation of memory cells during the primary response. Table 3-2 summarizes antigen antibody events in the immune response.

The cell-mediated immune system involves T-cell production and lymphokines. T-cells influence B-cell re-

sponses, a model of which is presented in Figure 3-1a. This system is responsible for rejection of organ transplantation, destruction of viruses and removal of early cancer cells (Hood, 1984) (the humoral immune system evolved before the cell-mediated system). There are several different types of T-cells: effector T-cells, suppressor T-cells and helper T-cells, which are interdependent immunocompetent cells. T-cells influence B-cell responses. Helper T-cells assist B-cells to produce immunoglobulins and switch IgM production to IgG whereas suppressor T-cells curtail or suppress Ab production by the plasma cells. The central regulatory role of T4 helper cells is depicted in Figure 3-1b. Therefore, cell mediated immune response (T-cells) also regulates the humoral immune system (B-cells). Effector T-cells inhibit viral multiplication through interferon production. The killer T-cells directly destroy antigens by lysis. T-cells exert great influence on the immune response through the production of lymphokines. Lymphokine production by T-cells is reviewed in Table 3-3.

In conclusion, three phases of the humoral response are components of the immune response: 1) the afferent phase, where there is recognition of antigen preceding antibody production, 2) the efferent phase, where there is Ag-Ab complex formation, and 3) antigen-antibody binding with subsequent localization and disposal of the antigen. During this last phase, there is development of memory that increases the number of clones of specific B-cells.

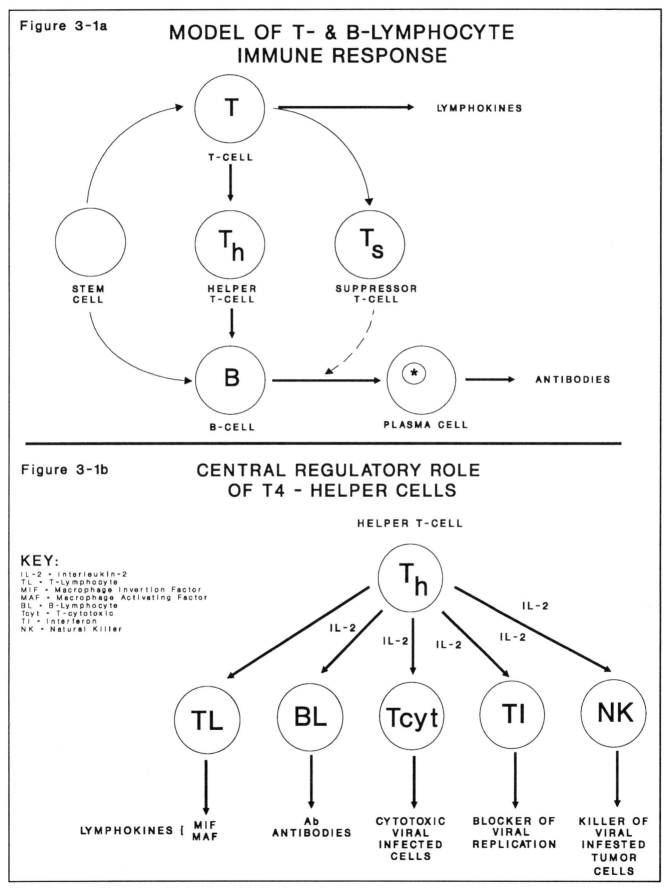

Figure 3-1a

MODEL OF T- & B-LYMPHOCYTE IMMUNE RESPONSE

Figure 3-1b

CENTRAL REGULATORY ROLE OF T4 - HELPER CELLS

KEY:
IL-2 = Interleukin-2
TL = T-Lymphocyte
MIF = Macrophage Invertion Factor
MAF = Macrophage Activating Factor
BL = B-Lymphocyte
Tcyt = T-cytotoxic
TI = Interferon
NK = Natural Killer

Figure 3-1. Generalized and specific functions of the T-cell in the immune response.

CONGENITAL IMMUNODEFICIENCIES

Certain hereditary conditions result in immunodeficiencies in the newborn of varying degrees of severity (Levy et al., 1989).

Bruton's infantile sex-linked agammaglobulinemia is a congenital X-linked hereditary condition characterized by a defect or blockage in the development of the B-cells. It occurs predominately in males. Germinal centers in the lymph nodes and spleen are absent or greatly reduced. The production of antibodies is severely decreased or absent. The condition usually does not become evident until the infant is about six months old. Maternal immunoglobulins are depleted from the infant's circulatory system at this time. Affected children are susceptible to pyogenic bacterial such as staphylococcus, streptococcus, and pneumococcus. They do not have a humoral immune system and usually die of massive bacteria infections.

DiGeorge syndrome (thymic hypoplasia, absent or rudimentary) is a congenital condition of unknown etiology whereby the child is born with a rudimentary or absent thymus; therefore, stem cells cannot differentiate into T-cells. The thymic-dependent paracortical areas in the lymph nodes and spleen thus are sparsely populated, whereas the germinal centers are intact. Affected children are susceptible to viral infections, such as measles and chicken pox, and to fungal infections. Parathyroid glands also are absent or hypoplastic, resulting in susceptibility for hypocalcemia to develop into tetany. These children do not have an adequate cell-mediated immune systems and are likely to develop severe viral and fungal infections, including cancer.

Swiss-type agammaglobulinemia (severe combined immunodeficiency) is another congenital condition in which stem cells cannot differentiate into T-cells or B-cells. It is inherited as an autosomal recessive. The lymph nodes and thymus are either missing or markedly reduced in size due to the lack of both germinal centers (B-cells) and the paracortical T-cells. These infants fail to develop both cellular and humoral responses. Until the 1980s, these children died within the first year of life from all forms of viral, fungal and bacterial infections.

ACQUIRED IMMUNODEFICIENCIES

Secondary immunodeficiencies are more common than hereditary disorders. They may be caused by diseases such as leukemia (cancer of the white blood cells) and Hodgkin's disease (cancer of the lymph nodes). Currently, the most important disease of epidemic proportions that is acquired and produces severe immunodeficiencies is AIDS (Robbins

Table 3-3
LYMPHOKINE PRODUCTION BY T-CELL TYPE FUNCTION

Type	Function
Macrophage-activating factor	Acts on macrophages to enhance phagocytosis
Transfer factor	Increases the number of lymphocytes sensitized to the foreign matter
Chemotactic factor	Several substances that selectively attract one of the various types of leukocytes (white blood cells)
Interferon	Prevents intracellular viral replication
Mitogenic factor	Stimulates mitosis and maturation of lymphocytic blast (stem) cells
Lymphotoxin	Destruction of cells
Skin reactions factor	Sensitivity

& Kunmar, 1987). The disease is characterized by profound immunosuppression associated with opportunistic infections. The responsible organism is a retrovirus, the human immunodeficiency virus (HIV).

PEDIATRIC AIDS

HIV infects several distinct cell types including T-cells, monocytes, agranular leukocytes and cells of the central nervous system in both adults and infants (Levy, J.A. et al., 1985). The earliest abnormality detected in infants with pediatric AIDS is hypergammaglobulinemia. It is postulated that B-cell activation may occur from the direct infection of the B-cell by the HIV or through viral stimulation of B-cells. The incubation period (exposure to onset) of HIV infection in pediatric AIDS is similar, but not synonymous to, that in adult patients. The HIV incubation period is 2 years for children under 5, and 8 years for older children. One of the major differences between pediatric and adult HIV cases is the high frequency of bacterial infection in children. It is probably due to low levels of acquired immunity in young people. An adult is undoubtedly protected from infectious diseases by the increase of immunoglobulins, especially IgA. (This represents an enhanced humoral immunity.)

During the first six months of life, infants are normally protected by the presence of maternal antibodies. IgG crosses the placental barrier in utero from mother to fetus to enhance the poorly developed fetal immune system. Immunoglobulins are also transported in human milk to the breast-feeding infant.

PATHOGENESIS OF HIV INFECTIONS

Viruses are one of the smallest microorganisms on earth. The viruses that cause disease in plants and animals are obligate intracellular parasites capable of multiplying only in living cells. Their specificity applies not only to the broad category of animals or plants but frequently to a specific cell organelle, namely the nucleus or cytoplasm in a specific cell type in a specific genus and species. An example is the hepatitis virus, which resides only in liver cells. Upon entry to the host cell, the virus uses the host cell's organelles for its own replication.

In humans, the HIV invades the lymphocytes (T-helper cells) of the white blood cell series first, followed frequently by the invasion of neuronal cells and macrophages. In AIDS, the major consequence of T-cell invasion is severe immunosuppression, whereas dementia results from neuronal cell invasion.

All of our cells contain DNA and RNA, known collectively as nucleic acids. The DNA is located in the cell nucleus, and the RNA is located generally in the cytoplasm of the cell. Viruses, on the other hand, contain only one of the nucleic acids. They are categorized by belonging to either the DNA or RNA group. Hence, there are DNA viruses and RNA viruses. Examples of DNA viruses are herpes and infectious mononucleosis. HIV and the viruses that cause measles and mumps are RNA viruses.

HIV is classified as a lentivirus, a subclass of retroviruses. Retroviruses contain the nucleic acid RNA. Consequently, when the RNA virus initiates replication in the living host cell, it must convert its RNA genetic information into a DNA template using the enzyme reverse transcriptase. HIV is classified as a lentivirus whose pathologic characteristics result in severe immunodeficiencies.

The immunodeficiency caused by HIV results primarily from the depletion of helper T-lymphocytes. Normally, there are twice as many helper T-cells (T4) as suppressor T-cells (T8), ie. T4/T8 = 2:1. Helper T-cell membranes are studded with glycoprotein cell markers called CD4. These surface glycoproteins act as receptor sites for HIV attachment. Suppressor T-cells are distinguishable from helper T-cells by their different glycoprotein cell markers called CD8. Since these two markers, CD4 and CD8, are located on

T-lymphocytes, the lymphocytes are also known as T4 and T8 lymphocytes, respectively. Hence, T4 cells are helper T-lymphocytes and T8 cells are suppressor T-lymphocytes.

In summary, a comparison of T- and B-cell immune systems reveals important differences. Receptor sites on T-cells for antigen recognition are now identified, albeit different types. T-cells produce lymphokines. B-cells produce antibodies (and some lymphokines). T-cells produce memory cells and effector cells. The properties of effector T-cells are known. They migrate to inflammatory foci where they kill foreign cells and produce lymphokines, which influence inflammatory reactions and activities of the macrophage-monocyte system.

Furthermore, T- and B-cell systems do not operate exclusively of each other. It is known that removal of the bursa in chickens abolishes the humoral response but leaves the cell mediated responses intact. Removal of the neonatal thymus, however, not only abolishes the cell-mediated immune responses, but also impairs humoral response. For most antigens, B-cells require help or collaboration from T-cells. During the primary antibody response, two phenomena occur for which there is yet no explanation, the switch from IgM to IgG antibody production and the curtailing of the antibody response once it has achieved an optimal effect. Recent investigation suggests that T-cells are involved in both these phenomena, helper T-cells and suppressor T-cells, respectively. The therapist guided by immunologic markers must be cognizant of the pathogenesis of HIV and opportunistic infections.

REHABILITATION ASPECTS

HIV and the Nervous System

From the beginning of the HIV epidemic, severe immune suppression was recognized, but reports of neurologic dysfunction also began to appear. Neurologic illnesses were shown to arise from both the opportunistic disease processes and directly by nerve cell invasion of the T-lymphocytes in the patient with AIDS. It is now well known that HIV targets both the immune system and the nervous system.

The central nervous system appears to be more frequently attacked by HIV than the peripheral nervous system. One study revealed that 75 percent of HIV patients experience nervous system involvement. Thus, it is important for the therapist to become familiar with the spectrum of symptoms associated with HIV. The two systems (immune and nervous) may be affected simultaneously or, more commonly, the immune system may be affected first followed by the nervous system. In one study, 10 percent of all HIV patients first presented with symptoms of neurologic involvement (Levy, R.M. et al., 1985).

Health care professionals must realize that their HIV patients may not only display symptoms of immune suppression but also of neurologic illness. The patient may be irrational, exhibiting wide mood swings, and may not always follow instructions. As the disease progresses, the destruction of both the central and peripheral nervous system continues along with the increased severity of the immunosuppression. The individual may develop altered mental status, sensory losses, parasthesias and visual disturbances. He or she may be unable to walk on the treadmill or bicycle because of the associated weakness and a disordered gait. Seizures may occur for the first time in the presence of the health care provider, which may be stressful to those present. These persons also frequently complain of headaches and dizziness. Aphasia can often occur.

HIV and Cell-Mediated Immune Suppression

Laboratory findings are important for health care workers to understand when dealing with HIV patients. The lymphocyte count most frequently is low (<500 m/L). T-cell counting is accomplished by the use of monoclonal antibodies directed at the T-cell surface antigens. The CD4 helper T-cells are markedly decreased. In normal persons, the ratio of helper/inducer (CD4) T-cells to suppressor/killer (CD8) T-cells is 1.5 or greater; in HIV patients, the ratio of CD4 helper T-cells to CD8 suppressor T-cells is 1.0 or less (often < 0.5). This ratio represents a severe deficiency in cell-mediated immunity, thereby making the HIV patient extremely susceptible to opportunistic infections.

Testing for the presence of the HIV virus is still in the experimental stage (Grossman & Jawetz, 1988). The presence of antibody to HIV is an indicator of infection; therefore, HIV infection is suspected by that demonstrate the presence of HIV antibodies, but the presence of HIV antibody also is not diagnostic of HIV. Seropositivity is determined by the ELISA test, but confirmation of the diagnosis is determined by the Western Blot test. Dual testing is performed to avoid false positives.

References

Golden, J.A. (1989). Pulmonary complications of AIDS. In Levy, J.A. (Ed.): *AIDS Pathogenesis and Treatment.* Philadelphia: W.B. Saunders.

Gowans, J.L., McGregor, D.D., Cowen, D.M., and Ford, C.E. (1962). Initiation of immune responses by small lymphocytes. *Nature.* 196:651.

Grossman, M., Schroeder, S.A., and Jawetz, E. (1988). Acquired immunodeficiency syndrome. In Schroeder, S.A. (Ed.): *Current Medical Diagnosis and Treatment.* Norwalk, CT: Appleton & Lange.

Hood, L.E., Weissman, I.L., Wood, W.B., and Wilson, J.H. (1984). *Antibodies. Immunology.*, 2nd ed. Menlo Park, CA: Benjamin/Cummings Publishing Co., Inc.

Levy, J.A., Shimabukuro, J., McHugh, T., et al. (1985). AIDS-associated retrovirus (ARV) can productively infect other cells besides T-helper cells. *Virology.* 147:141.

Robbins, S.L., and Kunmar, V. (1987). *Disorders of Immunity.*, Chapter 5. Basic Pathology, 4th ed. Philadelphia: W.B. Saunders.

Roitt, I.M. (1988). *The Basis of Immunology.* Essential Immunology, 6th ed. Oxford: Blackwell Scientific Publications. Blackwell/Year Book Medical Publishers, Inc.

Shearer, W.T., Ritz, J., and Finegold, M.J. (1985). Epstein-Barr virus—associated B-cell proliferations of diverse clonal origins after bone marrow transplantation in a 12-year-old patient with severe combined immunodeficiency. *New England Journal of Medicine.* 312:1151.

4

Infection Control

Tina Sweezey, MS, PT

There is nothing to fear but fear itself...

—*Franklin Delano Roosevelt*

INTRODUCTION

Universal concern about transmission of HIV is warranted because, to date, no one has demonstrated immunity to this virus. The intensity of this concern is magnified in health care workers and care givers due to the perceived risk of exposure and infection. Although current research places health care workers and care givers at very low risk for contamination, myths and misinformation remain a significant source of ineffective care giving. Health care professionals must be informed about infection control so that they may continue to provide optimal care to their HIV-infected patients.

TRANSMISSION OF HIV

HIV has been isolated from the following body fluids: blood, semen, breast milk, saliva, tears, vaginal secretions, urine, amniotic fluid and cerebrospinal fluid (Centers for Disease Control, 1987). Epidemiologic evidence has implicated only blood, semen, vaginal secretions, and possibly breast milk in the transmission of the virus (Centers for Disease Control, 1987). Transmission occurs either through specific behaviors or as consequences of other behaviors.

According to former Surgeon General C. Everett Koop (1987), HIV is transmitted primarily through two specific behaviors: sexual intercourse or the sharing of an intravenous needle with an infected individual. Sexual intercourse, particularly anal sex, is risky because of the possibility of tissue trauma, thereby providing a point of entry for the HIV into the bloodstream. Entry may also occur during vaginal sex when ulcerations or lacerations are present. The sharing of needles and syringes of intravenous drug users is another

behavior that increases the chance of transmission of the HIV. HIV is carried in contaminated blood left in the needle, syringe, or other drug implements; and the virus is injected into the new victim by reusing dirty syringes or needles. Even the smallest amount of infected blood left in a used needle or syringe can allow live HIV to be passed on to the next user of the dirty implement.

Two other methods of HIV transmission occur as a result of consequence, rather than behavior. These methods include blood transfusions and perinatal transmission. Blood transfusion was a common way of transmission before March 1985 due to lack of blood screening (Koop, 1987). Fortunately with routine testing of blood products, the number of new cases of HIV infection due to blood transfusion is decreasing. Unfortunately, perinatal transmission is not decreasing. Mothers with HIV can infect their newborn child, although the exact mechanism by which this occurs is unknown. It has been estimated that approximately one third of babies born to women infected with HIV will also be infected (Koop, 1987). Current evidence indicates that HIV is not transmitted through casual contact, although it may be transmitted through breaks in the skin or even more rarely through mucous membranes.

RISKS TO THE HEALTH CARE WORKER

Risk management of HIV infection and the health care worker begins by establishing a ratio of reported infections to reported exposures. The type of exposure as well as the variety and quantity of inoculum can then be determined by closer analysis of the documented cases.

Needlesticks appear to be the most common exposure,

Table 4-1
SUMMARY OF IMPORTANT RECOMMENDATIONS AND WORK RESTRICTIONS FOR PERSONNEL WITH INFECTIOUS DISEASES

DISEASE	RELIEVE FROM DIRECT PATIENT CONTACT	PARTIAL WORK RESTRICTION	DURATION
Conjunctivitis	Yes		Until discharge ceases
CMV	No		
Diarrhea	Yes		Until symptoms resolve and
Acute stage (diarrhea with other symptoms)			salmonella is ruled out
Convalescent stage (Salmonella [nontyphoidal])	No	Should not care for high-risk patients	Until stool is free of organism on two consecutive cultures not less than 24 hours apart
Other enteric pathogens	No		
Enteroviral infections	No	Should not care for infants	Until symptoms resolve
Group A streptococcal disease	Yes		Until 24 hours after adequate treatment is started
Hepatitis, viral			
Hepatitis A	Yes		Until 7 days after onset of jaundice
Hepatitis B			
Acute	No	Personnel should wear gloves for procedures involving trauma to tissues or contact with mucous membrane or broken skin	Until antigenemia resolves
Chronic antigenemia	No	Same as acute illness	Until antigenemia resolves
Non-A, Non-B	No	Same as hepatitis B	Period of infectivity has not been determined
Herpes simplex			
Genital	No		
Hands (herpetic whitlow)	Yes	Note: Not known whether gloves prevent transmission	Until lesions heal
Orofacial	No	Personnel should not care for high-risk patients	Until lesions heal
Measles			
Active	Yes		Until 7 days after rash appears
Postexposure (susceptible personnel)	Yes		From 5-21 days after exposure or 7th day after rash appears

continued ...

with lacerations and mucocutaneous, cutaneous, parenteral and noncontact modes less commonly reported. Blood and semen are comparatively high in viral concentration, with titers of HIV appearing much lower in urine, saliva and tears. The stage of infection will also determine the titer of HIV. The quantity of the virus found in the inoculum, along with the volume of titers, is thought to significantly affect the risk of transmission. Thus deep penetrations of large needles with blood inoculum are the most commonly reported needlestick accidents causing infections (Gerberding, 1990a).

The Centers for Disease Control (1988a) states that the risk of seroconversion following needlestick exposures to blood from HIV infected patients is less than 1.0 percent. The risk associated with the exposure of nonintact skin or mucous membranes would appear to be even less than those associated with needlestick exposures.

Another mode of possible transmission that has received

Table 4-1 (continued)
SUMMARY OF IMPORTANT RECOMMENDATIONS AND WORK RESTRICTIONS FOR PERSONNEL WITH INFECTIOUS DISEASES

DISEASE	RELIEVE FROM DIRECT PATIENT CONTACT	PARTIAL WORK RESTRICTION	DURATION
Mumps*			
Active	Yes		Until 9 days after onset of parotitis
Postexposure From 12-26 days after exposure and/or 5 days after onset of symptoms	Yes		
Pertussis			
Active	Yes		From beginning of catarrhal stage through 3rd week after onset of paroxysms, or until 7 days after start of effective therapy
Postexposure (asymptomatic personnel)	No		
Postexposure (symptomatic personnel)	Yes		Same as active pertussis
Rubella Active	Yes		Until 5 days after rash appears
Postexposure (susceptible personnel)	Yes		From 7-21 days after exposure or 5 days after rash appears
Scabies	Yes		Until treated
Staphylococcus aureus (skin lesions)	Yes		Until lesions have resolved
Upper respiratory infections (high-risk patients)	Yes	Personnel with upper respiratory infections should not care for high-risk patients	Until acute symptoms resolve
Varicella (chickenpox) Active	Yes		Until all lesions dry and crust
Postexposure	Yes		From 10-21 days after exposure or, if varicella occurs, until all lesions dry and crust
Zoster (shingles) Active	No	Appropriate barrier desirable; personnel should not take care of high-risk patients until lesions dry and crust	
Postexposure	Yes		From 10-21 days after exposure or, if varicella occurs, until all lesions dry and crust

*Mumps vaccine may be offered to susceptible personnel. When given after exposure, mumps vaccine may not provide protection. However, if exposure did not result in infection, immunizing exposed personnel should protect against subsequent infection. Neither mumps immunoglobulin nor immune serum globulin (USG) is of established value in postexposure prophylaxis. Transmission of mumps among personnel and patients has not been a major problem in patients in hospitals in the United States, probably due to multiple factors, including high levels of natural and vaccine-induced immunity. (*Used with permission. Institute for Immunological Disorders: Manual of Infection Control, Houston, Texas 1986.*)

much attention in the media is the aerosols of infected blood or saliva, which is commonly found in dentists' offices, operating rooms and laboratories. Small particles of blood, bone, saliva and other substances become aerosolized and are small enough to pass through the masks and other protective equipment. This mode of transmission has alarmed some health care workers, although, to date, no cases have been reported (Gerberding, 1990a).

In assessing the risk of HIV transmission to the health care worker cumulative effects must be considered. Along with the type and amount of inoculum on exposure, the overall risks increase with the number of exposures the worker encounters. Thus health care providers in frequent contact with the virus, such as nurses, dentists, surgeons, emergency care providers and rehabilitation specialists, are at greatest risk over a lifetime of practice (Grady et al., 1978; Werner & Grady, 1982).

Another consideration is the immunologic status of the health care worker. This factor could influence the possibility of transmission of HIV to the employee (Gerberding, 1990a). Although the risk of HIV transmission in a health care setting appears to be low, fear persists among many health care professionals. Much of this anxiety stems from lack of education and understanding of the disease process (Gerbert et al., 1988). The risk should be acknowledged and professionals encouraged to minimize it. The benefits and limitations of infection control need to be emphasized. In addition, authorities must give accurate information, clearly delineating what is known, what is unknown and what is reasonable speculation. The goal may not be to totally eradicate the fear but rather to prevent it from compromising the quality of patient care and health care professional's well-being (Gerbert et al., 1988).

PREVENTION FOR THE HEALTH CARE WORKER

Transmission of HIV in a health care setting can be minimized if health care workers are cautious when performing invasive procedures. Use of the universal precautions (Appendix B) should be implemented with all patients, not just those known to be infected. It is suggested that all health care workers obtain a copy of the universal precautions and that they be posted wherever applicable (Centers for Disease Control, 1987). Employers of health care workers have the responsibility of instructing health care workers about these universal precautions, providing equipment and supplies necessary to minimize the risk of infection and monitoring the workers' adherence to these precautions (Centers for

Disease Control, 1988a). Sterile surgical or nonsterile examination gloves made of vinyl or latex regulated by the FDA (Centers for Disease Control, 1988b) should be readily available. Masks, protective eye wear and gowns must also be easily accessible where and when appropriate. In case of emergency, ventilation devices should be available to decrease the need for mouth-to-mouth resuscitation.

No environmentally-mediated mode of HIV transmission has yet been documented. Sterilization and disinfection procedures for patient care equipment should be followed routinely for all patients. Studies have shown that commonly used germicides rapidly inactivate HIV, so standard procedures are adequate to sterilize items contaminated with blood or body fluids of persons with HIV (Centers for Disease Control, 1987). Calcium hypochlorite (household bleach) prepared daily in a 1:10 dilution is an inexpensive and effective germicide against HIV (Centers for Disease Control, 1987).

As stated previously, certain health care worker are at a greater risk than other for exposure to HIV. Allied health professionals, such as physical therapists and occupational therapists, are at decreased risk as compared to health care workers who are frequently in situations involving excessive blood or body fluids (Yohn, 1987). When treating HIV seropositive patients in the rehabilitation department, some general precautions should be taken (Hopp & Rogers, 1989). Gloves should be worn when in contact with blood or body fluids. Masks should be worn if the patient has a contagious opportunistic infection, or if the therapist is infected (eg. cold, flu). Personnel with infectious diseases should take into consideration certain work restrictions (Table 4-1). Patient care equipment should be cleaned with a bleach solution after use and linen and waste management policies implemented. HIV seropositive patients should not be treated in close proximity with severely immunosuppressed patients (eg. patients with cancer). On the other hand, it is important not to alienate the patient. Receiving treatment in an environment with other patients will help HIV patients deal with the psychosocial aspects of their chronic illness (see Chapter 15).

During physical therapy, exposure to blood occurs most often with whirlpool procedures. For this reason, therapists should consider all patients as potentially infected with HIV (Appendix B). Gowns, masks and gloves are recommended for wound care in the hydrotherapy department. Identified patients with HIV in need of whirlpool treatments should be scheduled at the end of the day (Appendix B). Hands should be washed immediately after gowns and gloves are removed. All scalpels used for debridement should be immediately disposed of in puncture-resistant containers. All soiled laundry, bandages and disposables containing drainage of any body fluid should be disposed of properly according to institutional policy. The whirlpool should be cleaned with the bleach solution and allowed to dry.

PSYCHOLOGICAL ISSUES CONCERNING HIV EXPOSURES

Whenever a case of transmission of HIV infection to a health care worker is reported, fear persists among the remaining professionals. Along with fear, many also experience denial, anger and depression (Gerberding, 1990a). It is important that the health care worker have a support system to rely on for counseling. This is especially true after accidental exposure to the virus. The University of San Francisco has provided a Counseling and Testing Service for all health care workers who have been exposed to the HIV virus. The University believes that a multidisciplinary approach to accidental exposures provides the psychological and medical care necessary for the health care worker (Gerberding, 1990b).

SUMMARY

Human immunodeficiency virus infection affects society at all levels. Education has been implemented on many levels and should be continued. Concerns about fear of contagion should be addressed at the initiation of treatment. Keeping an open dialogue facilitates communication about the level of comfort in treatment of an HIV-infected patient. No one is immune to infection and responsibility for the prevention of the spread of HIV is of primary importance of all.

Acknowledgment

The author would like to thank Rick Dellagatta, MEd, PT for manuscript editing.

References

Centers for Disease Control. (1983). Universal precautions. *Morbidity and Mortality Weekly Report.* 32:358.

Centers for Disease Control. (1987). Recommendations for prevention of HIV transmission in health-care settings. *Morbidity and Mortality Weekly Report.* 36:1S.

Centers for Disease Control. (1988a). Update: Acquired immunodeficiency syndrome and human immunodeficiency virus infection among health-care workers. *Morbidity and Mortality Weekly Report.* 37(17):229.

Centers for Disease Control. (1988b). Update: Universal precautions for prevention of transmission of human immunodeficiency virus, hepatitis B virus, and other bloodborne pathogens in health-care settings. *Morbidity and Mortality Weekly Report.* 37(24):377.

Gerberding, J.L. (1990a). Occupational HIV transmission: Issues for health care providers. In Sande M.A., and Volberding P.A. (Eds.) *The Medical Management of AIDS* (pp. 57-60). Philadelphia: W.B. Saunders.

Gerberding, J.L. (1990b). Managing HIV exposures in health care settings. *FOCUS: A Guide to AIDS Research and Counseling.* AIDS Health Project at the University of California—San Francisco.

Gerbert, B., Badner, V., Maguire, B., et al. (1988). Why fear persists: Health care professionals and AIDS. *Journal of the American Medical Association.* 260(23):3481.

Grady G.F., Lee V.A., Prince A.M., et al. (1978). Hepatitis B immune globulin for accidental exposures among medical personnel: Final report of a multicenter controlled trial. *Journal of Infectious Diseases.* 138:625.

Hopp, J.W., and Rogers, E.A. (1989). Increasing safety in health care settings. In *AIDS and the Allied Health Professions* (pp. 80-89). Philadelphia: F.A. Davis Co.

Koop C.E. (1987). *Surgeon General's Report on Acquired Immune Deficiency Syndrome.* Washington, DC: U.S. Department of Health and Human Services.

Werner B.J., and Grady G.F. (1982). Accidental hepatitis-B-surface antigen-positive inoculations: Use of antigen to estimate infectivity. *Annals of Internal Medicine.* 97:367.

Yohn, J. (1987). AIDS risk to PTs minimal with normal precautions. *Progress Report.* 16(9):1.

5

Adaptive Human Performance and HIV Infection: Considerations for Therapists

Michael Pizzi, MS, OTR/L

Human adaptation falters when meaning can not be derived from environmental interaction.

—Mary Reilly

INTRODUCTION

Rene Dubos (1978, p. 88) defines health as "primarily a measure of each person's ability to do what he wants to do and become what he wants to become. Good health implies an individual's success in functioning within his particular set of values, and as such it is extremely relative." At some point during their illness, persons living with HIV infection are unable to perform the activities of daily living. The ongoing process of living, namely activity and human movement, is the cornerstone to human performance and daily functioning, the basis on which one declares oneself in good health.

ADAPTIVE PERFORMANCE

After diagnosis of HIV infection, the affected person is confronted with an immediate need to change, restructure, reorganize and transform his or her life. Often, there is an urgent need to adapt to the new health status. The ability to adapt varies among individuals. Initially, adaptation is difficult as many persons living with HIV perceive the diagnosis as a "death sentence." With the increasing number of long-term survivors, HIV is now considered a chronic disease. In our death-denying culture, adaptation to

a chronic disease, although difficult, is often easier than adaptation to a "life-threatening" illness such as HIV.

Reilly (1974, p. 88) states that "human adaptation falters when meaning can no longer be derived from environmental interaction." Meaningful life activity (eg. walking, working, leisure, self-care, communicating) sustains life and living. It supports interactions with people and the physical environment. People living with HIV often require support to regain and restore life activity performance and environmental interaction. When support is not available but is required, or when support is not sufficient or is rejected, the person living with HIV may begin a maladaptive cycle of behavior. This cycle perpetuates the belief that one may hold about an inability to perform tasks, may prevent one from acquiring basic skills needed to achieve a more complex skill, and may likely result in failure of task performance in the future. The perpetuation of maladaptive behavior often occurs in people with life-threatening illness. Persons who enter this cycle of behavior may require extensive therapy.

Persons who develop adaptive skills, or an adaptive cycle of performance, generally believe in their abilities and have faith in future outcomes, explore new possibilities to acquire skills, and attempt tasks with the trust and encouragement of others. If they fail, they try again.

Benign (adaptive) and vicious (maladaptive) cycles involve both internal beliefs and external objective successes and failures. Internal convictions leading to success and failure in engaging the environment are only half the adaptive process. The second component of adaption is the internal pleasure or displeasure associated with success and failure. Thus, any view of adaptation includes meeting environmental requirements and yielding personal satisfaction (Kielhofner, 1980a, p. 733).

As has been noted, the mind-body-environment interaction that supports daily living is essential to examine and understand in relation to facilitating human adaptation for people living with HIV infection. Each domain (physical, psychosocial and environmental) affects the other and determines human performance and subsequent function. If dysfunction occurs in any domain, the other two will be affected. For example, Joe has severe myelitis secondary to HIV infection. He has subsequent lower extremity weakness and poor sensation, which limit standing and sitting balance. Bill has the same diagnosis and clinical presentation. Joe has a supportive relationship and has always created projects in his work and daily life that he readily accomplishes and completes, producing a great sense of satisfaction. Bill has been in and out of relationships, has been a substance abuser, and has held many different jobs. Joe begins to work readily with the health care team in developing strength, endurance, increased mobility, and more independence in self-care and work. He becomes functionally independent and mobile in a wheelchair in four weeks. Bill states that he is helpless, can never again be independent, and becomes dependent on his sister who reluctantly cares for him. Joe continues to create new projects in his work and develops a stronger bond with his partner and other relationships with family and friends. Bill dies within three months.

Even the most adaptive person may encounter a disruption of life-style if he or she is living with multiple opportunistic infections. However, the adaptive person may overcome even those obstacles more readily than persons in a maladaptive cycle, thus regenerating an already positive quality of life and attitude toward living. Health care professionals have an obligation to support and assist persons living with HIV to become as adaptive and functional as possible, thereby maximizing the meaningfulness in living and in the quality of living. Health care professionals must first understand the interrelatedness of the physical, psychosocial and environmental domains of human performance.

Physical Domain

Asymptomatic persons have few if any physical symptoms that impair function. Over time, physical considerations may take the form of fatigue, shortness of breath, visual impairments, peripheral and central nervous system

(CNS) damage, various forms of cancer (KS lymphoma) and opportunistic infections that compromise physical wellness. Other physical considerations include cardiac problems, the wasting syndrome and seizure disorders. Physical pain is often noted, especially in persons with peripheral nervous system damage. Neuropathies are common and are often evident in both the upper and lower extremities. Central nervous system damage results in dementia, spinal cord dysfunction and stroke. People with peripheral nervous system (PNS) and CNS damage show evidence of gait, balance and general mobility problems, as well as changes in muscle tone. Range of motion, strength and coordination are also compromised; sensation can also be affected. These areas of change result in mild to severe changes in function and human performance.

There is a vast continuum of function and dysfunction and independence and dependence, which is unique for each person living with HIV. For therapists, physical considerations must be noted with regard to human performance. Often, physical problems impede function in mobility, work, self-care and play/leisure performance. Daily routines are impaired, and it often takes longer to accomplish tasks, including walking to and from areas within the home and community. Because extra time must be allotted to accomplish these tasks, the person with HIV infection may experience anger and frustration. Physical considerations must be assessed and treated according to how they interface with the psychosocial and environmental domains of performance. Health care professionals must also assess the value, importance and meaning that restoration/maintenance of physical function has for each individual. They must be careful to balance their own health care values and goals with those of the patient. This show of respect for the patient's views will elicit greater cooperation and psychosocial benefit. The focus on function and adaptation of function is vital. Given the demands of our society for holism in health care (Ferguson, 1980), it is no longer sufficient to simply increase active range of motion or strength in the extremities.

Psychosocial Domain

HIV disease is often viewed as a catastrophic illness, although this view is changing with the increased numbers of longterm survivors. Persons living with AIDS (PLWA) can easily become immobilized by the diagnosis alone, resulting in a diminution of life activity performance, including mobility. PLWA may experience depression, anxiety and preoccupation with illness. They may experience anger about the disease, discrimination that usually accompanies it, the prospect of a lonely and painful death, the lack of currently available treatments, medical staff and themselves (U.S.D.H. & H.S., 1986).

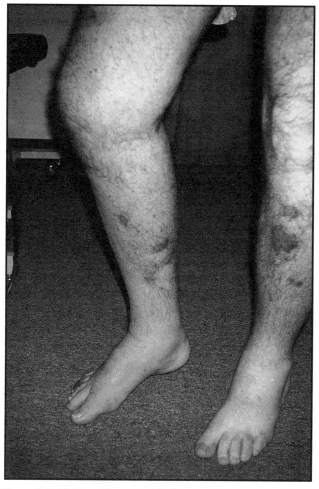

Figure 5-1. (a) Kaposi's sarcoma lesions, status post radiation and chemotherapy resulting in altered gait.

In many cases, patients develop guilt about the disease, past behaviors and the possibility of transmitting the disease to others. Health care professionals may observe depressive symptoms such as sadness, hopelessness, helplessness, withdrawal and isolation at various stages of illness. Suicidal ideation can occur, (see Chapter 11), most often due to perceived meaninglessness of life. Future goals are often shattered and require adaptation and restructuring. Anxiety may manifest as tension, stress, tachycardia, agitation, insomnia, anorexia and panic attacks.

Denial may alternate with realistic concerns about the outcome of illness. Concern can be replaced with hypochondriasis. Often people with HIV interpret any new symptom as bringing them closer to death. This behavior can perpetuate an already maladaptive cycle of behavior. In a majority of cases, there are neuropsychiatric sequelae. Symptoms may be seen as forgetfulness, lack of concentration, apathy and withdrawal, decreased alertness and diminished interest in familiar and pleasurable activity (see Chapter 11). In later stages of the illness, there is often severe confusion and disorientation (Institute of Medicine, 1986; Devita, et al., 1988; Vomvouras, 1989).

Given the physical disfigurement often caused by KS, patients often develop a problem with body image. Physical disfigurement, along with neuropsychiatric dysfunction, can lead the person with HIV to choose limited social and other familiar activity, which can then put the person at risk for future altered physical function. For example, Tim had noticeable KS lesions on his face and lower extremities; he often exercised at the gym and was a model for a fashion magazine. He ceased going to the gym and pursuing his career, even though he was a functional and productive

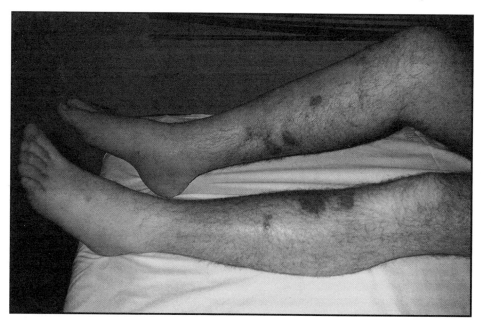

Figure 5-1. (b) Right lower extremity knee flexion contracture.

Figure 5-2. (a) Use of a Dynasplint to regain full range of motion.

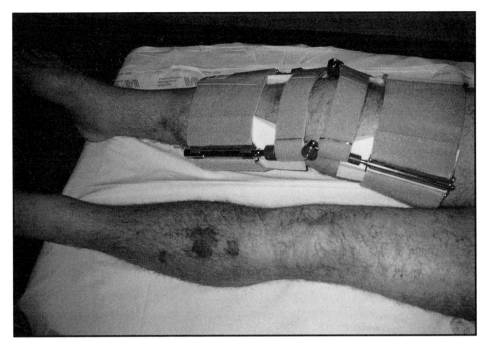

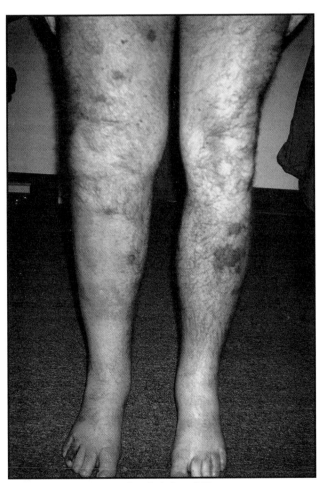

Figure 5-2. (b) Functional ambulation skills.

human being. He also placed limitations on friends visiting at home. In a short time, he began to experience decreased range of motion of right knee extension, with resultant gait and balance problems. This combination may have occurred as a direct result of psychological dysfunction related to a change of his physical appearance (Figure 5-1a and 5-1b). With appropriate rehabilitation, however, strategies, (the use of a Dynasplint range of motion exercises and transfer/gait training), Tim was able to achieve improvement in range and quality of ambulation, thus enhancing his self-image (Figures 5-2a and 5-2b).

From the time of diagnosis and throughout the course of illness, patients may experience a poor sense of control and perception of loss of mastery of the self in the environment. Persons with HIV often state that the disease controls choices of activity, including when and how tasks are performed. This contributes to a sense of helplessness and hopelessness.

A sense of incompetence can result in diminished task performance, which often leads to a withdrawal from activity. Having a sense of future or being able to establish future goals is perceived as being threatened. Current goals (eg. walking independently) often need to be adapted, revalued and redefined, in light of the disease process. Meaningfulness and what is valuable and important in one's life are more critically analyzed by the person living with HIV.

People with HIV who have high standards for performance or who organize time and activity rigidly are at high risk for psychosocial dysfunction (Pizzi, 1988). As physical function deteriorates, adaptability of one's standards and use of time is crucial. Also at risk for psychosocial dysfunction are those persons who have difficulty identifying interests or who may be termed "workaholic" with no other future goals. When one can no longer carry out work tasks, other activity and interests are needed to help that person organize time and a daily schedule (Pizzi, 1989a).

When physical function continues to deteriorate and roles (eg. homemaker, worker, hobbyist) can no longer be performed, adaptation of life roles and the commensurate physical skills to maintain function are needed. Health care professionals should also be acutely aware of the loss, grief and bereavement associated with loss of function and should be prepared, to some degree, to help patients cope with those issues.

Environmental Domain

The social, physical, cultural/subcultural and even economic environments of people with HIV must be considered as they affect function and life choices. Most people with HIV have already been stigmatized by society by the very nature of who they are as human beings. Gay and bisexual men and IV drug users comprise the majority of people with HIV and have had to contend with discrimination. When diagnosed with HIV, an added dimension of discrimination is often perceived. In the United States, antidiscrimination policies have been proposed, some of which are in effect in several states. Nevertheless, the personal value systems of noninfected persons may be in direct conflict with those of seropositive persons. Health care professionals must be aware of the stigma perceived by persons with HIV. This awareness and open and honest communication with the patient about the issue could provide a safe and comfortable therapeutic milieu (Pizzi, 1989b).

The social environment is defined as the people in a person's life. When a person is diagnosed with HIV disease, many times family members must cope not only with the person's disease but also with the fact that the person is gay or bisexual and/or an IV drug user. This social situation can lead to alienation bay family. In addition, significant others (spouse, lover, roommate) of the person living with HIV may leave the situation for any number of reasons (eg. fear, guilt, blame, the significant other also being seropositive, or perceived inability to care for the person). Finally, health care providers may have value systems that differ from that of the infected person and/or still suffer from irrational fear of HIV itself, thus alienating the person with HIV from the health care system. Health care workers must be aware of these possibilities as they impact on the rehabilitation process and on the person's overall function (Pizzi, 1989b). Persons with symptomatic and advanced HIV disease may have difficulty negotiating physical environments. Fatigue, shortness of breath, and CNS and PNS damage may affect

one's mobility in the community, at work or at home. Visual and sensory problems may also make it difficult to negotiate physical environments. Structural changes and adaptations of routines, roles and skills can assist persons in mastering their environments (see Chapter 18).

Economic loss experienced by one's inability to work can dramatically affect how one interacts with both the physical and social environments. The loss may be so profound that the person living with HIV/AIDS may need to find alternative housing or be faced with the possibility of being homeless. Loss of friends, due in part to the inability to manage financially (for movies, going to dinner, leisure trips), will alter socialization. Therapists should consider the economic situation of patients before making treatment recommendations, particularly if patients need to purchase equipment or materials to maintain function.

A MODEL OF CARE FOR PEOPLE WITH HIV

Human performance and one's ability to adapt in daily life can be viewed from an open system perspective. Open systems (eg. human beings) interact with environments and as a result constantly change and adapt. A model of care called the Model of Human Occupation (MOHO), based on open systems theory, can expand the already broad body of knowledge possessed by therapists working with people living with HIV. This model (Table 5-1) supports promotion of a global assessment and treatment of people with HIV and AIDS.

Kielhofner, who co-developed the model, aptly describes the model and its subsystems (Note: where *system* appears, substitute *person*).

> In this model, the volition subsystem is the highest level subsystem. Its function is to enact behavior. It guides the systems choices of action. Its structure involves three components: personal causation, valued goals, and interests. Personal causation refers to the individual's beliefs about the efficacy of action; it guides action according to the belief that a given action, or set of actions, is likely to achieve desired results or allow mastery over the world. Valued goals refer to those ends towards which the individual is willing to commit to sustained action. Interests refer to the disposition to engage in actions for their own sake and because of the pleasing results they can achieve. Personal causation, valued goals, and interests all contribute to the volition subsystem's influence over the propensity for action. In combination they determine what the system chooses

Table 5-1
The Model of Human Occupation

ENVIRONMENT
(physical, social, cultural)

VOLITION

Personal Causation
  Belief in skill
  Belief in efficacy of skill
  Expectancy of success/ failure
  Internal/ external control

Values
  Temporal orientation
  Meaningfulness of activity
  Occupational goals
  Personal standards

Interests
  Discrimination
  Pattern
  Potency

HABITUATION

Roles
  Perceived incumbency
  Internalized expectations
  Balance

Habits
  Degree of organization
  Social appropriateness
  Flexibility/rigidity

PERFORMANCE

Skills
  Interpersonal/communication
  Process
  Perceptual motor
  Symbolic
  Neurologic
  Musculoskeletal

From Kielhofner and Burke, 1980b

---

guides the output of action that does not need to be enacted through choice, action that is routine and largely out of consciousness. For instance, when behaviors originally energized by interest become routine, their organization becomes the function of the habituation subsystem.

Internalized roles refer to expectations from the environment for productivity that have been incorporated into the internal makeup of the system within the habituation subsystem. Internalized roles are important to the system's ability to meet demands from the environment for consistent performance. Habits are organized routines of behavior; they incorporate skills into patterns of action that can function automatically without the conscious attention of the actor.

The production/performance subsystem is the third and lowest level subsystem. The function of this subsystem is to produce action. Its structure consists of skills: social, cognitive, and/or physical actions organized to an end. A skill involves the integration of such diverse components as anatomy, neurological circuitry, and cognition. Skills organize components of the organism into patterns of action that achieve a given end under whatever conditions exist in the environment. Either the volition or habituation subsystems can trigger the system toward employment of a skill. Once the system is in action, this subsystem serves as a guide, controlling the quality of action and giving it that characteristic referred to as skill (Kielhofner, 1980c, pp 13-14).

The following is an example of how the motto can be used by health care professionals.

Tom, a 24-year-old wealthy white male who acquired HIV through IV drug use and/or through "a couple of gay experiences" presents in therapy with bilateral lower extremity weakness and mild neuropathy in both feet. He has unsteady gait and he fears falling. Also noted is upper extremity incoordination and atrophy and neuropathy in both hands. Tom, who has never worked, graduated from Harvard with a degree in liberal arts and lives alone in a penthouse in New York City. He is supported by a trust fund from his deceased father's estate. He went to college only to appease his mother.

Therapy recommendations include gait training with assistive device, upper and lower extremity strengthening, pain management, and activities of daily living adaptations, all of which are also his goals. During the first session, you are met with anger and verbal abuse and no cooperation after presenting Tom with treatment options. You can choose:

  1. to not treat because "I don't have to put up with abuse

---

to do. Since this subsystem determines what the individual finds pleasing and satisfying to do, it must be in harmony with other internal subsystems and with the environments' requirements. If there is a gap between the volition subsystem and the structure of another subsystem or in the requirements of the environment, disorganization can ensue.

The second subsystem is the habituation subsystem. Its structure is made up of habits and roles. It functions to maintain action. This subsystem from any patient" and discharge

2. to provide treatment recommendations, demonstrate for Tom despite his lack of cooperation, and discharge him

3. unfold with Tom what is really present (underneath the anger), which precludes his working with you at this moment

Option 1. When health care workers choose this option, they are playing "take away" games with the patient. That is, if a patient does not cooperate, they "take away" any hope or possibility for change for that person by denying therapy for what they say is a "very good reason"; the patient was verbally abusive. Patients living with HIV are often frightened of losing function. When the reality of this loss of function occurs, as in Tom's case, the patient may relate to anyone with anger, (acting out with abusive behaviors that can be short term) and needs understanding and a sensitivity to listening from therapists. Health care professionals often "play take away" because they feel personally threatened, but patients' reactions are rarely personal. Time spent exploring with patients where they are emotionally at any given moment in their illness can make the difference in a therapeutic relationship versus demanding cooperation with therapy. Should option 1 be chosen, health care workers must begin examining how to begin being proactive versus reactive in situations such as Tom's. Often, the situation to which health care professionals might react is rarely the underlying reason why they respond in this manner. Hypothetically, in Tom's case, one might be reacting from judgments one holds about "rich" people (like Tom). One might also have "secret" judgments about homosexuality or drug use that will alter the quality of care.

Option 2. For patients who have a strong internal sense of control or who perceive health care workers as "telling them" what to do (volition subsystem) (eg. this is how you walk with a walker), option 2 may be in the best interest of the patient. The health care worker may consider providing oral and written information and training and also demonstrations, even though patients may not appear to be interested. The contribution of the health care provider may not be immediately appreciated by the patient until after discharge from therapy.

Lack of cooperation and apathy may also be a secondary reaction to HIV encephalopathy. As HIV involves the brain, encephalopathy and subsequent neuropsychiatric sequelae may be apparent before any other symptom (see Chapter 11). Over 65 percent of patients will show some cognitive deficits eventually (Levinson & O'Connell, 1989). Awareness of these facts can enhance provided care and health care professionals can explain techniques and strategies in modified terms for both the patient and care giver.

Option 3. It is generally acceptable practice and often necessary to explore with patients what and how they are

Table 5-2 Assessment Battery for Adults with HIV	
Component	Assessment
VOLITION	
Personal Causation	Occupational history
	Occupational questions
	Psychological adjustment to illness scale
	Locus of control
Values	Occupational history
	Occupational questions
	Role checklist
	Time reference inventory
	Psychological adjustment to illness scale
Interests	Occupational history
	Occupational questions
	Psychological adjustment to illness scale
	Level of interest in particular activity
HABITUATION	
Roles	Occupational history
	Occupational questions
	Role checklist
	Psychological adjustment to illness scale
Habits	Occupational history
	Occupational questions
	Activities of daily living
	Activity record
	Interview
PERFORMANCE	
Skills	Occupational history
	Occupational questions
	Activities of daily living
	Activity record
	Clinical observation/ biomedical assessment
Environment	Occupational history
	Occupational questions
	Home assessments
	Social environment interview

From Pizzi, M. (1990). The model of human occupation and adults with HIV infection and AIDS. American Journal of Occupational Therapy 44(3):257. Used with permission.

Table 5-3
OCCUPATIONAL QUESTIONS

Evaluation of a person with HIV infection must consider total functioning. Looking at performance, or how one does a certain task, is not sufficient in assessing this population, given the scope and magnitude of occupational dysfunction already discussed. The following questions to support assessment are intended as a guide to screen for dysfunction due to HIV.

Does the person feel that HIV or other external forces are in control of the person's life or does the person feel in control?

Does the person identify skills?

Are these skills appropriate and relevant to the person's life situation?

Is there a sense of being effective at carrying out skills, or is there a sese of incompetence?

Does the person expect success/failure in carrying out skills?

Is there a past, present or future orientation?

How does the person believe time should be used?

What activities hold meaning for the person?

What are the person's goals?

Is the person able to identify goals?

What are the person's standards of performance?

Has the value or importance of certain activities, situations and/ or relationships altered since diagnosis with HIV?

How have they altered (positive or negative)?

Can the person identify interests?

Is there an abundance or scarcity of interests?

Is there a pattern of interests (eg. all physical activity)?

How often does the person engage in these interests?

In which life roles does the person identify himself/herself?

What roles are most and lease valuable?

Is there a balance of roles?

Conflict of roles?

Can the person describe a typical day, or how one uses time, from the time one rises until going to bed?

Is there an organized way in which one uses time?

Does the person allow flexibility in the routine or is the person rigid in time use?

What are the symbolic, neurologic and musculoskeletal limitations and abilities of the person (eg. range of motion, strength, endurance, coordination, cognition)?

How do these impede or enhance function?

Does the physical environment impede/enhance performance or acquisition of skill?

Does the social environment impede/enhance performance or acquisition of skill?

What factors of the person's culture/subculture need to be considered in evaluation, goal planning and treatment?

Other guiding questions that need to be considered include:
How, if at all, have these areas of functioning changed since being diagnosed with HIV?
In which areas of functioning does the person wish to remain most productive/ functional?
Can the person rank those areas of functioning (eg. self-care, relationships, work, leisure) in order of priority?

From Pizzi, M. (1989, February). Occupational therapy: Creating possibilities for adults with HIV infection, ARC and AIDS. AIDS Patient Care, 18-23. Used with permission.

feeling. Feedback about what may provoke certain reactions as they relate to the rehabilitation process can establish the patient-therapist partnership.

In the hypothetical case example, when the therapist sat and talked with Tom about how his lack of cooperation doesn't give room for helping him achieve his goals, Tom immediately began to cry. The heath care provider discovered that, for Tom, walking with any assistive device signaled lack of control, dependence, loss of function, and being "closer to death," all of which are unfamiliar to Tom. Socially, he feels he would be outcast from his wealthy

circle of friends who do not know he is ill with HIV. He fears that he has infected his girlfriend and he tells the health care provider of the guilt and shame he feels.

Being an avid tennis player and ranked number two in his country club, Tom discusses immediate changes he must make (and is not prepared to make) in his habits and roles. He also describes the many interests he has, all of which necessitate physical performance. The health care professional also realizes that Tom has always had to try to prove he was "good enough" to his father, which forced him to develop unrealistic standards and expectations of performance. In a physically debilitated condition, he realizes he can never prove anything to his father or anyone and states a total sense of helplessness and futility.

Based on the conversation with Tom, the health care professional develops a care plan. The occupational therapist evaluates Tom using a battery of assessments (Table 5-2) (Pizzi, 1990a). Social work is contacted to help Tom learn to cope with his losses, guilt, shame and fear. His program of care addresses role changes, development of interest and adapting performance for successful engagement in interests, and adaptive equipment/strategies for activities of daily living (ADL) performance. Also explored are Tom's values, goals, standards of performance, and the meaning Tom places on current and former activities.

In this brief case example and in the options for care presented, health care professionals can get a clear sense of the need to examine the patient's global function and underlying areas that can impede or enhance adaptive human performance. This case can also assist therapists in determining ways to modify treatment recommendations. For example, the care giver can discuss with Tom the psychological impact of assistive walking devices and can support him in determining ways to be independently mobile while coping with these issues. It can be emphasized that allied health professionals may incorporate and/or acknowledge the patient's goals, values, beliefs and attitudes about his or her own rehabilitation in order to appropriately assess and treat people living with HIV.

ASSESSMENT

Assessment begins with a basic screening tool that examines all areas of occupational functioning (Table 5-3) (Pizzi, 1989b). These occupational questions provide the therapist with a basic overview of the range of function and dysfunction and can dictate areas for further assessment. Treatment considerations can also be addressed from this tool.

Performance

Assessment and treatment of ADL should be performed at natural times in a normal routine and in the environment where the patient usually performs the activity. ADL encompasses physical, psychosocial, and environmental aspects of function. It incorporates areas of eating, transfers and mobility, bathing, dressing, grooming and general communication. Observation and interview are both used to assess ADL. Observational assessment should be used as time and environment permit. Health care workers should also obtain permission from the patient with respect to the patient's values and sense of privacy. An interview may not present a true picture of functional abilities. For example, answers in an interview may be skewed by impaired cognition, or the patient may state a certain degree of independence and not communicate that he or she receives assistance at home from a care giver. Interview, however, may be the only alternative should a patient refuse an observational assessment. The ADL checklist (Pizzi, 1989b) is designed as both an observational and interview assessment and can be used by any discipline (Appendix C). Health care professionals must consider performance of tasks; the routine in which tasks are performed; the environment in which tasks are performed; and the values, interests and choices of the patient with respect to ADL. The Functional Independence Measure (FIM) (Appendix C) is a tool that assesses ADL in several domains and is often used in rehabilitative settings.

It is also necessary to include the significant other in this type of interview assessment to gather data on the routine. This input can affect treatment recommendations if the significant other needs to assist the patient with ADL. Recommending ADL treatments commensurate with the patient's and significant other's former routines can decrease stress for the family system and result in greater productivity.

For example, health care professionals worked with pain management and gait training to a level where it would be manageable for Bill at home, with the support of his lover, John. At home, Bill remains in his wheelchair most of the day and only occasionally works with his therapeutic exercise and pain management regimen. Bill uses these programs to manipulate John, forcing him to interrupt his own daily routine, leave work and assist Bill in daily functioning. The pay off for Bill is having John around more often. The manipulation is also due to Bill's fear of being alone, even though he was independently mobile in the hospital. The cost to Bill in this situation may be loss of his relationship. Involvement of the health care team is vital.

Physical Assessment

The HIV Evaluation Form (Appendix C) is designed for the therapist in the rehabilitation setting. The following are assessed in relation to occupational role performance and in self-care, work and leisure. A general assessment should include the following.

1. Strength. usually evaluated via a manual muscle test in physical therapy, strength can also be assessed through functional activity

2. Range of Motion (ROM). Passive or active ROM. When documenting ROM, be specific as to passive range of motion (PROM) or active range of motion (AROM). This distinction can make a difference when planning treatment. Compromised ROM can be due to radiation necrosis for treatment of KS.

3. Coordination. Evaluated through observation of patient at rest and in activity. If HIV directly invades the cerebellar area, then tremor, dysdiadochokinesia, dysmetria and ataxia may be noted. If the basal ganglia are affected, tremor, athetosis, dystonia, chorea and hemiballismus may be present.

4. Muscle tone. Evaluation is through passive movement of extremities. Extremities may be rigid or flaccid or may present varying degrees of spasticity. Tone may fluctuate on a daily basis due to the neurologic sequelae of HIV.

5. Sensation. Assessment of sensation includes light touch, deep pressure, temperature, pain, proprioception, kinesthesia, two-point discrimination and stereognosis. A thorough assessment is necessary since many people with HIV present with neuropathies. Neuropathic pain can be so severe that it limits the performance of any activity.

6. Endurance. Most patients have endurance deficits. Endurance is the length of time or the number of repetitions for performance of an activity. Endurance can be observed during an ADL assessment or by walking with a patient. It is essential to determine the extent to which endurance interferes with occupational performance. Standing and sitting tolerance should also be evaluated in relation to performance of occupational tasks.

7. Cognition. Assessing cognitive areas such as short- and long-term memory, judgment, problem solving and decision making, sequencing, general orientation, and perceptual-motor is vital. Safety issues are important, especially with self-care, mobility, negotiating community and work environments, and home maintenance. The Mental Status Questionnaire (Kahn et al., 1960) can be used to determine orientation and is a short and easy interview. The Mini-Mental State (MMS) (Folstein et al., 1975) assesses five areas of cognition: orientation, memory, attention and calculation, recall and language. The FROMAJE Mental Status Evaluation (Libow, 1981) can also be used. The speech-language pathologist and neuropsychiatric staff may perform cognitive assessments; hence, a team approach can benefit the patient and care givers.

HABITUATION

Occupational Roles

Occupational roles are assessed by the Role Checklist (Appendix C) (Oakley et al., 1986). Occupational roles are assessed in terms of the value they hold for individuals, which is essential for treatment planning. It is important to

note that occupational roles serve as a source of identity. For people with HIV, it is essential to determine the value placed on particular roles, adaptation of roles, and the tasks necessary to carry out these roles. This may assist health workers in setting goals and planning treatments that are more likely to be continued by the patient when making the transition from hospital to community. For example, a person may note that the home maintainer role was performed, is being performed, and will be performed, although the individual does not value this role. Treatment planning may then incorporate adaptations of home maintenance and not make it a priority for treatment, given the low value placed on the role.

Ninety-eight percent of all reported cases of HIV and AIDS are people in the worker years, ages 20 to 60. Given the chronic and progressive nature of HIV, therapists should thoroughly assess the role of worker and develop creative treatment programs designed around work and productivity (Pizzi, 1989a).

Habits of Daily Living

Assessment of habits and functional routines of daily living is necessary when working with the person with HIV. Habits become dysfunctional when one no longer engages in productive and meaningful activity. This may occur due to medical problems (dementia, fatigue, neuropathy) or psychosocial problems (fear, anger, withdrawal, depression) that impede performance. Adaptation for individuals within their habit structure (eg. rigid or flexible) is also important to assess in view of the progressive nature of HIV, the occupational changes inherent in disease progression, and the need for flexibility in the daily routine. For example, a person who rigidly organizes the day is at greater occupational risk than one who is flexible and can adapt to changes such as fluctuations in fatigue that demand a change in the level of activity.

The Activity Record (Appendix C) is designed to collect information on the physically disabled. Information about the habit structure and volitional aspects of daily living (personal causation, values, interests) is gathered. The assessment assists health care workers in determining pain, level of difficulty, and fatigue in certain activities. These clinical data can be used in planning treatments, especially for developing an adapted routine of daily living (Pizzi, 1990b).

Volition

Several psychosocial/psychiatric tools are often used to assess areas of values and personal causation. Among those used are the Psychological Adjustment to Illness Scale (Morrow et al., 1978) and the Locus of Control Scale (Rotter, 1966). An important area to explore with patients is the area of interests.

Loss of interest in favored activities often occurs after diagnosis, and the amount of time spent in these pursuits also diminishes. Performance of an interest could be constrained due to the increased time required to complete the activity of interest (eg. hobby, reading, etc.), decreased mobility and decreased abilities. The environment, ie. a hospital bed or the hospital itself, also may be constricting. People with HIV may develop depressive symptoms and withdraw or have difficulty establishing or maintaining continuity of performance. Since at some point, most people with HIV can no longer work, other interests and roles need to replace work as a means of restructuring habits and maintaining productivity. The Level of Interest in Particular Activities (Appendix C) (Scaffa, 1981) assists the health care provider in identifying the level of interest during the past 10 years and past year, current participation and interest in future pursuit of the activity.

Treatment can be planned with the help of this assessment. For example, if a patient who developed myelopathy had previously focused only on physical activity, the obvious need to change would place the patient at higher risk for psychosocial dysfunction (ie. loss of meaningful activity and productivity). The health care professional can then plan treatment based on nonphysical interests, the value of these interests to the patient, and adaptation focused on performance of these interests (Pizzi, 1989).

Environment

The physical environment is assessed by either a home visit or interview with patient and significant other. The living space must be made accessible for performance of daily activities. The social environment (significant other, friends, co-workers, family) can also be assessed by the Social Environment Interview (Appendix C) (Pizzi, 1989b). The interviewer gathers data about the primary person involved with the care of the patient, which can help therapists explore ways to assist care givers in diminishing the stress of care giving, especially in latter stages of illness, while maintaining their own personal level of wellness.

It is essential for health care workers to recognize the impact of the environment on human activity and performance and the influence of the environment on the level of adaptability to illness. For example, stressed care givers may be forfeiting nights out with friends and may be taking much time off work to care for the patient. This routine may produce feelings of anger and frustration, resulting in less attention paid to bed positioning and drug administration. The level of care need not be compromised if health care workers can help care givers develop their own sense of well-being. Likewise, if doorways and halls in the home are inaccessible for wheelchairs, a patient may be relegated to one room for most of the day, far from the rooms of family

activity. This arrangement can heighten a sense of isolation and vulnerability. Health care professionals empower patients and care givers to regain control and mastery over the environment by involving them in the assessment of all areas of functioning and the development of strategies of care.

TREATMENT

Treatment is based on the data gathered from the screening and assessment of the patient and care giver(s). While the HIV seropositive person is asymptomatic, psychosocial interventions may take priority and can be provided individually or in groups. Role and habit changes and transitions are emphasized and occupational strategies to provide opportunities for more control and choice in the patient's life are recommended. Wellness programs that focus on productivity and maintaining a balance between work, rest, sleep and play and strategies that focus on contributions to others are examples of such an intervention (Pizzi, 1990a). As disease progression is noted, fatigue, neuropathies, dementia and other opportunistic infections alter human performance of daily living skills; impair work, play and ADL habits and roles; and can result in a sense of helplessness, hopelessness, and loss of control and meaning, thus altering the patient's perception of the future (Pizzi, 1989a). Treatments can include adaptive equipment for ADL, adaptation of occupational roles such as home maintainer and worker, habit retraining, energy conservation, development of leisure interests and their performance, environmental adaptations, general body strengthening, mobility training, pain management, imagery and visualization, myofascial release and craniosacral therapy. Care giver education should be incorporated in all treatment plans.

SUMMARY

Rehabilitation specialists may view patients as having physical, psychosocial and environmental dimensions of living and a need to restore these areas based on the patient's values, interests and choices. This chapter has served as a template for assessment and treatment of the person living with HIV and the effect of care givers and environment on the outcome of functional measures. Viewing the patient and care giver as vital partners in the rehabilitation process is the first step to achieving multifaceted results in quality care.

Acknowledgment

The author would like to acknowledge Mary Lou Galantino, MS, PT, for her support and encouragement in the writing of this chapter.

References

DeVita, V., Hellman, S., and Rosenberg, S. (1988). *AIDS: Etiology, Diagnosis, Treatment and Prevention* (2nd ed.). Philadelphia: J.B. Lippincott Co.

Dubos, R. (1978). Health and creative adaptation. *Human Nature*. 1:74. Ferguson, M. (1980). *The Aquarian Conspiracy*. Los Angeles: J.P. Tarcher.

Folstein, M.F., Folstein, S.E., and McHugh, P.R. (1975). Mini-mental state: A practical method for grading the cognitive state of patients for the clinician. *Journal of Psychiatric Research*. 12:189.

Institute of Medicine. (1986). *Confronting AIDS: Directions for Public Health, Health Care and Research*. Washington, DC: National Academy Press.

Kahn, R.L., Goldfarb, A.I., Pollack, M., and Peck, A. (1960). Brief objective measure for the determination of mental status in the aged. *American Journal of Psychiatry*. 117:326.

Kielhofner, G. (1980a). A model of human occupation: Part 3, Benign and vicious cycles. *American Journal of Occupational Therapy*. 34(11):731.

Kielhofner, G., and Burke, J.P. (1980b). A model of human occupation: Part I, Conceptual framework and content. *American Journal of Occupational Therapy*. 34:572.

Kielhofner, G., Burke, J.P., and Igi, C.H. (1980c). A model of human occupation: Part 4, Assessment and intervention. *American Journal of Occupational Therapy*. 34(12):777.

Levinson, S.F., and O'Connell, P.G. (1989). Update on the epidemiology and treatment of HIV infection and AIDS. Course supplements of the joint annual meetings of the American Academy of Physical Medicine and Rehabilitation and the American Congress of Rehabilitation Medicine, November, pp. 1302-1313.

Libow, L.S. (1981). A rapidly administered, easily remembered mental status evaluation: FROMAJE. In Libow, L.S., and Sherman, F.T. (Eds.). *The Core of Geriatric Medicine: A Guide for Students and Practitioners*. St. Louis: CV Mosby.

Morrow, G., Ciarello, R., and Derogatis, L. (1978). A new scale for assessing patients' psychosocial adjustment to medical illness. *Psychological Medicine*. 8:605.

Oakley, F., Kielhofner, G., Barris, R., and Reichler, R.K. (1986). The Role Checklist: Development and empirical assessment of reliability. *Occupational Therapy Journal of Research*. 6:157.

Pizzi, M. (1988, August 18). Challenge of treating AIDS patients includes helping them lead functional lives. *OT Week*. 6-7, 31.

Pizzi, M. (1989a, February). Occupational therapy: Creating possibilities for adults with HIV infection, ARC and AIDS. *AIDS Patient Care*. 18-23.

Pizzi, M. (1989b). *HIV infection and AIDS: Transformation of an Illness: The Manual*. New York: Mary Ann Liehert, Inc. Available from Michael Pizzi, 8201 16th Street #1123 Silver Spring, Maryland 20910.

Pizzi, M. (1990a). The model of human occupation and adults with HIV infection and AIDS. *American Journal of Occupational Therapy*. 44(3):257.

Pizzi, M. (1990b). HIV infection, AIDS and occupational therapy. In Munkind, J. (Ed.): *AIDS and Rehabilitation*. New York: McGraw-Hill.

Reilly, M. (1974). *Play as Exploratory Learning*. Beverly Hills: Sage Publications. Rotter, J. (1966). Generalized expectancies for internal versus external control of reinforcement. *Psychological Monograph*. 80:1.

Scaffa, M. (1981). Temporal adaptation and alcoholism. Unpublished master's thesis, Virginia Commonwealth University, Richmond, VA.

Task Force for Development of a Uniform Data System for Medical Rehabilitation. The Functional Independence Measure is copyrighted by the State University of New York Foundation, 1990.

United States Department of Health and Human Services (1986). *Coping with AIDS*. DHHS Publication No. (ADM) 85-1432.

Vomvouras, S. (1989). Psychiatric manifestations of AIDS spectrum disorders. *Southern Medical Journal*. 82(3):352.

6

Nutritional Assessment and Management

Richard C. Elbein, MS, RD, LD

*The fundamental precept of fight for longevity is avoidance of satiation.
One must not lose desires; they are mighty stimulants to creativeness, to
love, and to long life.*

—Alexander A. Bogomoletz
Russian doctor, scientist, 1881-1946

INTRODUCTION

HIV directly and indirectly affects the digestive system and overall nutritional status of infected individuals. Progressive HIV infection is associated with weight loss, cachexia, nutrient deficiencies, and protein-calorie malnutrition (Jansen, 1988; Colman & Grossman, 1987).

The majority of persons with AIDS experience malnutrition (Pan American Health Organization, 1989). Their morbidity and mortality rates are directly related to their nutritional status (Sato & Mirtallo, 1987). Nutrient-related immunodeficiencies can combine with HIV-related immunodeficiencies to hasten the development of AIDS in malnourished HIV-infected persons (Jain & Chandra, 1984). AIDS, when accompanied by nutritional complications, further compromises the patient's quality of life (Clinical Nutrition Cases, 1988).

Malnutrition in patients with chronic symptomatic HIV disease is seen as a wasting disease with a loss of overall weight and muscle tissue. This type of wasting is due to an inadequate supply of energy and protein and is referred to as protein calorie malnutrition (PCM). Psychological and physical manifestations of PCM can be observed in AIDS patients (Kotler, 1989). These changes, such as lethargy, apathy, decreased sociability, and disinterest in self-care, exacerbate nutrient deficiencies by creating a worsening cycle of malnutrition (Solomons & Allen, 1983).

Nutritional intervention at all stages of HIV infection may prevent or postpone PCM and improve quality of life. Some AIDS-related symptomatology may be prevented by good nutritional support, which could also provide protection from exacerbation of the disease (Jain & Chandra, 1984). Aggressive nutritional intervention in malnourished AIDS patients may improve disease symptoms (American Family Physicians, 1989). For these reasons, nutritional status is an important consideration in maintaining the health of HIV-infected individuals and in responding to the changing needs of AIDS patients. This chapter reviews basic nutrition and applies a model of nutritional care for HIV-infected clients.

BASIC NUTRITION

The standard human diet provides nutrients essential for survival, maintenance and growth. These nutrients are found in all foods and beverages, regardless of their cultural diversity. Due to the widely divergent food choices of different cultural groups, nutrition must be understood by its basic component. Nutrition can best be discussed by identifying the six basic nutrients: water, protein, carbohydrate, fat, vitamins and minerals.

Calories

A *calorie* is the amount of energy that can be derived from food. Proteins, carbohydrates and fats are the food components that provide calories; vitamins, minerals and water have no caloric or energy value. The *basic metabolic rate* (BMR) is the energy (calories) needed to drive basic bodily functions such as heart, lungs, and digestion. Energy required for activity is added to the BMR to determine the total daily energy requirements. Activities that increase caloric needs include sitting, walking, jogging and eating. These energy needs can be met only by eating combinations of proteins, carbohydrates, and fats to provide adequate energy.

When the energy intake is different from the body's energy needs, weight fluctuations occur. Weight gain occurs when the caloric intake is greater than the caloric need. During growth and development, that weight gain may occur as muscle tissue or bone growth. Weight gain may be due to increased numbers and/or size of fat cells. During weight loss the opposite situation occurs. Inadequate intake creates a negative calorie balance with a related loss of fat, muscle tissue or both. That loss may be intentional (as in the case of weight reduction diets) or unintentional (as in the case of cancer and other chronic diseases).

Water

Water normally constitutes about 60 percent of human body weight. Water balance is maintained by a combination of kidney function and the thirst mechanism and is achieved by matching the water losses (through sweat, respiration, urine, feces, and bleeding) with water repletion (from liquids and solid foods). The daily water requirement ranges from two to four liters. Starvation, carbohydrate restriction, inadequate fluid intake and fever increase fluid needs and generally produce dehydration. Water deficiency is the most fatal of the nutrient deficiencies.

Protein

Protein, available from both plant and animal sources, is used for numerous body systems, processes and functions. Proteins are made up of amino acids. Essential amino acids are the protein components that cannot be manufactured by the human body and must be obtained from foods. Proteins that provide all of the essential amino acids are referred to as complete. Only complete proteins can be effectively used for protein-related functions or structures. Animal products, with few exceptions (gelatin), are complete proteins and are excellent sources of all the essential amino acids. Plant proteins provide some essential amino acids, but must be combined to create a complete protein (eg. beans and rice). Proteins are used to maintain organs and tissues and to manufacture enzymes and hormones. All cells and cell processes require amino acids, which are obtained from digestion and utilization of protein from foods. Excess protein is catabolized for energy to supply a portion of the

BMR and activity energy requirement. Nitrogen released from protein catabolism is converted into nitrogen, producing compounds such as nucleic acids, creatinine and porphyrins.

The body is constantly synthesizing and breaking down protein within the cells and organs. This process of protein replacement, called protein turnover, affects the daily protein and amino acid requirement. Protein and amino acid requirements are also affected by the physiologic state of the individual. Requirements for amino acids and protein increase during trauma, diseases and infection.

Carbohydrates

Carbohydrates are the main source of energy in the human diet. The brush border of epithelial cells in the intestinal mucosa break carbohydrates down into sugar. Carbohydrates are present in the diet in three major forms: complex, simple and nondigestible. Complex carbohydrates are starchy foods such as breads, cereals, grains and pastas. Simple carbohydrates, usually called simple sugars, are sweet foods like sucrose (table sugar), fructose (fruit sugar), lactose (milk sugar), maltose (beer sugar), and mixed sugars found in syrups and honey. Nondigestible carbohydrates, commonly called bulk or fiber, are plant products that cannot be broken down by human digestive enzymes. Fiber, therefore, remains intact as it passes through the digestive tract. Fiber is often broken down by microflora of the digestive tract, with flatus as a by-product. Dietary fiber is important because it affects transit time, gastric emptying, absorption and mineral and electrolyte availability.

Carbohydrate-rich foods are excellent sources of the vast majority of the vitamins and minerals. For this reason, as well as the importance of carbohydrates as an energy source, they are a vital part of the human diet.

Fat

Fat is a poorly understood nutrient, which receives generally poor press. Fat, like carbohydrate, is a major energy source. In the diet, fat is present mainly in the form of triglycerides and fatty acids. The structure of fatty acids determines whether the fat is saturated (solid fats such as shortenings and lard) or monounsaturated and polyunsaturated (liquid fats such as corn, safflower, and olive and soy oil). Two polyunsaturated fatty acids are considered essential for cell growth and development. The essential fatty acids cannot be produced by the body and must be supplied by the diet.

Fat is important for a number of reasons. First, it is an important source of concentrated energy, both fat from the diet and that stored in the body. Fat provides 35 percent of the calories in the average American diet. Body fat stores may be used during negative calorie balance to supply the deficient calories. Second, it improves the palatability of foods and helps hunger/satiety responses. Finally, the fat soluble vitamins are richly available from the fat components of food. Dairy products supply the fat soluble vitamins A and D, and vegetables provide vitamins E and A.

Vitamins

Vitamins are organic compounds used for maintenance and growth of cells and to promote organ functions; they are not sources of energy nor are they used for cell structure. Since they cannot be produced by the body, vitamins must be supplied by the diet or by bacteria that inhabit the gastrointestinal (GI) tract. Vitamins promote cell processes such as nutrient metabolism, cell replication, and antioxidant functions. Some vitamins are present in the water-based food compartments (B-complex and C), whereas others are present in the fat-soluble food compartments (A, D, E and K). Vitamins A, D and K are used in cell replication and differentiation processes. Vitamins E and C are antioxidants and protect lipids from free radical formation. The B vitamins are precursors for coenzymes in enzyme systems, such as metabolism and energy utilization (of carbohydrates, protein and fat), formation of cell constituents, repair, and defense mechanisms. Vitamin requirements depend on their availability from foods in digestion, absorption, transportation and elimination by the body. Specific guidelines for vitamins based on age and sex are provided by the National Research Council as the Recommended Dietary Allowances (RDA). RDA values represent the average daily nutrient intake over time for a population to meet or exceed their nutrient requirements. They are not designed to be used for the specific individual. The United States Recommended Daily Allowance (U.S. RDA) was established to assist consumers to identify how their needs are being met. U.S. RDAs are commonly used on nutrition labels on food and vitamin/mineral supplements. Table 6-1 supplies U.S. RDA for vitamins. They may be seen as a percentage of the daily recommended allowances for men.

Minerals

Minerals are naturally occurring inorganic nutrients. Nineteen of the 25 minerals are considered essential for normal human growth and maintenance. They have a wide array of functions within the body. Calcium and phosphorus act as structural components in bone. Sodium, potassium, chloride, calcium and magnesium act as charged ions that facilitate muscle contractions and neuromuscular transmissions. Magnesium and manganese are charged ions that facilitate energy metabolism. Other minerals, such as iron in hemoglobin, copper in ceruloplasmin and selenium in glutathione peroxidase are components of enzymes or proteins. Minerals may play roles in other important small

Table 6-1
U.S. RDA FOR VITAMINS / MINERALS

NUTRIENT	U.S. RDA	SIGNIFICANT SOURCES
WATER-SOLUBLE VITAMINS		
Vitamin C	60 mg	Citrus fruits, tomato, greens, potato, strawberries
Thiamin	1.5 mg	Meat whole grains, nuts, legumes, fortified grains
Riboflavin	1.7 mg	Milk, yogurt, meat, fortified grains, cottage cheese
Niacin	20 mg	Meat, poultry, fish, liver, fortified grains
Folic Acid	0.4 mg	Liver, green leafy vegetables, legumes
Vitamin B_6	2.0 mg	Meat, poultry, fish, whole grain, legumes, green and leafy vegetables
Vitamin B_{12}	6.0 mcg	Meat, fish, poultry, eggs, dairy products
Biotin	0.3 mg	Organ meats, milk, fresh vegetables, egg yolks
Pantothenic Acid	10 mg	Meats, organ meats, milk, egg yolks, legumes, whole grains
FAT-SOLUABLE VITAMIN		
Vitamin A	5000 IU	Liver, butterfat, egg yolk, carrots, leafy green vegetables, yellow vegetables
Vitamin D	400 IU	Fortified margarine, fortified dairy products, fish oils, egg yolks
Vitamin E	30 IU	Vegetable oil, margarine, green and leafy vegetables

molecules, such as cobalt in B-12 and chromium in glucose tolerance factor.

Mineral needs depend on bioavailability and individual health factors. Competing compounds in mineral-rich foods may impair absorption. For example, calcium absorption from green, leafy vegetables is interrupted by the presence of oxalic acid, rendering the calcium unavailable. These antagonistic relationships also exist with iron and zinc in some foods.

An inadequate supply of minerals can cause deficiency

Table 6-2
U.S. RDA FOR VITAMINS / MINERALS

NUTRIENT	U.S. RDA	SIGNIFICANT SOURCES
MINERALS		
Calcium	1 g	Milk and milk products, green leafy vegetables, citrus fruits, dried beans and peas
Iron	16 mg	Meat, liver, egg, yolk, fish, green leafy vegetables, whole grains, dried beans and peas, dried fruit
Phosphorus	1.0 g	Meat, poultry, fish, eggs, whole grains
Iodine	150 mcg	Seafood, ocean products, iodized salt
Magneseum	400 mg	Whole grains, nuts, dried beans and peas
Zinc	15 mg	Meat, liver, eggs, oysters, seafood, milk
Copper	2.0 mg	Organ meats, shellfish, nuts, legumes, raisins, chocolate

states with developmental, structural or metabolic impact. Deficiencies in iron lead to deficiencies in anemia; deficiencies in zinc lead to arrested sexual development; calcium deficiencies lead to decreased bone density. Excess intake of minerals may also adversely effect overall health. For example, sodium may increase blood pressure and fluid retention. Fluorine may cause defects in the formation of tooth enamel. Mineral intakes should remain within the upper and lower limits of safety. RDAs and U.S. RDAs have been established for minerals. Table 6-2 supplies U.S. RDA values for minerals.

Digestive Tract

A discussion of nutrition in HIV infection requires a basic understanding of the digestive tract. The GI tract is a system of related organs. Their main function is to process food and extract the nutrients. Each organ's role in the system represents a unique aspect of the digestive process.

Food enters the GI tract through the mouth. The teeth and tongue reduce solid food to smaller pieces and mix it with saliva. Saliva eases the food's movement and begins carbo-

hydrate breakdown. The esophagus moves food from the mouth to the stomach. In the stomach, food is mechanically mixed with digestive enzymes that break down proteins. Food is slowly released from the stomach into the small intestine. The small intestine moves this dispersed liquid by peristalsis while exposing it to numerous enzymatic processes to release nutrients. Carbohydrates, proteins, fats and vitamins are absorbed in the small intestine. As digestive materials pass through the large intestine (colon), water, electrolytes (minerals), biotin and vitamin K (a by-product from bacterial metabolism) are absorbed.

Functional disturbances of organs in the GI tract can produce identifiable symptoms and nutrient deficiencies. If food enters the small intestine too rapidly due to the lost regulation of gastric emptying, it produces abdominal pain and diarrhea. An interruption of peristalsis in the small intestine can produce pain, distension and vomiting. Damage to endothelial cells in the intestinal tract compromises absorption and prevents adequate nutrient availability. Because the integrity of the GI tract is critical to the adequate supply of nutrients, it is often the focus of dietary intervention. Nutritional support often focuses on correcting GI disturbances and nutrient malabsorption.

NUTRITION AND IMMUNE FUNCTION

The effectiveness of the immune system and its susceptibility to infections is altered by malnutrition (Probart, 1989). Malnourished individuals develop infectious complications more quickly than well-nourished individuals (Probart, 1989). Poor nutritional status is the most common cause of secondary immunodeficiency (Chandra, 1981). Many nutrients directly influence immune function, GI function, susceptibility to infection and cancer risk. Specific nutritional deficits can impair immune response by altering cell-mediated immunity, bactericidal functions of neutrophils, the complement system, and secretory IgA antibodies (Mosesen et al., 1989).

Malnourished patients routinely have impaired T- and B-cell functions (Nwiloh et al., 1988). Nutritional repletion improves these patients' immune functions (Nwiloh et al., 1988). Inadequate or excess intake of certain vitamins or minerals is known to alter specific organ or system functions. For example, PCM and deficiencies of iron, zinc, pyridoxine, folic acid and vitamins B-12 and A are associated with compromised immune function (Moseson, et al., 1989). A variety of nutrients can affect immune function. Appropriate nutritional therapy addresses these issues by preventing deficiencies, as well as excess intake. Table 6-3 summarizes nutrient impact on immune function. As previously discussed, some changes in the immune system from HIV infection mirror changes that occur from nutritional deficiencies and imbalances. Because malnutrition generally precedes infection, nutrition may be a cofactor that influences the development of AIDS in HIV-infected individuals (Moseson, et al., 1989). Just as nutritional deficits impair immune response, optimal nutrition may influence lymphocyte and immune function. Therefore, nutritional support is likely to affect immune abnormalities from HIV infection and enhance resistance to opportunistic infections (Hyman & Kaufman, 1989).

PROTEIN CALORIE MALNUTRITION

The simultaneous deficiency of energy and protein is known as protein calorie malnutrition (PCM). When expenditures of energy exceed their availability in the body, the result is a loss of body cell mass (Nutrition Reviews, 1988). Poor intake and malabsorption have the same effect in limiting the protein and energy available to the body *Nutrition Reviews*, 1988. PCM is characterized by severe weight loss and depletion of somatic and visceral proteins *Journal of the American Dietetic Association*, 1989). Furthermore, PCM is generally associated with depletion of body minerals and water- and fat-soluble vitamins, such as folate, thiamine, riboflavin, nicotinic acid, pyridoxine, ascorbic acid and vitamin A (Rudman, 1980).

The immunologic abnormalities seen in patients with PCM are similar to those seen in HIV infection, including depressed T-cell number, reduced T-helper cell function, reduced secretory IgA, and impaired primary and secondary delayed cutaneous hypersensitivity responses (Cunningham-Rundles, 1982). Atrophy of the thymus, among other organs, has been observed in children with PCM (Linder, 1987). This adaptive response creates major immunologic manifestations including impaired T-cell function such as delayed hypersensitivity, lymphokine production and cell killing (Hughes et al., 1974). PCM is believed to be an important factor in the development of PCP pneumonia in children with cancer (Chelluri & Jastremski, 1989). PCP is also a common complicating factor in HIV infection.

PCM is almost always present in AIDS (Rudman et al., 1980). Decreased intake and malabsorption associated with HIV infection contribute to the development of malnutrition and onset of PCM (Hickson & Knudson, 1988). PCM increases HIV-infected individuals susceptibility to opportunistic infectious organisms and increases their morbidity and mortality from common infections (Cunningham-Rundles, 1982). Patients with PCM enter a cycle of worsening malnutrition with associated severe weight loss, diarrhea

Table 6-3
NUTRIENT IMPACT ON IMMUNE FUNCTION

ITEM	EFFECT
Malnutrition	-Impaired T- and B-Cell function, which improves with repletion -Low levels of secretory IgA in infants -Decreased efficiency of lymphocytes to locate in mucosal tissue
Vitamin A Deficiency	-Reduced protective goblet cells in GI epithelium -Decreased efficiency of lymphocytes to locate in mucosal tissue -Increased susceptibility to respiratory and GI infections -T-cell depletion in rats -Rise in lymphocyte count in rats when repleted with retinoic acid
Vitamin C	-Depression of leukocyte activity with daily 2g supplement -Increase in serum IgG, IgM, and immune complex component C3 with daily 1g supplement -Increased proliferative response of T lymphocytes with 500mg daily supplement -Megadoses (over 2g daily) cause GI disturbances, rise in serum cholesterol, destruction of vitamin B12
Vitamin D	-Suppresses CD4+ cell numbers -Reduces synthesis of IgG and IgM
Vitamin B_6	-Deficiency reduces functional cytotoxic T-lymphocytes
Zinc	-Deficiency associated with susceptibility to infections -Zinc repletion alleviates clinical symptoms of acrodermatitis enteropathica (characterized by GI malfunction, bacterial, fungal, viral, and yeast infections) -Deficiency impairs T-helper cell function -Excess dietary zinc may enhance or inhibit tumor growth
Iron	-Deficiency depresses numbers of peripheral lymphocytes -Iron repletion in anemic patients with *Candida* infection improves both conditions -Iron therapy improves lymphocyte counts
Fatty Acids	-Polyunsaturated fatty acids suppress IgG and IgM plaque forming cell responses -Saturated fatty acids increase IgG and IgM plaque forming cell responses -High-fat diets are associated with increased incidence of carcinogenesis and tumor development

and intestinal damage. During anorexic periods, skeletal muscle tissue may play a greater role as an energy source for patients with AIDS than for healthy persons on self-induced starvation diets (Masur, 1983). This phenomenon suggests that AIDS patients are physically stressed, as well as being starved (Masur, 1983). Whereas HIV infection worsens nutritional status by altering metabolism and absorption, the resulting PCM promotes a rapid deterioration in overall health and progression of AIDS (Probart, 1989). The impact of PCM on overall health in HIV infection illustrates the importance of nutritional support in AIDS treatment.

Changes in Body Composition

Malnutrition and PCM cause physiologic and metabolic changes in persons with HIV infection. Depletion of body cell mass (wasting) is a common and devastating complication of AIDS (Kotler, 1989). Wasting, caused by alterations in food intake, nutrient absorption, metabolic rate, and regulation, is the most significant change in body composition (Dworkin et al., 1986). One study of body weights in AIDS patients observed an average weight loss of just over 35 pounds. In another study, every patient hospitalized with AIDS and PCP was malnourished at the time of admission (Chelluri & Jastremski, 1989). Some studies have documented a 10 percent loss of body weight in over 60 percent of persons with HIV (O'Sullivan et al., 1985); others have documented a 20 to 30 percent loss of usual body weight (Probart, 1989). Losses of more than 30 percent of usual body weight can be fatal (Probart, 1989).

Homosexual HIV patients are observed to have reduced levels of body fat, serum albumin, potassium, retinol-binding protein, and iron-binding proteins when compared to homosexual norms (Kotler et al., 1985). Kotler describes a significant depletion of IgA- producing plasma cells in intestinal biopsies from homosexuals with HIV, which is not present in HIV-negative homosexuals (Kotler et al., 1987). IgA-deficient individuals have an increased prevalence of mucosal infections (Ernst et al., 1987). This secretory IgA prevents bacterial attachment to mucosal cells, which is believed to be important in retarding colonization of mucosal surfaces (such as those of the GI tract) (Drutz & Mills, 1987). These GI mucous membranes are in constant contact with a wide number of pathogens and toxins because they interface between the internal and external environments (Kotler, 1989). The GI luminal membrane forms an excellent chemical barrier but a poor one to water-soluble materials. Therefore, the proliferating epithelial cells of the GI tract are extremely vulnerable to infection (Kotler, 1989). Any changes in the epithelial cells of the GI tract may contribute to opportunistic infections and malabsorption seen in HIV seropositive patients.

Lipid metabolism also changes with HIV infection (Grun-

feld et al., 1989). Hypertriglyceridemia exists in both HIV-infected and AIDS patients (Grunfeld et al., 1989). The cytokines released during immune responses may decrease clearance of lipoproteins and increase hepatic lipid synthesis (Grunfeld et al., 1989), thus explaining the hyperlipidemia observed in bacterial and parasitic infections. Serum triglycerides in HIV-infected individuals clearly indicate changes in lipid metabolism. These changes in serum triglycerides may drastically underestimate the overall disturbances in lipid metabolism due to HIV infection (Grunfeld et al., 1989).

Changes in Absorption

Many HIV-infected individuals report changes in bowel habits, including less formed stools and increased passage of mucus. These problems may exist for months or years before the diagnosis of AIDS and before other manifestations of immune dysfunction become apparent (Kotler, 1989). As previously discussed, changes in epithelial cells of the GI tract contribute to problems of malabsorption. For example, T-lymphocyte depletion causes alterations in lymphoid composition of the intestinal mucosa in AIDS patients (Rodgers et al., 1986). The decreased secretory immunity alters mucosal permeability and increases uptake of macronutrients (Hickson & Knudson, 1988). Rapid growth rates of epithelial cells in the gut also interferes with absorption by interrupting the development of the enzyme lactase, which breaks down lactose (milk sugar). Without the development of lactase, milk is poorly absorbed, contributing to the development of bloating and diarrhea in HIV patients.

Increased mucosal infections lead to malabsorption in these patients, which can in turn result in malnutrition. Infectious diseases influence nutrient requirements by altering absorption efficiency, rate of tissue metabolism, and efficiency of nutrient utilization. Acute intestinal disturbances such as diarrhea cause malabsorption of sugar, nitrogen, protein, amino acids, fat, vitamin A, B-12 and folate (Rosenberg et al., 1977). Chronic intestinal diseases can lead to vitamin and mineral deficiencies, especially if significant malabsorption is present (Figure 6-1) (Moseson et al., 1989). The intestinal damage from opportunistic infections is responsible for enteric protein losses (Kotler et al., 1984). These losses might explain the hyperalbuminemia observed in HIV patients (Kotler et al., 1984).

OPPORTUNISTIC INFECTIONS OF GI

The entire digestive tract is susceptible to AIDS-related diseases, including involvement of the oral cavity, esophagus, stomach, liver and small and large intestines (Crocker,

1989). The associated opportunistic infections create pain, nausea, vomiting and diarrhea. These intestinal disturbances cause weight loss, dehydration and electrolyte imbalances (Probart, 1989). GI infections often damage the mucosal lining and result in impaired nutrient absorption. A variety of pathogenic agents (viruses, bacteria and protozoa) are normally present in the GI tract but are controlled by the immune system. As the immune system fails, these agents may become acute or chronic infections, producing progressive tissue depletion (wasting) (Kotler, 1989). Opportunistic GI infections such as these are a major source of morbidity and mortality in HIV infection (Kotler, 1989).

Infections of the oral cavity that affect the ability to eat are experienced by 94 percent of AIDS patients (American Family Physicians, 1989). Oral candidiasis (a thin film on the tongue), KS ulcers, CMV that produces indolent ulcers and oral herpes create pain during chewing and swallowing (American Family Physicians, 1989). Patients often respond to oral discomforts by restricting their intake. The resulting decreased intake promotes weight loss and PCM.

Infections of the small and large intestines are responsible for digestive disorders and malabsorption. The diarrhea commonly observed in HIV may be due to bacterial infections *Cryptosporidium, Isospora belli, Giardia lamblia, Mycobacterium avium-intracellulare* [MAI]); viral infections (CMV, HIV); protozoal infections (microsporidia); or lesions and tumors from KS, cancers or lymphomas (Kotler, 1989; Probart, 1989). These infections raise the metabolic rate, alter energy metabolism, increase losses from the body and cause morphologic changes (Kotler, 1989). The morphologic changes observed in the GI tract may result from toxins produced by the infecting organism or by direct invasion of the mucosa. Insufficiencies of secretory antibodies allow invading bacteria to adhere to the luminal membrane in increased numbers (Kotler, 1989). In addition to the bacterial overgrowth and damage to cell or brush border membranes, this invasion may complicate the secretory immunodeficiencies seen in HIV (Crocker, 1989). The resulting cellular changes and related diarrhea promote malabsorption and malnutrition.

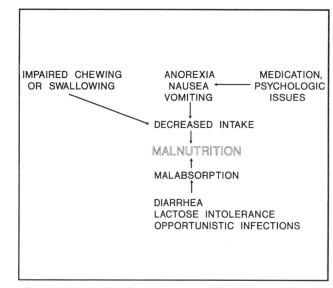

Figure 6-1. Causes of malnutrition. (From Moseson, M., Zuleniuch-Jacquotte, A., Belsito, D.V., et al. (1989). Relationships between muscle potassium and total body potassium in infants with malnutrition. *Journal of Pediatrics* 74:49.) Used with permission.

support (Winick et al., 1989). Any potentially drug-induced nutritional disorders should be documented and monitored. Table 6-4 lists some common drugs used in HIV infection and the associated GI disturbances.

Some commonly prescribed drugs used in HIV treatment promote changes in nutritional status. The toxicity of AZT to bone marrow is associated with a decreased level of serum vitamin B-12 (Barbaro, 1986). Pentamidine, used in the treatment of PCP pneumonia, produces unpredictable hypoglycemia, perhaps due to its toxicity to the beta islet cells in the pancreas (Stahl-Bayliss et al., 1986). This hypoglycemia is associated with IV, but not aerosol, administration of pentamidine (Corkery et al., 1988). Many of the drugs used in HIV treatment have side effects of anemia and neutropenia (Crocker, 1989). Nutritional status must be monitored during drug therapies for AIDS to prevent nutrient deficiencies.

DRUG THERAPIES AND NUTRITION

Some disturbances in absorption and GI function can be attributed to AIDS treatments and therapies. The proliferation of drug treatments, diverse drug tolerances and unique ailments demand responsiveness to drug-nutrient interactions and specific somatic complaints. Persistent medication-related anorexia, nausea, vomiting for more than two weeks, or weight loss indicate the need for nutritional

PSYCHOSOCIAL IMPACT ON NUTRITION

The changes in physical status, quality of life and daily activities often cause depression and reduced appetite in the HIV- infected patient. Furthermore, HIV patients experience social changes (due to the reactions of peers, colleagues and family), economic hardships (associated with illness and medication costs), and distress (from the realization of having a chronic illness). The resulting anxiety and depression may contribute to anorexia. Fear of painful eating or

Table 6-4
NUTRITION-RELATED PROBLEMS FROM
DRUG THERAPIES FOR AIDS

DRUG THERAPY	TREATMENT FOR	GI IMPACT OF DRUG
Acyclovir	Herpes	Diarrhea, nausea, vomiting
Adriamycin	KS	Nausea, vomiting, diarrhea, stomatitis, esophagitis
Amphotericin B	Meningitis	Anorexia, weight loss, nausea, vomiting, diarrhea
AZT, retrovir	HIV	Nausea, vomiting, anemia
Bactrim	PCP	Nausea, vomiting, thrush
Bleomycin	KS	Nausea, vomiting, diarrhea, anorexia, stomatitis
Clotrimazole	Candida	Nausea, vomiting
DFMO	PCP, *Cryptosporidium*	Diarrhea
DHPG	CMV	Nausea, vomiting
Ethambutal MCL	MAI	Nausea, vomiting, anorexia
Ethionamide	MAI	Anorexia, nausea, vomiting, metallic taste
Ketoconazole	*Candida*	Nausea, vomiting, diarrhea constipation
Pentamidine IV	PCP	Hypoglycemia, diarrhea dysgeusia
Pyrimethamine	Toxoplasmosis	Diarrhea, vomiting, anorexia
Vincristine	KS	Weight loss, dysphagia nausea, vomiting, stomatitis anorexia, constipation

diarrhea may cause persons with HIV to self-limit their dietary intake. Medications for treatment or products of the disease syndrome may produce anorexia. All of these situations interfere with an adequate dietary intake.

The mild-to-moderate disinterest in foods and eating can carry over into food acquisition, meal preparation and restaurant dining. HIV seropositive individuals often suffer from fatigue, making shopping and food preparation exhausting. Dementia affects 60 percent of AIDS patients (Barbaro, 1986; Christ & Wiener, 1985). It causes confusion, disorientation and short-term memory loss. Dementia complicates shopping, cooking and eating. Whatever the reason, failure to eat can be a self-imposed death sentence for HIV-infected individuals. The presentation of quick foods that require minimal preparation can facilitate adequate dietary intake. For that reason, patients living with HIV need the availability of convenience foods, meals on wheels and easily prepared foods.

Food also provides emotional support. Although there is a pervasive loss of appetite in HIV infection, some foods may provide psychological comfort. Patients in the end stages of HIV infection may be too ill to consume appreciable amounts of food (Hickson & Knudson, 1988). Even so, food can be used to gratify their desires. These patients may request hamburgers, hot dogs, pizza and milk shakes (O'Sullivan, 1988). The presentation of preferred foods to patients, especially as the disease progresses, contributes to an atmosphere of dignity before death.

EVALUATION OF NUTRITIONAL STATUS IN HIV INFECTION

Proper nutrition is critical in the treatment of HIV infection. During all stages of the disease, nutritional status and the success of nutritional intervention should be monitored. When one approach to nutritional intervention becomes less effective, other, often more aggressive, techniques should be included. The process of monitoring the success and appropriateness of nutrition interventions is accomplished by nutritional assessment and diet modification.

All members of the treatment team need a working knowledge of nutrition, assessment techniques and nutrition interventions. This working knowledge is not meant to substitute for the active participation of a registered dietitian or carefully chosen nutritionist. Clients seen in a clinic or out-patient setting often depend on treatment team members other than a dietitian to help them identify potential nutritional deficiency states. Patients and physicians need to be alerted to potential changes in nutritional status. When changes in nutritional status are identified, patients should be referred to a dietitian. The dietitian is the team member trained, licensed and appropriate to accept liability for nutritional interventions.

Nutritional Assessment Techniques

A nutritional assessment done at the time of initial diagnosis is the most helpful assessment in long-term treatment of HIV infection (Probart, 1989; Winick et al., 1989). This assessment provides a set of baseline values, which are useful to evaluate changes. Later, assessments can be compared with the baseline values. HIV seropositive patients require a periodic review of their nutritional status (Probart, 1989; Crocker, 1989; Winick et al., 1989). These routine evaluations of nutritional status ensure nutritional support at the earliest opportunity to postpone or prevent onset of nutritional deficiencies and malnutrition.

The need for routine nutrition intervention parallels the need for nutrition assessments. Nutrition intervention and education are necessary at diagnosis and throughout the course of the disease. Nutritional counseling and education empowers the person living with HIV by giving him or her dietary control. The well-informed patient may have enough information to identify overt changes in nutritional status and to make appropriate changes in dietary habits.

The currently accepted nutritional assessment parameters, excluding the use of total lymphocyte count and skin hypersensitivity, can be used appropriately in nutritional evaluation of HIV-infected patients (Kotler et al., 1985). A routine nutritional assessment should include the following: diet history, calculation of nutrient intake, anthropometric measurements, laboratory tests, and functional measurements (Winick et al., 1989).

Diet histories and calorie counts are useful for a number of reasons (Crocker, 1989; Winick et al., 1989). They document the food selections and help identify nontraditional diets (eg. macrobiotics, herbal remedies, megadoses of vitamins) that may negatively impact nutritional status (Crocker, 1989). Diet histories can be used to determine the adequacy of meals and intake. Changes in food selections may occur as the disease progresses and may explain some nutritional deficiencies. This kind of information facilitates identification of inadequate intakes before they manifest as deficiencies. Calorie counts are used to determine current intake and, when compared with weight changes and laboratory values, help establish the calorie needs of the patient. The complete calculation of nutritional intake includes protein, vitamins and minerals in addition to calories.

Anthropometric measurements help identify nutrition-related physical changes. These parameters include height and weight, midarm muscle circumference, and triceps skinfold (Table 6-5). Rapid shifts in body water content from HIV infections make the usefulness of body weight somewhat problematic (Kotler et al., 1989). Many patients with PCM have elevated total body water and extracellular water volumes (Pierson et al., 1974). The progressive

Table 6-5
ANTHROPOMETRIC MEASUREMENTS

WEIGHT

Ideal Body Weight (IBW) Provides pounds for base height plus additional pounds for additional height.
As Follows:

MEN - 160 # First 6 feet
16 # each additional inch
WOMEN - 100 # First 5 feet
5 # each additional inch

(Add 10% for large frame, subtract 10% for small frame)
Usual Body Weight (UBW)
Normal pre-illness adult weight

% Change of UBW
Identifies potential malnutrition. To monitor % change, use the formula as follows:

$$\frac{UBW - ACTUAL\ WEIGHT}{UBW} \times 100 = \%\ change$$

2% loss in 1 week →
5% loss in 1 month → Indicates malnutrition
10% loss in 6 months →

TRICEPS SKINFOLD (TSF)
Measured with a skinfolds caliper, readings are evaluated with a standard table.
Referencing from chart provides percent body fat (energy stores).

MIDARM MUSCLE CIRCUMFERENCE (MAMC)
First midarm circumference (MAC) must be taken by measuring the circumference of the upper arm in centimeters. The MAC measures skeletal and fat stores. In addition to MAC, TSF must also be done to determine MAMC, using the following formula:

$$MAMC\ (cm) = MAC\ (cm) - (0.314 \times TSF\ (cm))$$

wasting of PCM may go unrecognized when body weight alone is used as the nutritional assessment tool. For this reason, other anthropometric measurements must also be used. Midarm muscle circumference measures the somatic protein stores, and triceps skinfold measures body fat. Monitoring these two anthropometric measurements can help identify changes in lean body tissue and energy stores that may be missed by monitoring weight only.

The body weights of HIV-seropositive infected individuals may be lower than the parameters included on height/weight charts that use national norms (Crocker, 1989). Therefore, the use of pre-illness usual body weight, instead of ideal body weight, can more accurately be used to identify

Table 6-6
LABORATORY TESTS*

MEASUREMENT	NORMAL LEVELS	COMMENTS

Serum Albumin	3.5 - 5.0 g/dL	Measures long-term PCM levels under:
		   3.5 indicate depletion
		   2.8 indicate severe depletion
		
		Poor indicator of short-term protein losses
		   affected by plasma volume, malabsorption

Hemoglobin	14 - 18 g/dL (Men) 10 - 16 g/dL (Women)	More direct measure of iron deficiency than hematocrit (Hct) Levels under 12 indicate iron deficiency anemia or PCM Dehydration may mask deficiencies or cause elevated levels
TIBC (total iron binding capacity)	250 - 350 mcg/dL	Indicates total amount of iron that can be carried in the blood transferrin Levels under 200 indicate PCM, B_{12} or folate deficiency anemias Levels over 400 occur with hepatitis, blood loss and iron deficiencies

*Values commonly used in nutritional assessment of HIV infected patients.

weight changes throughout the disease process (Table 6-5) (Crocker, 1989). Although changes in body weight can be deceiving, the following weight losses are indicative of malnutrition: two percent in one week, five percent in one month, ten percent in six months.

Laboratory tests are another nutritional assessment tool. Serum levels of albumin, hemoglobin, total iron binding capacity (TIBC), vitamin B-12 status, zinc and selenium should be monitored. Table 6-6 provides information on laboratory values commonly used in nutritional assessment of the HIV-infected patient. Low serum levels of vitamins and minerals, particularly B12, zinc and selenium, are also indicative of nutritional deficiencies.

Measurements (ie. range of motion, manual muscle tests), determine overall function of an individual (eg. Appendix C). This assessment tool can be used by a physical or occupational therapist. The information can be used to support the dietitian's evaluation of the wasting syndrome and PCM.

Malabsorption can be evaluated with techniques that determine severity and extent. Fecal fat excretion is used to measure the absorption of fats, and d-xylose absorption measures the absorption of carbohydrates. Both of these tests help pinpoint the kind of malabsorption being experienced.

Evaluation of Intake

Monitoring the nutrient intake of HIV-infected patients facilitates early identification of nutrient deficiencies or inadequate dietary consumption. Generally, a diet history will readily provide the information necessary to evaluate the adequacy of a patient's intake. Some HIV complications interfere with the accurate recording of dietary intake. Dementia can make information gathering difficult or impossible (Hyman & Kaufman, 1989). Under these conditions, the accuracy and reliability of the information is often doubtful. Dementia also interferes with nutrition counseling and intervention.

IDENTIFICATION OF
OPPORTUNISTIC INFECTIONS

Often the first symptoms causing HIV infected individuals to seek medical advice is weight loss and diarrhea (Crocker, 1989). Diarrhea is the most common GI symptom of HIV infection. Other common GI complaints include steatorrhea, lactose intolerance, anorexia, nausea, vomiting, abdominal pain, taste alteration and dysphagia (Gelb & Miller, 1986). The following discussion of common symptoms from opportunistic infections may be helpful in identifying them.

The oral cavity and esophagus often are affected by creamy white patches or a curd-like covering of the mouth and tongue (Crocker, 1989). Caused by *Candida*, this oral thrush causes pain and difficulty in chewing; in the esophagus it may cause severe dysphagia (Kotler, 1989; Crocker,

1989). The appearance of oral *Candida* is a marker for the presence of esophageal *Candida* (Crocker, 1989). Candida infection can be a significant cause of poor dietary intake. KS invades the GI tract in about 50 percent of HIV patients (Brinson, 1985). Although some GI lesions from KS are asymptomatic, more commonly there is pain, hemorrhaging and obstruction (Bernstein et al., 1987; Friedman et al., 1985; Lustbader & Sherman, 1987). Esophageal KS can interfere with swallowing (Kotler, 1989; Garcia et al., 1987). KS in the small and large intestines can disrupt motility and cause organic obstructions. These KS lesions may be partly responsible for the inflammation and edema seen in HIV patients (Crocker, 1989). KS is not usually responsible for the diarrhea that is usually present.

Cryptosporidium is a chronic, protracted, debilitating infection in HIV patients (Kotler, 1989). It may appear as mild, self-limiting diarrhea. More often, it is a severe and massive secretory diarrhea of up to 10 liters of watery stool per day (Kotler, 1989; Crocker, 1989). These nonbloody bowel movements, which are larger after food intake, are more frequent at night or early in the morning. The associated cramping from *Cryptosporidium* diminishes after a bowel movement. The organism causes slow weight loss and fat depletion due to malabsorption and may produce dehydration and hypokalemia (Kotler, 1989).

MAI is responsible for much of the diarrhea and steatorrhea seen in HIV disease (Crocker, 1989). Symptoms from MAI range from mild to severe abdominal pain with persistent diarrhea. MAI causes GI dysfunction, liver enlargement, fever and malaise. Often patients with MAI infection limit their food intake to avoid the pain and diarrhea. Weight loss in these patients may be rapid because they are hypermetabolic with energy requirements up to 60 percent higher than the predicted basal metabolic rate (Kotler, 1989).

CMV also produces watery diarrhea, abdominal pain, weight loss and fever (Crocker, 1989). The diarrhea from CMV may or may not contain blood. The abdominal pain is associated with marked distension and rebound tenderness. CMV directly damages the mucosa and causes malabsorption. CMV-infected patients may experience multiple small mucoid bowel movements throughout the day and night. These patients are weak and anorectic and generally look and feel sick.

HIV enteropathy is a syndrome of persistent diarrhea, weight loss, malabsorption and malnutrition without an identifiable organism or neoplasm (Kotler et al., 1984). HIV enteropathy can produce intestinal damage, including villous atrophy, crypt hyperplasia, and increased intraepithelial lymphocytes. The diarrhea is generally unrelated to intake, so appetite is usually preserved. The weight loss and malabsorption in HIV enteropathy is not as severe as in

other opportunistic infections.

This discussion of GI infections is not exhaustive. GI complaints may originate from numerous other sources. Salmonella and shigella bacteria may produce abdominal cramps, diarrhea and colitis (Kotler, 1989). Herpes and other ulcerations can produce difficulty in swallowing (Winick et al., 1989). Many epigastric complaints may be related to ulcerations from CMV or lymphoma, and dyspepsia may result from medications. Preventing or diminishing the effects of malnutrition due to opportunistic infections can be accomplished only by responding to the specific symptoms and complaints and identifying the infections when possible.

Body Weight and Composition

The effect of malabsorption from opportunistic infections and physical changes in the digestive tract is malnutrition. Decreased appetite from dementia, depression or medications may also produce a malnourished state. The resulting malnourished state, often PCM, creates dramatic changes in body weight and composition.

The average weight loss seen in HIV patients is 25 pounds (Chelluri & Jastremski, 1989). That amount of weight loss usually represents a depletion of protein tissue. Whether produced by infectious agents, metabolic changes or decreased intake, the resulting changes in body weight and composition must be addressed to effectively provide nutritional support.

NUTRITION INTERVENTION

Given the many factors that impact nutritional status in HIV patients, the interventions for them should meet some general criteria. The Task Force on Nutrition Support in AIDS was organized to set primary goals for nutrition management of HIV infection (Winick et al., 1989). The goals are as follows:

1. preserve lean body mass
2. provide adequate levels of all nutrients
3. minimize symptoms of malabsorption.

These three basic goals are addressed by the interventions that follow.

General Nutrition Requirements

Nutrition support should be given to patients living with HIV before they become malnourished. The support provided will minimize weight loss and prevent nutrient deficiencies (Probart, 1989). Intervention should also relieve the associated disease symptoms. During asymptomatic periods of HIV infection, nutrition support should promote

Table 6-7
ENERGY AND PROTEIN REQUIREMENTS

BASAL ENERGY EXPENDITURES (BEE)

Determines the energy requirement of the resting individual The formula is as follows:

MEN —   BEE = 66 + (13.7 X WT) + (6 X HT) - (6.8 X AGE)

WOMEN —   BEE = 655 + (9.6 X WT) + (1.6 X HT) - (4.7 X AGE)
           WT — weight in kg
           HT — height in cm
           AGE — age in years

BEE is increased by the following:
    infection
    trauma
    cancer
    surgery
    starvation

TOTAL ENERGY EXPENDITURES (TEE)

Total energy requirements are influenced by the following:

Increase TEE	Decrease TEE
Activity (5-20%)	Sleeping (9%)
Fever (7% per degree)	Age (7% per decade over 25)
Growth	Hypothermia (15-40%)
Surgery (5-20%)	Starvation (15-30%)
Stimulants (drugs)	Fasting Smoking Weight loss (10-30%)
Infections (15-60%)	Depressants (drugs)

TEE = BEE X Activity Factor X Stress Factor

Activity Factor:	Confined to bed	1.2
	Ambulatory	1.3
Stress Factor:	Surgery	1.2
	Sepsis	1.2 - 1.6
	Trauma	1.1 - 1.6
	Burn	1.5 - 1.9

PROTEIN NEEDS

Allow 1.5 g of protein per kg of body weight per day. Protect protein with 40 - 50 calories/kg body weight per day.

an adequate balanced diet. The diet should maintain weight, provide generous protein, and prevent vitamin and mineral deficiencies (Probart, 1989; *Journal of the American Dietetic Association,* 1989; Staff, 1987). Its adequacy can be assured by providing nutrition information about food groups and energy requirements. Providing a meal plan can

stimulate intake and help patients set goals.

Adequate calories and protein should be supplied to prevent wasting and improve quality of life. The calories and protein necessary are based on age, weight, height, sex, and degree of metabolic stress (Weaver, 1987). Muscle wasting can be reduced by a high-protein diet (Staff, 1987). The suggested allowance for protein is 1.5 g/kg body weight (Staff, 1987; Weaver, 1987). Protein must be protected by a sufficient calorie intake of 40 to 45 kcal/kg body weight (Weaver, 1987). If the protein is not adequately protected, it may be catabolized for energy. Some studies suggest intake of up to 50 kcal/kg body weight to prevent weight loss (Weaver, 1987). Table 6-7 provides formulas for determining energy and protein requirements for these patients.

Each meal should provide at least one third of the RDA for calories, vitamins and minerals (Food and Nutrition Board, 1980; Food and Nutrition Service, 1980). Energy intake should be enhanced by any means, including the use of sugar, fat and cholesterol-rich foods (McCaffrey, 1987). Foods should generally be energy dense so that patients do not become full on low-calorie foods such as salads, broths, tea or coffee. Carbohydrate-rich foods should also be encouraged. Because the typical dinner for the American male contains 1080 calories (Staff 1987), the target meal for HIV patients should provide one-third of the RDA for energy, or 1000 calories (Staff, 1987; Recommended Dietary Allowances, 1980; Menu Planning Guide for School Food Service, 1980).

The loss of fluids and electrolytes must be considered in addition to protein and calories (Crocker, 1989). At least eight cups of fluids should be taken each day. The replacement of electrolytes can be facilitated by routine consumption of fruit juices, particularly nectars and citrus juices.

The goals for nutrition intervention in asymptomatic HIV infection and early-to-advanced disease are similar. First, the diet must be adequate to prevent weight loss. Second, the protein intake needs to be generous and of high quality. Third, the overall intake needs to meet or exceed the RDA for vitamins and minerals. Finally, education about the disease and its nutrition implications cannot be overemphasized. The better understanding the patient has about HIV disease, the more prepared they will be to respond to nutritional concerns and inadequacies.

Goal setting for meals can best be accomplished with the use of the four basic food groups. Using this educational tool makes nutrition readily available and understandable. It is the best way to engage the patient living with HIV. The four basic foods simplify nutrition into a system of counting groups for nutritional adequacy. The milk/dairy group provides protein, calcium, phosphorus and vitamins D and A. The meat group provides protein, iron, manganese, magnesium, zinc, B6, and B12. The fruits and vegetables group, which should include a daily citrus fruit and leafy green vegetable, is a rich source of vitamins C and E and minerals. Breads and cereals provide calories, B-vitamins and minerals. Table 6-8 provides minimum serving requirements for the four food groups. Table 6-9 provides modifications of the four basic food groups for vegetarians who eat eggs and dairy products. Table 6-10 provides a modified basic four food groups model for strict vegetarians. The vegetarian modifications include other groups that provide adequate B12 (brewer's yeast) or complete protein (legumes and nuts/seeds).

Eating foods from the four basic food groups and drinking at least eight cups of liquid provide the foundation for adequate nutrition. The presence of infection or fever increases the need for additional calories, protein, vitamins, minerals and fluids.

Vitamin and Mineral Supplements

The diminished intake and malabsorption states of HIV seropositive patients are partially responsible for their compromised vitamin and mineral nutritional status. Changes in metabolism may also be responsible for low or deficient serum vitamin or mineral status in these patients. Deficiencies of protein; the vitamins A, C, and B-complex; and the minerals zinc and iron affect nutritional status, cause damage to the intestinal mucosa and lead to skin lesions (Robinson et al., 1986). Vitamin deficiencies can also cause significant disturbances in normal immune responses. Disturbances in serum vitamin levels, either high or low, may interfere with other vitamins and with immune functions. Mineral deficiencies can also significantly impair immune functions (see Table 6-3 and *Nutrition and Immune Function* for a review of both vitamin and mineral information). Zinc deficiency and iron deficiency anemia are related to opportunistic infections such as *Candida* (Beach & Laura, 1983). Zinc and selenium deficiencies are common in HIV infection (Crocker, 1989). Zinc is known to play a major role in immune function, and zinc deficiency may exacerbate impaired immune function (Gillin et al., 1985). In patients with long-term HIV disease, diminished T-cell helper cells respond to selenium supplementation (Dworkin et al., 1986). Patients studied with iron deficiency anemia, *Candida* lesions, and low numbers of peripheral lymphocytes responded well to ferrous sulfate supplementation (Moseson, et al., 1989). Supplements of 200 mg of ferrous sulfate, two times per day, normalized hemoglobin, serum iron, and total iron binding capacity (Moseson, et al., 1989). Additional responses to iron treatments include rapid improvement of *Candida* infection and a rise in numbers of peripheral lymphocyte counts. The correction of mineral deficiency states may improve immune responses.

Table 6-8
MINIMUM FOOD GROUPS FOR HIV INFECTION MIXED DIET

FOOD GROUPS	NUMBER OF SERVINGS	SOURCES/ SERVING SIZE
Milk	2 - 4	1 cup milk or yogurt 1 oz. cheese
Meat	2 - 3	2 eggs 3 oz. meat, poultry, fish 5 oz. tofu 1 cup dried beans, lentils, peas 4 Tbsp peanut butter
Fruits	3 or more	1 average fresh 1/2 cup canned or juice
Vegetables	3 or more	1/2 cup cooked 1/2 cup juice 1 average fresh
Breads/cereals	5 or more	1 slice bread 1/2 cup cooked cereals (rice or grain) 1/2 cup noodles 1/2 - 1 cup dry cereal 1 muffin, roll, biscuit
Fats/oils	1 - 2	1 Tbsp oil 1 Tbsp butter/oleo

Homosexual men with HIV infection are generally taking dietary supplements with high, sometimes toxic, levels of vitamins, minerals, and other nutrients according to numerous studies (Fordyce-Baum et al., 1988). Asymptomatic HIV patients have low or deficient serum levels of the following vitamins and minerals: B6, B12, zinc, selenium, iron, and retinol binding protein (Beach & Lefkowitz, 1989). These deficiencies suggest the need for reasonable vitamin/mineral supplementation. A reasonable supplement provides the nutrients at adequate levels that are not toxic and do not interfere with each other's effectiveness. Patients with compromised nutritional status may require two to three times the RDA for vitamins and minerals (Food and Nutrition Board, 1980; Dionigi et al., 1979). Therefore, the

Table 6-9
MINIMUM FOOD GROUPS FOR HIV INFECTION LACTO-OVO VEGETARIAN

FOOD GROUPS	NUMBER OF SERVINGS	SOURCES/ SERVING SIZE
Milk (A)	2 - 4	1 cup milk or yogurt
Cheese (A)	1	2 oz.
Eggs (A)	1 optional	1 egg 2 egg whites
Legumes (B)	2	1 cup cooked dried beans, peas, lentils 4 Tbsp peanut butter 5 oz tofu
Nuts/seeds (C)	2	3 Tbsp almonds, beans, sesame seeds, etc.
Breads/cereals (C)	6 or more	1 slice bread 1/2 cup cooked cereal (rice or grain) 1/2 cup cooked pasta 1/2 - 1 cup dry cereal 1 muffin, roll or biscuit
Fruit	3 or more	1 average fresh 1/2 cup canned or juice
Vegetables	3 or more	1/2 cup cooked 1/2 cup juice 1 average fresh
Fats/oil	1 - 2	1 Tbsp oils 1 Tbsp butter/oleo

Complete protein from (A) alone, or (B) + (C) together

Table 6-10
MINIMUM FOOD GROUPS FOR HIV INFECTION, STRICT VEGETARIAN

FOOD GROUPS	NUMBER OF SERVINGS	SOURCES/ SERVING SIZE
Soy milk (A)	4	1 cup enriched soy milk
Legumes (A)	2	1 cup cooked dried beans, peas, lentils 4 Tbsp peanut butter 5 oz. tofu
Nuts/seeds (B)	2	3 Tbsp almonds, sesame seeds, pecans, etc
Breads/cereals (b)	8 or more	1 slice bread 1/2 cup cooked cereal (rice or grain) 1/2 cup cooked pasta 1/2 - 1 cup dry cereal 1 muffin, roll or biscuit
Fruit	6 or more (3 citrus)	1 average fresh 1/2 cup canned or juice
Vegetables	2 or more	1/2 cup cooked 1/2 cup juice 1 average fresh
Dark green leafy vegetables	2	1 cup spinach, greens, broccoli, etc
	1 - 2	Brewers yeast 1 Tbsp powder
Fats/oils	1 - 2	1 Tbsp oil 1 Tbsp butter/oleo

Complete protein from (A) + (B) together

RDAs should be viewed as floor levels of intake for early or midstage HIV patients (Hickson & Knudson, 1988).

The current recommendations for vitamin-mineral supplementation are as follows: three times the RDA for all vitamins and minerals as an oral supplement (a prenatal vitamin/mineral supplement is ideal), additional daily oral intake of 20 mg of vitamin B6, and monthly intramuscular injection of 1200 mg of vitamin B12 (Beach & Lefkowitz, 1989; Beach & August, 1989; Beach, September, 1989). The additional supplement of vitamin B6, 10 times the RDA, is a response to the significantly lower serum levels seen in HIV infection. The additional vitamin B12 is also a response to the depressed serum levels, further aggravated by bone marrow destruction from AZT use. Vitamin B12 injections are preferred over oral supplementation because intestinal damage and interruption in normal GI function severely limit absorption of the vitamin. The administration of vitamin/mineral supplements can be viewed as an insurance policy for patients, which may help limit progression of HIV disease (Hickson & Knudson, 1988).

Boosting Intake with Snacks

HIV-seropositive patients often have difficulty consuming adequate calories. This problem becomes acute during periods of anorexia, nausea, depression or general apathy. Patients must be educated about the relative nutritional values of different foods. Within the context of a meal or snack, they should be taught what foods to eat first to provide maximum calories and nourishment. Then, even if their appetites diminish rapidly, they would have gained the most nourishment possible. Healthful, nutritionally dense snacks are far more desirable than low-calorie snacks. Table 6-11 provides examples of calorically dense versus hollow foods.

Patients with HIV infection must receive adequate calories and protein, especially because PCM is such a common complication. Adequate calorie intake protects protein. Some of the foods suggested are very different from those encouraged by the American Heart Association or the American Cancer Society. The use of the "Healthy Heart Diet" is not necessarily appropriate for patients fighting to maintain body weight.

Each individual should be encouraged to view eating as an opportunity to boost their protein and calorie intake. High-fat foods may be used as a source of calories, except when contraindicated by diarrhea or malabsorption (steatorrhea). If the patient is able to digest them, fats should be liberally added to foods, especially when the patient is hypermetabolic or running a fever. Carbohydrate-rich foods are also good sources of calories. Sweets are a reasonable addition to the diet unless *Candida* or thrush is present.

In addition to food, beverages are easily tolerated sources of calories. Drinking large quantities of coffee or tea and substituting milk, fruit and vegetable juices, and flavored drinks such as Kool-Aid can dramatically boost calorie intake. A 12-ounce glass of apple juice provides 175 calories, whereas the same size glass of tea with sugar would provide only 30 calories and none of the vitamins or minerals. If bloating and gastric pain are not a problem, carbonated beverages (not diet drinks) are also a good source of calories, although they do not provide the vitamins or minerals associated with milk or juices.

Good snack items are those that are readily available and can be eaten without much preparation. Fresh or dried fruits are rich sources of calories, vitamins and minerals. Fresh

---

Table 6-11
FOODS FOR HIV INFECTION
CALORICALLY DENSE FOOD

—Dried fruit, nuts, granola

—Ice cream

—Peanut butter

—Breaded and fried meats

—Whole milk, cream, half & half, in cooking, on cereals

—Add butter to cooked items—vegetables, rice, noodles, etc.

—Add cheese to items

—Add whipped toppings, frostings to desserts

—Add gravies to meats, vegetables, starches

—Keep meat salads (tuna, chicken) for snacks with crackers or bread

—Add dry milk powder to mashed potato, soup, ground beef, eggs, hot cereal, milk

—Use honey on toast, cereal, rolls

—Liberally use jellies, jams, preserves

—Add chopped hard boiled egg to salad, vegetables, starches

—Drink milk or juice in place of tea, coffee, or diet soda

—Drink instant breakfast for snacks

---

vegetables, on the other hand, are nutrient dense but calorically hollow. As such, they satiate quickly while providing relatively few calories, making them a great diet food but a poor calorie-boosting food. Breads, cereals, and crackers are good carbohydrate snack foods. Protein snack foods such as nuts, pasteurized cheeses, hard-cooked eggs, peanut butter, and yogurt provide good calorie and protein sources. Because snacks can provide a significant portion of the daily nutrient intake, their selection should be deliberate and careful.

Enteral and Parenteral Feeding

Meals and snacks may not meet the protein and energy requirements of patients living with HIV disease as absorption and intake drop and metabolism increases. For this reason, nutritional support may be offered as a supplement to or a replacement for meals. Nutritional support may be provided to boost protein and calorie intake or may replace feedings completely. Support is administered orally, as in enteral feeding, or directly into the blood supply, as in parenteral feeding.

Enteral feedings are always the preferred method of nutritional support and repletion if the GI tract is functioning. Enteral feedings help maintain the structural and functional integrity of the GI mucosa (Probart, 1989; *ASPEN Board of Directors*, 1987). Enteral formulas are complete liquid nourishment containing complex nutrients that require digestion. Enteral feedings are most commonly polymeric formulas, which have complex carbohydrates and proteins, moderate fat levels, and differing caloric densities and osmolarities. They may be administered as a supplement when intake is suboptimal (due to anorexia or disinterest in food) or as a complete food replacement. Medical and dietary supervision should be provided to assure that the individual needs of the patient are met. When GI complications exist, an elemental enteral formula may be used (Probart, 1989). Elemental formulas require minimal digestion because they are composed of predigested nutrients (free amino acids, essential fatty acids, oligosaccharides) in a low-fat, lactose-free matrix, which promotes maximum absorption. They may be taken orally (often with the addition of flavor packets to improve acceptability), transnasally via a nasogastric (NG) tube (which allows intermittent or nocturnal use), or through a surgically placed percutaneous endoscopic gastrostomy (when long-term feeding is indicated but oral or esophageal complications would preclude NG feeding). Modular, or single-nutrient, formulas may be used to modify other enteral formulas to meet the specific nutritional needs of the patient. The selection and use of an enteral formula considers GI function, financing, patient acceptance and formula tolerance (American Family Physicians, 1989). All enteral possibilities should be exhausted before the use of parenteral nutrition in HIV patients is initiated.

Parenteral nutrition is used as a last resort. Parenteral nutrition allows rapid calorie administration. It may be used in combination with enteral feedings to preserve lean body mass during short hospital stays (American Family Physicians, 1989; Winick et al., 1989). When used in this capacity, it is administered through a peripheral vein and is referred to as peripheral parenteral nutrition (PPN). Central parenteral nutrition (CPN) is delivered via a central vein and is used when the GI tract does not function or to meet extraordinary caloric needs of hypermetabolic patients (when it may be combined with enteral feeding). In total parenteral nutrition (TPN) the only nutrition being received by the patient is via parenteral feeding. Since parenteral nutrition totally bypasses the GI tract, there is a risk of atrophy (American Family Physicians, 1989; Probart, 1989). The risk of catheter-related infection is also present during use of any parenteral nutrition intervention. The criteria for parenteral nutrition in HIV are as follows: loss of 20 percent of reference weight, intolerance to enteral feeding, partial or complete bowel obstruction, or cryptosporidium enteropathy (Nutrition Reviews, 1988; American Family Physicians, 1989; Crocker, 1989; Winick, et al., 1989). Parenteral nutrition is an important option, which should be reserved as a final solution after all enteral routes have failed.

Management of GI Complications

Patient care and long-term management of GI complaints in HIV-seropositive patients must focus on fluid and electrolyte balance, nutritional support, and symptom control (Nutrition Reviews, 1988; American Family Physicians, 1989). Treatment of GI diseases are complicated by GI pathologies, increased metabolic demands, and decreased food intake (creating malaise and fatigue) (Crocker, 1989). GI complaints that lead to decreased dietary intake and protein catabolism increase metabolic needs for protein, calories and micronutrients (Hyman & Kaufman, 1989; Crocker, 1989). Weight loss and diarrhea often continue as predominant clinical problems of patient management for HIV-infected patients (Crocker, 1989). Responding to GI complaints by making changes in meal times, food temperatures and dietary composition may diminish the number and duration of the complaints (Journal of the American Dietetic Association, 1989).

When specific opportunistic infections have been identified, the course of treatment may include medical and nutritional support. For example, in dealing with *Cryptosporidium*, where the therapeutic options are limited, parenteral nutrition, maintaining fluid and electrolyte balance, and providing antidiarrheal agents are the only appropriate interventions (Nutrition Reviews, 1988). In many other GI complications that occur, from opportunistic infections or medications, treating the complication is often the most appropriate method of nutrition intervention. Table 6-12 provides specific complaints, possible causes and recommended interventions.

ALTERNATIVE NUTRITION THERAPIES

Evaluation of Products and Remedies

The chronic nature of HIV infection and the perception that it cannot be cured make HIV disease a prime target for nontraditional medical approaches. Patients often seek alternative therapies as a cure because the traditional medical model does not offer one (Hyman & Kaufman, 1989). Alternative therapies include a variety of unconventional or nonwestern traditions, such as yoga, visualization, acupuncture and herbology (Frutchey, 1987). Although some may be helpful adjunct therapies to the traditional medical model,

Table 6-12			
NUTRITION MANAGEMENT OF GI COMPLICATIONS			
SYMPTOM	INTERVENTION	SYMPTOM	INTERVENTION
Fatigue	Prepare extra food when feeling well Rest before eating (nap improves appetite) Use ready-to-eat foods (tuna, hot dog, etc.) Use fast food or take-out Use disposable plates, cups, pans Use convenience appliances (microwave, etc.) Drink lots of nutritious beverages Solicit assistance from others	Lactose intolerance	Try using yogurt or buttermilk Use soy-based milk formulas Use Lactaid tablets or milk additive
		Change of taste	Use poultry, fish, egg, dairy Marinate foods in sweet juice or wine Eat protein foods at room temperature Liberally use flavorings and spices Use sauces, mayonnaise, cream, appetite (improves ability to taste in liquid or moist foods) Use good oral hygiene Mints and gum mask bitter mouth tastes
Anorexia	Eat small meals Eat only calorically dense foods Eat whenever appetite is up Eat with other people when possible Walk before eating to increase appetite Dine in pleasant surroundings Indulge in your favorite foods		
		Feeling full	Eat small meals Avoid fatty or dry foods Eat high carbohydrate foods Eat nutritionally dense foods Drink beverages either before or after meals by about 1 hour
Sore mouth/throat	Use soft foods without need to chew Consume high-calorie beverages Avoid acidic foods and juices Avoid spicy, salty, dry or coarse foods Liberally use sauces and gravies Consume foods at room temperature Avoid smoking and alcohol Use straw when possible	Difficulty breathing	Eat soft moist foods, ground meats/gravies Eat high-calorie beverages via a straw Eat small frequent meals Replace whole milk with skim milk Avoid salty foods and adding salt
Diarrhea	Consume 12 cups or more of fluid daily Avoid fiber-rich foods (whole grains, etc) Avoid high-fat foods Avoid skins of fresh fruits Grate raw vegetables Consume high-carbohydrate foods (breads) Do not chew gum or smoke Eat potassium-containing foods (bananas) With cramping, avoid carbonated beverages	Chronic fever	Increased need for fluid and calories Drink juice, soda, gatorade, popsicles Eat broth with added pureed baby food Consume calorically dense foods/beverages
Nausea/vomiting	Eat soft/bland foods Eat foods at cold or room temperature Eat in well-ventilated area Rest after meals without lying down Do not eat favorite foods Do not mix liquid and solid foods Avoid strong smelling foods Eat dry foods before getting out of bed Tart/sour foods more tolerated than sweet Avoid spicy, hot, or greasy foods		

others may be harmful. They may be marketed as a substitute and a cure for AIDS or HIV infection.

The danger in claims made by alternative therapies is that many of them cannot be substantiated. Often they do not distinguish between cause and effect versus mere coincidence (Herbert, 1986). The substantiating research for these products or services is often not objective, reliable and reproducible; and it is unlikely to be reviewed by a peer

---

Table 6-13
FOOD SAFETY RECOMMENDATIONS

—Avoid raw and unpasteurized milk or dairy products
—Avoid raw or uncooked beef, pork, eggs, seafood
   (Including sushi, oysters on a half shell)
—Eat only pasteurized cheeses
—No raw eggs (Exclude hollandaise, Caesar salad, home
   made ice cream or eggnog)
—Precook poultry prior to grilling or BBQ
—Thoroughly wash all produce, especially if eaten raw
—Throw out leftovers if unsure of safety
—Look for sell-by dates (throw out after expired)
—Protect hands from raw foods when cuts or open sores are
   present
—Wash hands and surfaces between each use
—Protect surfaces and other foods from raw meat contact
—Avoid use of wooden or cracked utensils or bowls
—Immediately refrigerate leftovers in small covered
   containers
—Follow directions for microwave use including standing
   time

---

review committee (Herbert, 1966). All of this is not to suggest that alternative therapies lack merit, but rather that they must be closely scrutinized with a knowledgeable and open mind.

A helpful approach in evaluating an alternative product or therapy is to use the three-pronged evaluation technique. First, determine if there is any reason to believe the product may be harmful. Reliable information about product safety cannot be gathered from individuals promoting, selling or using the product or service. When the product's safety has been determined, proceed to the second question: "Will the product or service help?" Again, reliable information cannot be obtained from individuals involved in the product. Even without proven therapeutic benefits, as long as the product is not harmful, consider the third question. The third question has to do with the expense of the product or service and its relative value. The cost must take into account the person's finances. Proven therapies should not be compromised to use the alternative therapies, nor should patients endure financial hardships to use them. This evaluation technique eliminates all but the most promising alternative therapies as viable options.

Neutral and Dangerous Nutrition Therapies

In the last few years, products targeted toward the immunocompromised person have proliferated. That trend is likely to continue, especially if new and more effective

medical treatments are not identified. Many of those treatments may be neutral, as identified in the three-step approach mentioned in the last section. Many others may directly compromise the health of the HIV population. (Journal of the American Dietetic Association, 1989; Dwyer, 1988). As the use of these products becomes more widespread, public health agencies will make policy statements regarding their safety.

One effective method for identifying dangerous diets is to evaluate whether any food groups are being eliminated or whether meeting nutritional requirements is made more difficult. Macrobiotics, for example, limit the availability of proteins, which can aggravate PCM conditions in patients with HIV disease. The "Fit for Life Diet" asserts that certain foods cannot be eaten together and discourages dairy products. Limiting what and when foods may be eaten may decrease overall intake and exacerbate conditions of malnutrition. The "Yeast Connection Diet," much like the others already mentioned, eliminates many bread and cereal products and fermented dairy products. Limitations such as these may restrict intake further and complicate adequate nutrition. Patients should be encouraged to consult dietitians and public health services to gather information about new diets, dietary supplements or nutrition products.

FOOD-BORNE INFECTIONS

HIV-seropositive patients are at a much greater risk of food-borne infection than is the general population (Taber-Pike et al., 1987). Changes in GI physiology and immune status provide a susceptible environment to microorganisms and toxins, which can cause severe infections and GI disturbances. These food-borne microorganisms can lead to infections or death (Profeta et al., 1985). Education about proper food preparation, selection, cleaning and storage can help prevent food-borne infection and food poisoning. Table 6-13 provides appropriate general food guidelines for individuals to follow.

SUMMARY

The nature of HIV infection requires constant monitoring of patients' on-going health status. Some changes in health status are directly related to individual dietary intake or absorption. Other aspects of health status are affected by metabolic changes that increase energy needs, reduce vitamin and mineral levels, and increase demands for protein. Medications designed to improve or correct one somatic complaint frequently create others. Often the side effects of these medications impact GI function or appetite.

HIV infection, its complications and treatment, dramatically changes the nutritional status of the individual. For these reasons, nutrition education and intervention should be available to every patient at diagnosis and throughout their treatment. Nutrition education and intervention will improve the quality and quantity of life while reducing many of the symptoms.

References

A.S.P.E.N. Board of Directors. Guidelines for the use of enteral nutrition in the adult patient. (1987). *Journal of Parenteral and Enteral Nutrition*. 11:435.

American Dietetic Association, The (1989). Nutrition intervention in the treatment of human immunodeficiency virus infection. *Journal of the American Dietetic Association*. 89:839.

American Dietetic Association, The (1988). *Manual of Clinical Dietetics*. Philadelphia: W.B. Saunders.

Barbaro, D. (1986). Nutrition for AIDS patients. *Directions in Applied Nutrition*. 1:4.

Battan, R., Pablos-Mendez, A., Aceves-Casillas, P., et al. (1989). Infections associated with Hickman catheters in patients with acquired immunodeficiency syndrome. *The American Journal of Medicine*. 86:780.

Beach, R.S., and Laura, P.F. (1983). Nutrition and the acquired immunodeficiency syndrome. *Annals of Internal Medicine*. 99:565.

Beach, R., and Lefkowitz, M. (1989, November/December). Nutritional aspects of HIV infection. *PAACNOTES*. 1:221.

Beach, R. (1989, September). Unpublished data. The Second Annual Nutrition AIDS Conference, Stanford, CA.

Bernstein, M.A., Hollerman, J.J., and Fenczko, P.J. (1987). Gastrointestinal complications of AIDS: Radiologic findings. *Henry Ford Hospital Medical Journal*. 35:20.

Brinson, R.R. (1985). Hypoalbuminemia, diarrhea, and the acquired immunodeficiency syndrome. *Annals of Internal Medicine*. 102:413.

Campbell, S.M. (1984). *Practical Guide to Nutritional Care: For Dietitians and Other Health Care Professionals*. Birmingham, AL: University of Alabama.

Chandra, R.K. (1981). Immunodeficiency in undernutrition and overnutrition. *Nutrition Reviews*. 39:225.

Chelluri, L., and Jastremski, M.S. (1989). Incidence of malnutrition in patients with acquired immunodeficiency syndrome. *Nutrition in Clinical Practice*. 4:16.

Christ, G.H., and Wiener, L.S. (1985). Psychosocial issues in AIDS. In Devita, V., Hellman, S., Rosenberg, S.A.,(Eds.): *AIDS: Etiology, Diagnosis, Treatment and Prevention*. Philadelphia: J.B. Lippincott Co.

Clinical Nutrition Cases. (1988). Severe malnutrition in a young man with AIDS. *Nutrition Reviews*. 46:126.

Colman, N., and Grossman, F. (1987). Nutritional factors in epidemic Kaposi's sarcoma. *Seminars in Oncology*. 14:54.

Corkery, K.J., Luce, J.M., and Montgomery, A.B. (1988). Aerosolized pentamidine for treatment and prophylaxis of *pneumocystis carinii*. pneumonia: An update. *Respiratory Care*. 33:676.

Crocker, K.S. (1989). Gastrointestinal manifestations of the acquired immunodeficiency syndrome. *Nursing Clinics of North America*. 24:395.

Cunningham-Rundles, S. (1982). Effects of nutritional status on immunological function. *American Journal of Clinical Nutrition*. 35:1202.

Dionigi, R., Gnes, S., Bonera, A., Dominioni, L. (1979). Nutrition and infection. *Journal of Parenteral and Enteral Nutrition*. 3:62.

Drutz, D., and Mills, J. (1987). Immunity and infection. In Stites, D.P., Stobo, J.D., and Wells, J.V. (Eds.): *Basic and Clinical Immunology*. Norwalk, CT: Appleton & Lange.

Dworkin, B., Rosenthal, W.S., Wormser, G.P., and Weiss, L. (1986). Selenium deficiency in acquired immunodeficiency syndrome. *Journal of Parenteral and Enteral Nutrition*. 10:405.

Dwyer, J.T. (1988, March/April). Unproven therapies for AIDS: What is the evidence? *Nutrition Today*. 25.

Ernst, P., Underdown, B., and Bienenstock, J. (1987). Immunity in mucosal tissues. In Stites, D.P., Stobo, J.D., and Wells, J.V. (Eds.): *Basic and Clinical Immunology*. Norwalk, CT: Appleton & Lange.

FDA/CDC-Office of Public Affairs. (1989, September). *Eating Defensively: Food Safety Advice for Persons with AIDS*. Videocassette. Distributed by National AIDS Information Clearinghouse.

Food and Nutrition Board. (1980). *Recommended Dietary Allowances*, 9th revised edition. Washington DC: National Academy of Sciences.

Food and Nutrition Service. (1980). *Menu Planning Guide for School Food Service*. Washington, DC: U.S. Department of Agriculture.

Fordyce-Baum, M., Matero-Atienza, E., Crass, R., et al. (1988, June 12-16). Toxic levels of dietary supplementation in early HIV infection. *Proceedings of the IVth International Conference on AIDS (Stockholm), Book 2*. 305.

Friedman, S.L., Wright, T.L., and Altman, D.F. (1985). Gastrointestinal Kaposi's sarcoma in patients with acquired immunodeficiency syndrome. *Gastroenterology*. 89:102.

Frutchey, C. (1987). Choosing alternative therapies. In Moffatt, B., Spiegel, J., Parrish, S., et al. (Eds.): *AIDS: A Self Care Manual.* Santa Monica, CA: IBS Press.

Garcia, M.E., Collins, C.L., and Mansell, P.W.A. (1987). The acquired immune deficiency syndrome. *Nutrition and Clinical Practice.* 2:108.

Gelb, A., and Miller, S. (1986). AIDS and gastroenterology. *American Journal of Gastroenterology.* 81:619.

Gillin, J.S., Shike, M., and Alcock, N. (1985). Malabsorption and mucosal abnormalities of the small intestine in the acquired immunodeficiency syndrome. *Annals of Internal Medicine.* 102:619.

Good, R., and Lorenz, E. (1988). Nutrition, Immunity, Aging and Cancer. *Nutrition Reviews.* 46:311.

Grunfeld, C., Kotler, D.P., Hamadeh, R., et al. (1989). Hypertriglyceridemia in the acquired immunodeficiency syndrome. *The American Journal of Medicine.* 86:27.

Herbert, V. (1986). Unproven (questionable) dietary and nutritional methods in cancer prevention and treatment. *Cancer.* 58:1930.

Hickson, J.F., Jr., and Knudson, P. (1988). Optimal eating: nutritional guidelines for People with AIDS. *AIDS Patient Care.* 2:28.

Hughes, W., Price, R., and Sisko, F. (1974). Protein-calorie malnutrition: A host determinant for *Pneumocystis carinii.* infection. *American Journal of Diseases in Children.* 128:44.

Human Nutrition Information Service. (1984). *Nutrient Intakes: Individuals in 48 States, Year 1977-1978.* Washington DC: U.S. Department of Agriculture.

Hyman, R.D., and Kaufman, S. (1989). Nutrition impact of acquired immune deficiency syndrome: A unique counseling opportunity. *Journal of the American Dietetic Association.* 89:520.

Jain, V.K., and Chandra, R.K. (1984). Does nutrition deficiency predispose to acquired immunodeficiency syndrome? *Nutrition Research.* 4:537.

Jansen, D.D. (1988, March). Nutrition and the AIDS patient. *Minnesota Pharmacist.,* 6. Kotler, D.P. (1989). Intestinal and hepatic manifestations of AIDS. *Advances in Internal Medicine.* 34:43.

Kotler, D.P., Gaetz, H., Lange, M., et al. (1984). Enteropathy associated with the acquired immunodeficiency syndrome. *Annals of Internal Medicine.* 101:421.

Kotler, D.P., Scholes, J., and Tierney, A. (1987). Intestinal plasma cell alterations in acquired immunodeficiency syndrome. *Digestive Disease Sciences.* 32:129.

Kotler, D.P., Tierney, A.R., Altilio, D., et al. (1989). Body mass depletion during ganciclovir treatment of cytomegalovirus infections in patients with acquired immunodeficiency syndrome. *Archives of Internal Medicine.* 149:901.

Kotler, D.P., Wang, J., and Pierson, R.J. (1985). Body composition studies in patients with the acquired immunodeficiency syndrome. *American Journal of Clinical Nutrition.* 42:1255.

Linder, J. (1987). The thymus gland in secondary immunodeficiency. *Archives of Pathology and Laboratory Medicine.* 111:1118.

Lustbader, I., and Sherman, A. (1987). Primary gastrointestinal Kaposi's sarcoma in a patient with acquired immunodeficiency syndrome. *American Journal of Gastroenterology.* 82:894.

Masur, H. (1983). The acquired immunodeficiency syndrome. *Disease Month.* 29:2.

McCaffrey, E.A. (1987, September). Meeting nutritional needs: Stimulating appetite and maximizing caloric intake. *AIDS Patient Care,* 28.

Moseson, M., Zuleniuch-Jacquotte, A., Belsito, D.V., et al. (1969). Relationship between muscle potassium and total body potassium in infants with malnutrition. *Journal of Pediatrics.* 74:49.

Nwiloh, J., Freeman, H., and McCord, C. (1988). Malnutrition: An important determinant of fatal outcome in surgically treated pulmonary suppurative disease. *Journal of the National Medical Association.* 81:525.

O'Sullivan, J. (1988, February). AIDS Overview. *Dieticians in Nutrition Support Newsletter,* 13.

O'Sullivan, P., Linke, R.A., and Dalton, S. (1985). Evaluation of body weight and nutritional status among AIDS patients. *Journal of the American Dietetic Association.* 85:1483.

Pan American Health Organization. Symposium on nutrition and AIDS. (1989). *Pan American Health Organization Bulletin.* 23:206.

Pasternack, B. (1989). The potential role of nutritional factors in the induction of immunologic abnormalities in HIV positive homosexual men. *Journal of Acquired Immune Deficiency Syndromes.* 2:235.

Pierson, R.N., Jr., Lin, D.H.Y., and Phillips, R.A. (1974). Total body potassium in health: Effects of age, sex, height, and fat. *American Journal of Physiology.* 226:206.

Probart, C.K. (1989). Guidelines for nutrition support in AIDS. *Journal of School Health.* 59:170.

Profeta, S., Forrester, C., Eng, R.H.K., et al. (1985). Salmonella infections in patients with acquired immunodeficiency syndrome. *Archives of Internal Medicine.* 145:670.

Robinson, C.H., Lawler, M.R., Chenoweth, W.L., and Garwick, A.E. (1986). *Normal and Therapeutic Nutrition.* New York: MacMillan.

Rodgers, V.D., Fassett, R., and Kagnoff, M.F. (1986). Abnormalities in intestinal mucosal T-cells in homosexual populations including those with the lymphadenopathy syndrome and acquired immunodeficiency syndrome. *Gastroenterology.* 90:552.

Rosenberg, I., Solomons, N., and Schneider, R. (1977). Malabsorption associated with diarrhea and intestinal infections. *American Journal of Clinical Nutrition.* 30:1248.

Rudman, D. (1980). Protein-energy undernutrition. In Isselbacher, K.J., Adams, R.D., Braunwald, E., et al. (Eds.): *Harrison's Principles of Internal Medicine*, 9th ed. New York: McGraw-Hill.

Sato, S.J., and Mirtallo, J.M. (1987). Nutritional support for the AIDS patient. *US Pharmacist.* 2.

Solomons, N.W., and Allen, L.H. (1983). The functional assessment of nutritional status. *Nutrition Review.* 41:33.

Stahl-Bayliss, C.M., Kalman, C.M., and Laskin, O.L. (1986). Pentamidine induced hypoglycemia in patients with the acquired immune deficiency syndrome. *Clinical Pharmacology and Therapeutics.* 39:271.

Special Medical Reports. (1989). Task force sets nutrition guidelines in HIV infection. *American Family Physicians.* 39:376.

Staff. (1987, June). AIDS news: Important nutritional facts for patients. *HIV Infection Aspects of Human Sexuality*, 134.

Taber-Pike, J., Schlanger, D., and Horn, B. (1987). *Nutrition and AIDS: Guidelines for PWA's/PWARC's.* Campbell, CA: The ARIS Project.

Weaver, C. (1987). *Care and Management of the AIDS Patient*: Postgraduate course Number 5 (12th Clinical Congress). Silver Spring, MD: American Society for Parenteral and Enteral Nutrition.

Winick, M., Andrassy, R.J., Armstrong, D., et al. (1989). Guidelines for nutrition support in AIDS. *Nutrition.* 5:39.

7

Exercise and Health Maintenance in HIV

Arthur LaPerriere, PhD
Michael Antoni, PhD
Mary Ann Fletcher, PhD
Neil Schneiderman, PhD

What doth not destroy me, maketh me stronger....

—Friedrich Nietzsche

INTRODUCTION

The rise of chronic disease as the major cause of death in recent decades emphasizes the importance of preventive medicine and health promotion. The Surgeon General in 1979 reported the necessity to adopt a more healthy life-style, including an increased focus on behavioral aspects of disease prevention (USDHEW, 1979). Much evidence links behavioral factors with improvements in health status and disease prevention (Matarazzo et al., 1984). One of the major advantages of a healthy life-style is a concomitant reduction in the risk for chronic disease (Ockene et al., 1988). In fact, by modifying a few simple personal behaviors (eg. smoking, drinking, diet, sleep and exercise) a healthier lifestyle can be achieved (USDHEW, 1979), thereby decreasing the risk associated with many chronic diseases and providing a longer, healthier and more enjoyable life (Gatchel et al., 1989).

Exercise training, well known to increase physical fitness levels (Fox et al., 1971; Kannel & Sorlie, 1979), can also be an effective therapeutic technique for many patients throughout the clinical course of certain chronic diseases (Goldstein, 1989; Painter & Blackburn, 1988). For instance, aerobic exercise training is an important component in cardiac rehabilitation programs as outlined by the American College of Cardiology (Parmley, 1986). Other clinical

therapeutic applications for exercise are indicated in the treatment of essential hypertension (Duncan et al., 1985; Jennings, et al., 1987), diabetes mellitus (Vranic & Berger, 1979; Richter et al., 1981), end-stage renal disease (Painter & Zimmerman, 1986), chronic respiratory disorders (Belman & Mittman, 1980; Unger et al., 1980) and obesity (Goldstein, 1989). Exercise has also recently been suggested as a possible therapeutic approach to manage diseases such as cancer (Eichner, 1987) and AIDS (LaPerriere et al., 1989a).

AIDS is characterized by progressive decrements in immunity, which may be associated with clinical disease progression and the appearance of overt physical symptomatology occurring over an extended period of time (Donegan et al., in press; Klimas et al., in press). Because an individual may be infected with the human immunodeficiency virus-type 1 (HIV-1), the etiologic agent of AIDS, and remain asymptomatic for as long as 15 years (Munoz et al., 1988), AIDS should be viewed as a chronic disease (Antoni et al., 1990). Pharmacologic treatments proposed for HIV-infected individuals include interferon (IFN) and azidothymidine (AZT) regimens, although producing improvements in cellular immunity (Fischl et al., 1987) provides somewhat less than optimal results and often have undesirable physiologic (Richman et al., 1987) and psychologic (Solomon & Mead, in press) side effects. Therefore, it would appear to be useful to develop behavioral-based alternative and adjunct thera-peutic approaches, such as exercise training, for a more effective management of HIV-infection progression. Ongo-ing research is attempting to elucidate how exercise effects both the physiologic and psychologic components of HIV infection, in addition to addressing the need to develop effective exercise evaluation and training protocols for HIV seropositive individuals (Spence et al., 1990; Rigsby, et al., 1989; LaPerriere, et al., 1988, 1989b, 1989c, in press).

This chapter provides an up-to-date report of the accumu-lating scientific information that establishes a rationale for the use of exercise training as a therapeutic health mainte-nance technique in HIV. A brief review of the immunologic and psychologic sequelae of HIV infection serves as the backdrop against the development of a working heuristic model of how HIV infection progression may be accelerated by stressor effects on psychosocial, neuroendocrine and immunologic factors. Exercise training is offered as one possible psychoneuroimmunologic therapeutic intervention designed to decelerate the progression of HIV. A synopsis of three research programs investigating the different types of exercise training and their relationship to HIV infection is presented. Finally, some suggestions and recommendations for implementing exercise training as a treatment for HIV are offered.

HIV INFECTION

Immunologic Sequelae

HIV directly infects helper/inducer (CD4) cells, the major regulatory cell of the immune response, by attaching to a surface-membrane receptor (Fauci et al., 1983) followed by virus assimilation into the DNA material of the cell. Consequently, the regulatory and effector functions of CD4 cells are severely impaired (Fauci, 1984) until eventually cell necrosis takes place. The ubiquitous nature of the immunologic deterioration seen in HIV seropositive indi-viduals is the result of these quantitative and qualitative effects of HIV-1 on the CD4 cells (Fauci, 1984, 1988). Among these secondary effects is a decrease in the cytotoxic function of suppressor/cytotoxic (CD8) cells (Fauci, 1984) which may be mediated by a reduction in the inducer subset of CD4+ (CD45RA+CD4+) cells as HIV infection proceeds over time (Raise et al., 1988). In fact, a decline in CD45RA+CD4+ has been implicated as a contributing factor in accelerating HIV progression (DeMartini et al., 1988). (Chapter 3 presents an in-depth review of immunol-ogy.)

Psychosocial Sequelae

In addition to the pervasive immunologic deterioration reported earlier, recent evidence has identified interrelation-ships among several psychosocial variables and HIV infec-tion. These psychosocial sequelae include mild to severe affective adjustments to receiving notification of a positive serologic test for HIV, psychosocial disruption precipitated by the need for immediate and stringent behavior change (eg. cessation of IV drug abuse, practicing safer sex), excessive demands on coping resources necessary for deal-ing with the uncertainty of the disease's clinical course, and adjustments to potential social isolation (see Chapter 15). Reactions to HIV, which include depression, anger, sadness, fear of illness, dependency, death, loss of bodily control, pain and disfigurement, resemble those of newly diagnosed cancer patients (Solomon & Mead, in press).

Ironson et al. (1988, 1990) noted that the psychologic impact of a positive serologic diagnosis for HIV resulted in increased anxiety and depression, as well as intrusive thoughts and avoidant behaviors related to HIV. Perceived and actual social isolation have also been reported as consequences of receiving a positive HIV diagnosis and may be the result of fear of infecting loved ones, loss of social support from significant others, lowered self-esteem and stigmatization by society (Morin et al., 1984).

Elevations in anxiety and depression appear to vary in severity throughout the clinical course of HIV infection (Goodkin, 1988; Temoshok et al., 1987; Tross, 1987; Tross et al., 1987). Persons with chronic symptomatic HIV disease, using general and AIDS-specific measures of distress, have scored higher on tests of anxiety and depres-sion than those with AIDS (Tross et al., 1987). These differences may be attributed to the greater degree of uncertainty present in the lives of the HIV patient who is mildly symptomatic with ARC (Tross, 1987). In addition, the uncertain future of HIV seropositive individuals, who are at present asymptomatic and relatively healthy, may increase unmanageable anxiety (Morin et al., 1984).

These findings indicate that the HIV-seropositive person experiences affective and behavioral changes that are espe-cially evident at certain disease-related periods (eg. prediag-nosis, postdiagnosis and emerging symptoms).

MODEL FOR ACCELERATED HIV DISEASE (THE PROBLEM)

The underlying reasons for extreme variability in the progression of HIV infection from an asymptomatic rela-tively healthy stage, through immunologic decrements, to the emergence of clinical symptomatology are not yet fully understood. Repeated exposure to HIV, other concurrent viral infections, substance abuse, age and nutrition have been suggested as possible cofactors in the clinical decline of HIV infection (Beech et al., in press; Fletcher et al., 1989). Several investigators have also proposed that psychosocial stressors may act as catalysts for accelerating HIV disease progression (Antoni et al., 1990; Cecchi, 1984; Coates et al., 1984; Donlou et al., 1985; Fletcher et al., 1989; Ironson et al., 1990; LaPerriere et al., 1989c). The exact functional mechanistic links between psychosocial stressors and HIV infection progression are unknown. However, a compendium of psychoneuroimmunologic literature suggests a model (Figure 7-1) for stressor-related immunomodulatory effects (Antoni et al., 1990). This model may be conceptualized as 1) stressor effects on the autonomic nervous system (ANS), neuroendocrines, and neuropeptides; and 2) effects of these ANS, neuroendocrine, and neuropeptide agents on the immune system of a compromised host. These immunomodulatory changes could then serve to accelerate the progression of the disease in HIV-infected persons.

Stressor Effects

McCabe and Schneiderman (1985) have reported that the way in which an individual perceives a stressor or the style of coping response used in attempting to manage the stressor may decide which specific ANS, neuroendocrine and neuropeptide changes occur. Coping strategies that are readily available and potentially sufficient to meet the stressful demands are usually associated with active coping. During active coping episodes, the sympathoadrenomedullary (SAM) system is actively releasing epinephrine (E) and norepinephrine (NE) into systemic circulation, which prepares the individual for stressor confrontation. If, however, the stressful situation is uncontrollable, unpredictable, or unrelenting and coping responses are unavailable or inadequate, then another physiologic pattern appears to be dominant. This pattern, characterized as behavioral inhibition associated with hypervigilance, lack of adequate coping resources and conservation-withdrawal (often termed passive coping), activates the hypothalamic-pituitary adrenocortical system (HPAC). HPAC activation begins a sequence of hormonal release of corticotropin-releasing hormone (CRH) and adrenocorticotropin hormone (ACTH), which results in the release of corticosteroids such as cortisol (McCabe & Schneiderman, 1985).

In summary, active and passive coping strategies activate discrete neuroadrenal systems that stimulate the release of different neuroendocrines and neuropeptides. The next section highlights the different immunomodulatory effects of these substances, thereby indicating that the coping style a person uses may in fact play an important role in determining the degree to which a stressor effects the immune system.

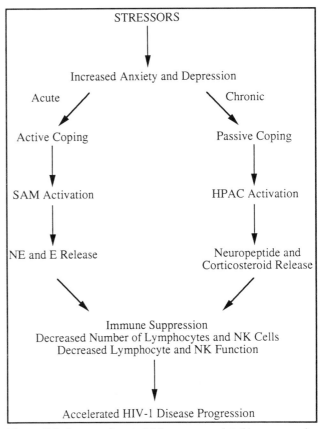

Figure 7-1. A suggestive model for stressor-related immunomodulatory effects.

Neuroimmune Effects

A number of studies have shown that an elevation in peripheral NE and E is capable of suppressing immune function (eg. decreasing natural killer [NK] cell-killing activity and T-lymphocyte proliferation) apparently by beta-adrenergic receptors on lymphocytes (Felten et al., 1985; Hadden, 1987; Hatfield et al., 1986; Livnat et al., 1985; Plaut, 1987). These immunomodulatory effects, at least in part, appear to be mediated by increases in intracellular levels of cyclic adenosine monophosphate (cAMP) Katz, et al., 1982; Plaut, 1987). Similarly, corticotropin-releasing hormone has been shown to inhibit human NK cell cytotoxicity, ostensibly by stimulating cAMP in large granular lymphocytes (Pawlikowski et al., 1988). In addition, ACTH and corticosteroids appear to impair several components of cellular immunity, including T-lymphocytes (Cupps & Fauci, 1982; Felton, et al., 1985), macrophages (Hall & Goldstein, 1981; Monjan, 1981), and NK cell activity (Heberman & Holden, 1978; Levy, et al., 1987). ACTH may interfere with intracellular levels of calcium, an important second messenger for T-cell activation (Kavelaars et al., 1988); and corticosteriods have been shown to impair production of essential soluble mediators, such as the cytokine interleukin-1 (IL-1), (Cupps & Fauci, 1982). A recent study reported that the ability of HIV to infect normal human lymphocytes is enhanced by adding corticosteroids to the cell culture (Markham et al., 1986). Therefore, glucocorticoid secretions during stress may augment the viral susceptibility of these lymphocytes and could lead to a quicker immunologic deterioration and earlier emergence of opportunistic infections.

This stressor-to-disease model provides the foundation for a framework of the possible underlying mechanisms by which a psychosocial stressor may accelerate HIV infection. In addition, this model indicates that passive coping strategies 1) are chronic, 2) activate the HPAC system, and 3) may result in more severe and longer lasting deleterious effects on immunity. By elucidating these psychoneuroimmunologic interrelationships, effective interventions can be developed.

MODEL FOR DECELERATING HIV SPECTRUM DISEASE (A SOLUTION)

The rationale for the use of exercise training to decelerate the progression of HIV spectrum disorders is suggested by studies that have documented relationships between 1) exercise and stress reduction, 2) exercise and endogenous opiates, and 3) exercise and immunity.

Exercise and Stress Reduction

Exercise training has been advanced as one behavioral technique for reducing the association between stress and illness by attenuating the organismic strain produced by stressful events (Kobasa et al., 1985). One possible explanation for this buffering effect is that aerobic exercise training reduces the psychologic and physical consequences of unavoidable or unmanageable stress (Roth & Holmes, 1985). It is possible, therefore, that aerobic exercise reduces the impact of chronic stress by adapting active coping strategies that enable each stressor to be more effectively managed, and thus limiting the activation of the HPAC system and favoring activation of the more acute and adaptive SAM network. Evidence demonstrates that aerobic exercise provides a spectrum of significant psychologic benefits. Many studies have established that both a single bout of exercise (Bahrke & Morgan, 1978; Morgan, 1985; Raglin & Morgan, 1985) and more prolonged aerobic exercise training (Goldwater & Collis, 1985; Raglin & Morgan, 1985) are associated with increased perceptions of well-being (Goldwater & Collis, 1985; Morgan, 1985) and reductions in anxiety

(Bahrke & Morgan, 1978; Goldwater & Collis, 1985; Morgan, 1979; Morgan, 1985; Raglin & Morgan, 1985).

Exercise and Endogenous Opiates

The euphoric feeling reported after aerobic exercise, which has been termed "runner's high," is similar to the euphoria produced from the injections or ingestion of various opiate-like drugs (Pargman & Baker, 1980; Sachs, 1984). In fact, the release of endogenous opiates after aerobic exercise may account in part for these affective benefits. Evidence from several laboratories has documented an increase in serum concentrations of endogenous opiates, including beta-lipotrophin, met-enkephalin, and beta-endorphin after aerobic exercises (Berk et al., 1981; Bortz et al., 1981; Carr et al., 1981; Colt et al., 1981; Farrell et al., 1982; Sutton et al., 1982. Carr et al. (1981) reported higher levels of serum concentrations of beta-endorphin in persons after an eight-week aerobic exercise training program consisting of cycling and running as compared to pretraining levels. This augmented release of beta-endorphin observed in the aerobically fit individual may indicate that those who maintain their aerobic fitness may also maintain higher levels of some endogenous opiates.

Endogenous opiates, besides the likely beneficial affective changes, have been documented as having direct effects on immunity. As early as 1979, Wybran et al. (1979) noted met-enkephalin receptors on the surface of human T-lymphocytes. The presence of such receptors implied a functional role. More recent investigations have in fact demonstrated increased active T-cell rosetting in peripheral blood lymphocytes in patients with lymphoma (Miller et al., 1983) as well as normal subjects (Miller et al., 1984) who receive met-enkephalin regimens. In addition, met-enkephalin has also been shown to enhance in vitro NK cell cytotoxicity (Faith et al., 1984; Mathews et al., 1983; Wybran, 1985). Recently, met-enkephalin protocols, because of the apparent capability to modify a variety of immune parameters, have been investigated in HIV disease. A 21-day treatment regime of intravenous met-enkephalin in mildly symptomatic (ARC) HIV patients showed an increase in numbers of OKT3 and OKT4 lymphocytes, production of interleukin-2 (IL-2), and lymphocyte proliferation response to plant mitogen phytohemagglutinin (PHA) (Wybran et al., 1987). Wybran et al., (1987) also noted a threefold increase in PHA response after a single injection of met-enkephalin in one person with AIDS and retrogression of KS lesions after four weeks of met-enkepalin treatments in another. These results, although exceedingly preliminary, suggest some potential for beneficial effects of met-enkephalin treatment regimens on both immunity and physical symptomatology in persons with HIV.

Exercise and Immunity

Several studies have documented immunomodulation after episodes of acute aerobic exercise (Brahmi et al., 1985; Hanson & Flaherty, 1981; Hedefors, et al., 1983; Targan, et al., 1981). The consensus of these studies is that acute aerobic exercise of moderate intensity appears to increase the numbers of T- and B-lymphocytes, as well as some functional indices of lymphocytes (Simon, 1984), including augmented cytotoxic activity. In one study, which investigated the immunologic effects of maximal exertion aerobic exercise, both trained and untrained individuals showed NK cytotoxicity values that increased immediately on completion of the exercise, decreased to a low point two hours later, only to return to baseline values within 20 hours (Brahmi et al., 1985). Another study, however, showed similar increases in NK cytotoxicity after only five minutes of moderate aerobic bike riding (Targan et al., 1981), suggesting that exercise to exertion may not be necessary to induce immunomodulatory effects. In a study of well-conditioned runners Hanson & Flaherty (1981), showed increases in antibody-dependent cellular cytotoxicity after a moderate intensity routine eight-mile training run. Interestingly, cytotoxic activity levels remained elevated for 24 hours. Watson et al. (1986) investigated the effects of an endurance exercise program on cellular immunity in previously inactive but young and healthy males. After several weeks of moderate aerobic exercise training, an increase in the percentage of T-lymphocytes was noted.

EXERCISE TRAINING RESEARCH PROGRAMS

These psychoneuroimmunologic effects of exercise have served as the foundation in the development of a heuristic model designed to demonstrate how exercise training may decelerate the progression of HIV spectrum disorders (Figure 7-2). From this model it can be seen that exercise training reduces negative effect, increases endogenous opiate release, and reduces HPAC activation, thereby enhancing immunity. An important element of this model may be the adoption of a more active coping strategy, exercise training. Three exercise training research programs have been used with HIV patients: 1) aerobic exercise training, 2) progressive resistance exercise (PRE) training, and 3) a combination program of flexibility, cardiovascular endurance, and muscle strength training in HIV seropositive individuals and patients with AIDS.

Aerobic Exercise Training Program

The purpose of this study was to investigate the efficacy of an aerobic exercise training program as a psychoneuroim-

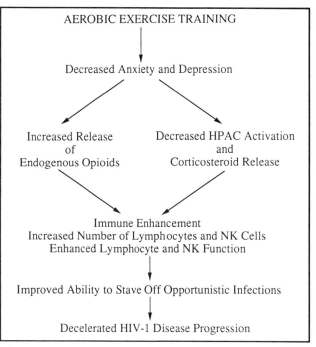

Figure 7-2. Heuristic model demonstrating how exercise training could possibly decelerate progression of HIV disease.

munologic intervention for gay males at risk for AIDS (LaPerriere et al., in press). One primary aim was to determine the effects of aerobic exercise training on the immune system in both HIV-negative and positive individuals. Because these individuals are at risk for a disease that attacks the immune system, it was important to document that moderate aerobic exercise was not adversely influencing immunity. A second aim was to determine if aerobic exercise training would attenuate the negative effect and immunologic compromise accompanying receipt of a positive HIV diagnosis. In fact, this study has shown that individuals who are simply at risk for HIV or already infected but still asymptomatic and at a very early stage in the HIV infection process can benefit, both physiologically and psychologically, from regular, moderate exercise.

Study Population. Fifty homosexual males who had never been tested for HIV and, therefore, did not know about their HIV serologic status entered the study following a complete physical examination, including a cardiovascular fitness evaluation and a medical history questionnaire. Individuals were excluded from the study for any of the following: 1) a diagnosis for either AIDS-related complex (ARC; CDC stage 3) or AIDS (CDC stage 4) as defined by the Centers for Disease Control (Center for Disease Control, 1987), 2) exhibiting any signs or symptoms suggestive of AIDS, 3) unexplained weight loss (greater than 10 percent or 15 pounds within the previous three months), 4) fever or diarrhea, 5) generalized lymphadenopathy, 6) oral candidiasis, 7) or herpes zoster within the previous year. Also excluded were those with a history of drug or alcohol abuse and individuals who reported use of anabolic steroids or regular use of antihistamines. Subjects were also not entered into this study if they routinely participated in regular aerobic exercise or showed a pretest estimated maximum oxygen consumption (VO^2max) greater than 53 mg/kg/min for ages 18 through 29 or 49 mg/kg/min for the age range of 30 to 40. It was intended that such a rigorous pretreatment evaluation targeting numerous exclusion criteria could help in establishing a relatively homogeneous study sample. The importance of methodologic considerations in psychoneuroimmunologic research has been pointed out by others as well (Kiecolt-Glaser & Glaser, 1988).

Study Design. Subjects were randomly assigned either to a 10 week aerobic exercise training or to a measurement-only control group. The aerobic exercise training involved 45 minutes of stationary bicycle ergometry three times per week, with the intensity maintained between 70 and 80 percent of age-predicted maximum heart rate (220 minus each subject's age). Each subject (whether exercise training or control) was evaluated for cardiovascular fitness by riding a stationary bicycle ergometer for five minutes at a fixed resistance of 150 watts and a constant pedal speed of 50 revolutions per minute. This procedure produced a fifth minute submaximal heart rate (HRSUB) which was then substituted into the Fox equation (6.3 minus 0.0193 times HRSUB/weight in kg) to yield a predicted VO^2max (PVO^2max) (Fox et al., 1973). VO^2max is considered to be the best overall indicator of aerobic fitness level (Saltin & Astrand, 1967).

This study incorporated four measurement time points: baseline (entry into the study), week five (72 hours before HIV serologic status notification), week six (72 hours after HIV serologic status notification), and week ten (conclusion of the study). Fitness status, control variables (eg. sleep behavior, physical activity, serum concentrations of albumin and hematocrit), immunologic panel (eg. CD4, CD8, CD45RA+CD4+, and NK cell enumerations), and the Profile of Mood States (POMS) (McNair et al., 1981) were assessed at baseline, week five and week ten. Immunologic and psychologic parameters were also collected at week six to determine the effects of exercise training on the stress accompanying serologic status notification.

Results. After five weeks of aerobic exercise training, both seronegative and seropositive subjects showed significant increases in PVO^2max, which were maintained for the remaining five weeks of the study. Individuals in the control group displayed no similar changes in PVO^2max.

Both HIV seropositive and seronegative subjects showed an increase in CD4 cells, however, the magnitude of change was greater in the seronegative group (220 vs 115 cells/mm$_3$; LaPerriere et al., in press). A CD4 cell increase of this size is comparable to that seen in clinical trials of the HIV drug AZT (Fischl et al., 1987) but without the accompanying side effects. A similar trend was also seen in the CD45RA+CD4+ cells. A significant increase in the anxiety and depression subscales of the POMS was observed in the seropositive control subjects at week six, after receiving a positive HIV serologic status notification. Seropositive exercisers, however, did not show any increases in anxiety or depression after receiving news of their seropositivity. This exercise training-induced buffering effect on affective mood states was accompanied by a similar attenuation of a cellular deficit in response to a positive diagnosis. Seropositive control subjects showed a significant 170 cells/mm$_3$ decrease in NK cells after notification of seropositivity, whereas seropositive exercisers displayed only a nonsignificant 38 cells/mm$_3$ decrease after receiving a similar diagnosis (LaPerriere et al., 1990).

Conclusions. This study documented that a 10-week program of aerobic exercise training increases cellular immunity while buffering the affective and immunologic deficits that accompany a stressful event. If the progressive decrement in immune function that normally occurs during the course of HIV spectrum disorders can be slowed by a continued program of exercise training, aerobic exercise training may prove to be an effective means of slowing the progression of HIV disorders.

Progressive Resistance Exercise Training Program

One major complication observed in HIV patients is a substantial wasting of body tissue (Kolter et al., 1984). This wasting includes muscle atrophy (Cornblath et al., 1987; Eidelberd et al., 1986; Elder et al., 1986), as well as a significant depletion of plasma volume and intracellular potassium concentrations (Kolter et al., 1985). PRE training has been shown to enhance muscle function and induce muscle hypertrophy in both healthy (Saltin & Golnick, 1983) and diseased (McCartney et al., 1988) and unhealthy individuals.

The purpose of this study was to investigate the effects of a PRE training program in HIV patients with the hope of observing improved muscle function (Spence et al., 1990). In addition, the influence of PRE training on body weight and dimensions was also examined.

Study Population. Twenty-four male, outpatient volunteers, ages 23 to 46, recovering from one episode of PCP, but with no other AIDS-defining opportunistic infections were enrolled into the study. All subjects were at least two weeks post-therapy for their acute PCP and remained on an AZT protocol throughout this study.

Study Design. Subjects were randomly assigned to either a six-week PRE training or a control group. The PRE training group exercised three times per week during the study period for a total of 18 PRE training sessions. In contrast, the control group did not engage in any exercise activity (except usual daily living activities) during the same time period.

PRE training was conducted on the total power hydraulic resistance unit (Peterson & Bell, 1987), which provides both bidirectional, concentric muscle contractions, and bilateral movement throughout the entire range of motion. Over the course of the six-week training program, the resistance load was uniformly increased from one set times 15 repetitions at the minimal setting to three sets times 10 repetitions at the maximal setting.

Before training, subjects were evaluated for muscle function and anthropometric measurements taken. Data on three components of muscle function (force, power, work) were collected for three muscle regions (thighs and legs, chest and arms, shoulder and arms) under low- and high-resistance conditions. Anthropometric measurements consisted of body weight, girth and skinfold thickness. This evaluation panel was repeated after PRE training.

Results. The prestudy evaluation showed no significant differences between those subjects assigned to PRE training and control subjects on any of the muscle function or anthropometric measures. After six weeks of PRE training, experimental subjects showed a significant improvement on virtually all of the muscle function tests. In contrast, control subjects displayed no increases on any muscle function test and, in fact, showed a significant decrease on several tests, resulting in significant post-study differences between groups on all but one muscle function measurement (Spence et al., 1990).

Similarly, no differences were observed between the experimental and control group at study entry on any of the three anthropometric measures. After six weeks of PRE training, however, body weight and girth measurements in the experimental group increased, while the control subjects displayed significant decreases on these variables (Spence et al., 1990).

Conclusions. This study documented improved muscle function and anthropometry following six weeks of PRE training in persons with HIV. Spence, Galantino and

colleagues theorize that similar effects may also be seen in asymptomatic HIV seropositive individuals and in symptomatic patients. Thus PRE may provide one way of retarding the wasting syndrome which accompanies HIV infection and improves the quality of life for these individuals.

Combination Strength Training and Aerobic Exercise Program

The purpose of this study was to investigate the effects of a combination of strength training and aerobic exercise on psychologic and immunologic parameters individuals with HIV (Rigsby et al., 1989).

Study Population. Thirty-seven HIV positive and eight HIV-negative individuals volunteered for this study. The HIV-positive subjects spanned the range of HIV disorders from asymptomatic to a diagnosis of AIDS.

Study Design. Subjects were randomly assigned either to a 12-week exercise training group or a counseling control. The exercise training group met for approximately one hour three times per week. Each training session consisted of 15 minutes of light stretching, 25 minutes of stationary bicycle ergometry, and 20 minutes of muscular strength training. The control group met once a week for an hour and received counseling. Before training, all subjects were evaluated for muscular strength using the Total Power hydraulic resistance unit (Peterson & Bell, 1987). Cardiovascular endurance was assessed by recording resting heart rate. Immunologic measures included numbers of CD4 and CD8 cells; the Beck Depression scale was used to assess affect. These evaluations were repeated after exercise training.

Results. Subjects in the exercise training group displayed a significant reduction in resting heart rate indicating an improvement in cardiovascular fitness. Subjects in the control group showed no similar changes. Both the exercise training and counseling groups showed a significant decrease in Beck Depression scores after 12 weeks of participation in the study (Rigsby et al., 1989).

The exercise training group showed a trend toward increased CD4 and CD8 cell numbers while effecting no change to the CD4/CD8 ratio. Similar changes in cellular immunity were not observed in control subjects (Rigsby et al., 1989).

Conclusions. Rigsby et al. concluded that exercise training can improve physiologic (increased cardiovascular endurance), psychologic (decreased depression) and immunologic (increased numbers of CD4 cells) measures in HIV-seropositive individuals.

Table 7-1
TYPICAL AEROBIC EXERCISE PROGRAM
(Six Steps)

Step 1 - Warm-up
A five-minute period that includes slow static stretching of the major muscles involved in the selected activity

Step 2 - Type of Training
Any activity that uses large muscle groups in continuous, rhythmic and dynamic nature, such as brisk walking, jogging, running, biking, swimming, etc

Step 3 - Frequency of Training
A minimum of three times per week (some individuals exercise five times or more per week)

Step 4 - Duration of Training
Usually 30 - 45 minutes of continuous aerobic exercise; however, duration is related to intensity; the higher the intensity the shorter the duration

Step 5 - Intensity of Training
Recommended target exercise range is between 20% - 80% of predicted maximum heart rate (PMHR); to calculate PMHR range, subtract age from 220 and multiply by .70 for lower limit and .80 for upper limit

Step 6 - Cool Down
A five-minute period of reduced intensity exercise (eg. walking after jogging), followed by slow static stretching of the major muscles involved in the activity

---

training would appear to provide a potentially promising therapeutic intervention for HIV seropositive individuals.

Some recommendations for prescribing exercise training as an intervention in HIV-infected persons would appear to be appropriate. Exercise prescriptions for all HIV-seropositive persons (regardless of stage of infection) should be made individually and only after intensive initial screening. Individuals with HIV disease, as all persons beginning an exercise program, should undergo initial screening, which includes a symptom-limited graded exercise test such as a modified Balke protocol (Protas & Galantino, 1989) or the previously described Fox Equation (Fox et al., 1973). These tests allow the therapist 1) to determine the safety of vigorous exercise; 2) to provide norms against which to measure cardiovascular progress; and 3) to prescribe an exercise program of the appropriate frequency, duration, intensity, and type (American College of Sports Medicine, 1986). However, in the case of the HIV-infected person, additional disease specific assessment is required to determine an exercise prescription.

The process of developing a successful exercise prescription entails creating a balanced program designed to increase aerobic capacity, muscle function, and flexibility of specific individuals. Table 7-1 provides easy-to-follow steps of a typical aerobic exercise session. The same techniques of warm up, training and cool down should also be followed for weight training as well.

EXERCISE TREATMENT FOR HIV SEROPOSITIVE INDIVIDUALS

Appropriately supervised moderate exercise training does not appear to adversely affect individuals with HIV disease. Furthermore, empirical evidence provides support for the use of exercise training in the treatment of HIV disease. The preliminary findings suggest that exercise training may help in slowing the progression of HIV spectrum disorders. If exercise training can keep individuals in the early stages of this disease free of overt symptoms, then relatively good health should be maintained longer than if exercise training is not undertaken. In addition, the research programs have documented the beneficial effects of various types of exercise training on physical, psychologic and immunologic parameters associated with HIV disorder progression. Although further research is needed to fully understand the complex interrelationships between exercise and health maintenance in a dynamic disease such as AIDS, exercise

SUMMARY

The available evidence suggests that an integrated exercise training program that includes both an aerobic and weight-training component could help maintain the psychologic and physical health status of individuals living with HIV. In the absence of a known cure for HIV disease disorder, a number of palliative measures would appear to be appropriate. One of these would seem to be pharmacologic management such as provided by AZT. Another would appear to be behavioral management. Among behavioral management interventions, programs involving aerobic exercise and strength training appear to be particularly promising.

Acknowledgment

The preparation of this chapter was facilitated by NIMH grant #P50MH4355. Address correspondence to: Arthur LaPerriere, Center for Biopsychosocial Studies of AIDS, Department of Psychiatry, University of Miami School of Medicine, 1425 N.W. 10th Avenue, Suite 302, Miami, FL 33136.

References

Antoni, M.H., Schneiderman, N., Fletcher, M.A. (1990). Psychoneuroimmunology and HIV-1. *Journal of Consulting and Clinical Psychology.* 58:38.

American College of Sports Medicine. (1986). *Guidelines for Exercise Testing and Prescription,* 3rd ed. Philadelphia: Lea & Febiger.

Bahrke, M.S., Morgan, W.P. (1978). Anxiety reduction following exercise and meditation. *Cognitive Therapy and Research.* R 2:323.

Beech R., et al. (in press). Vitamin B6 levels and immune function in early HIV infections. *J AIDS.*

Belman, M.J., and Mittman, C. (1980). Ventilatory muscle training improves exercise capacity in chronic obstructive pulmonary disease patients. *American Review of Respiratory Disease.* 121:273.

Berk, L.S., et al. (1981). Beta-endorphin response to exercise in athletes and non-athletes. *Medical and Science in Sports and Exercise.* 13:134.

Bortz, W.M., et al. (1981). Catecholamines, dopamine and endorphin levels during extreme exercise. *New England Journal of Medicine.* 305:446.

Brahmi Z., et al. (1985). The effect of acute exercise on natural killer-cell activity of trained and sedentary human subjects. *Journal of Clinical Immunology.* 5:321.

Carr D.B., et al. (1981). Physical conditioning facilitates the exercise-induced secretion of beta-endorphin and beta-e liptrophin in women. *New England Journal of Medicine.* 305:560.

Cecchi, R.L. (1984). Stress: Prodrome to immune deficiency. *Annals New York Academy of Science.* 437:286.

Centers for Disease Control. (1987). Revision of the CDC surveillance case definition for acquired immune deficiency syndrome. *Mortality and Morbidity Weekly Report.* 36:

Coates, T.J., Temoshok, L., and Mandel, J. (1984). Psychosocial research is essential to understanding and treating AIDS. *American Psychologist.* 39:1309.

Colt, E.W.D., Wardlaw, S.L., and Frantz, A.G. (1981). The effects of running on plasma beta-endorphin. *Life Sciences.* 28:1637.

Cornblath, D.R., McArthur, J.C., Kennedy, P.G., et al. (1987). Inflammatory demyelinating peripheral neuropathies associated with human T-cell lymphotrophic virus Type III infection. *Annals of Neurology.* 21:32.

Cupps, T., and Fauci, A. (1982). Corticosteroid-mediated immunoregulation in man. *Immunological Reviews.* 65:133.

DeMartini, R.M., Turner, R.R., Formenti, S.C., et al. (1988). Peripheral blood mononuclear cell abnormalities and their relationship to clinical course in homosexual men with HIV infection. *Clinical Immunology and Immunopathology.* 46:258.

Donegan, E., Stuart, M., and Niland, J.C., et al. (1990). Clinical outcome and laboratory findings for recipients of blood components from donors positive for antibody to Human Immunodeficiency virus type 1 at the time of blood donations. *Annals of Internal Medicine.* 113:733.

Donlou, J.N., Wolcott, M.S., Gottlieb, M.S., et al. (1985). Psychosocial aspects of AIDS and AIDS-related complex: A pilot study. *Journal Psychosocial Oncology.* 3:39.

Duncan, J.J., Fark, J.E., Upton, S.J., et al. (1985). The effects of aerobic exercise on plasma catecholamines and blood pressure in patients with mild essential hypertension. *Journal American Medical Association.* 254:2609.

Eichner, E.R. (1987). Exercise, lymphokines, calories, and cancer. *Physician and Sports Medicine.* 5:109.

Eidelberd, D., Sotrel, A., Vogel, H., et al. (1986). Progressive polyradiculopathy in acquired immunodeficiency syndrome. *Neurology.* 36:912.

Elder, G., Dalakes, M., Pezeshkpour, G., et al. (1986). Ataxic neuropathy due to ganglioneuritis after probable acute human immunodeficiency virus infection. *Lancet.* 2:1275.

Faith, R.E., Liang, H.J., Murgo, A.J., et al. (1984). Neuroimmunomodulation with enkephalins: Enhancement of human natural killer (NK) cell activity in vitro. *Clinical Immunology and Immunopathology.* 31:412.

Farrell, P.A., Gates, W.K., Morgan, W.P., et al. (1982). Increases in plasma B-EP and B-LPH immunoreactivity after treadmill running in humans. *Journal of Applied Psychology.* 52:1245.

Fauci, A.S., Macher, A.M., and Longo, D.L. (1983). Acquired immunodeficiency syndrome: epidemiologic, clinical, immunologic, and therapeutic considerations. *Annals of Internal Medicine.* 100:92.

Fauci, A.S. (1984). Immunologic abnormalities in the acquired immunodeficiency syndrome (AIDS). *Clinical Research.* 32:491.

Fauci, A.S. (1988). The human immunodeficiency virus: infectivity and mechanisms of pathogenesis. *Science.* 239:617.

Felten, D. Felten, S., Carlson, S., et al. (1985). Noradrenergic and peptidergic innervation of lymphoid tissue. *Journal of Immunology.* 135:755s.

Fischl, M.A., Richman, D., Grieco, M., et al. (1987). The efficacy of azidothymidine (AZT) in the treatment of patients with AIDS and AIDS-related complex. *New England Journal Medicine.* 317:185.

Fletcher, M.A., MD, Ironson, G., LaPerriere, A., et al. (1989). *Immunological and Psychological Predictors of Disease Progression in Gay Males for AIDS.* Proceedings of the V International Conference on AIDS, Montreal, Canada, p. 382.

Fox, S.M., Naughton, J.P., and Haskell, W.L. (1971). Physical activity and prevention of coronary heart disease. *Annals Clinical Research.* 3:404.

Fox, E., Billings, C., Bartels, R., et al. (1973). Fitness standards for male college students. *International Zeischrift Fuer Angewandte Physiologie Einschliesslich Arbeitsphysiologie.* 31:231.

Gatchel, R.J., Baum A., and Krantz, D.S. (1989). *An Introduction to Health Psychology,* 2nd ed. New York: Random House, p. 290.

Goldstein, D. (1989). Clinical Applications for Exercise. *The Physician and Sports Medicine.* 17:83.

Goldwater, B.C., and Collis, M.L. (1985). Psychologic effects of cardiovascular conditioning: A controlled experiment. *Psychosomatic Medicine.* 47:174.

Goodkin, K. (1988). Psychiatric aspects of HIV infection. *Texas Medicine.* 84:55.

Hadden, J. (1987). Neuroendocrine modulation of the thymus-dependent immune system. *Annals of the New York Academy of Sciences.* 496:39.

Hall, N., and Goldstein, A. (1981). Neurotransmitters and the immune system. In Ader, R. (Ed.): *Psychoneuroimmunology.* New York: Academic Press, pp. 521-543.

Hanson, P., and Flaherty, D. (1981). Immunological responses to training in conditioned runners. *Clinical Sciences.* 60:225.

Hatfield, S., Petersen, B., and DiMicco, J. (1986). Beta adrenoreceptor modulation of the generation of murine cytotoxic T lymphocytes in vitro. *Journal of Pharmacology and Experimental Therapeutics.* 239:460.

Heberman, R., and Holden, H. (1978). Natural cell-mediated immunity. *Advances in Cancer Research.* 27:305.

Hedefors, E., Holm, G., Ivansen, M., et al. (1983). Physiological variation of blood lymphocyte reactivity: T-cell subsets, immunoglobulin production, and mixed-lymphocyte reactivity. *Clinical Immunology and Immunopathology.* 27:9.

Ironson, G., O'Hearn, P., LaPerriere, A., et al. (1988). News of HIV antibody status and immune function in healthy gay males. *Proceedings of the Ninth Annual Scientific Sessions of the Society of Behavioral Medicine.* Boston: Society of Behavioral Medicine, p. 55.

Ironson, G., LaPerriere, A., Antoni, M., et al. (1990). Changes in immune and psychological measures as a function of anticipation and reaction to news of HIV-1 antibody status. *Psychomatic Medicine.* 52:247.

Jennings, S.L., et al. (1987). Long-term effects of exercise on blood pressure, sympathetic activity, and left ventricular hypertrophy in essential hypertension. Pre-

sented at the American Heart Association 41st Annual Fall Conference and Scientific Session, New Orleans.

Kannel, W.B., and Sorlie, P. (1979). Some health benefits of physical activity: The Framingham Study. *Archives of Internal Medicine.* 139:857.

Katz, P., Zeytoun, A., and Fauci, A. (1982). Mechanisms of human cell-mediated cytotoxicity: I. Modulation of natural killer cell activity by cyclic nucleotides. *Journal of Immunology.* 129:287.

Kavelaars, A., Ballieux, R.E., and Heijnen, C. (1988). Modulation of the immune response by pro-opiomelanocortin derived peptides. *Brain Behavior Immunity.* 2:57.

Kiecolt-Glaser, J.K., and Glaser, R. (1988). Methodological issues in behavioral immunology research with humans. *Brain Behavior and Immunity.* 2:67.

Klimas, N.G., Baron, G.C., and Fletcher, M.A. (in press). The Immunology of HIV-1 infection. In McCabe, P., Field, T., Schneiderman, N. (Eds.): *Stress, Coping and Disease.* Hillsdale, NJ: Lawrence Erlbaum Associates, Inc.

Kobasa, S., Maddi, S., Purcetti, M., et al. (1985). Effectiveness of hardiness, exercise, and social support as resources against illness. *Journal of Psychosomatic Research.* 29:525.

Kolter, D.P., Wang, J., Pierson, R.H. Jr., et al. (1984). Enteropathy associated with the acquired immunodeficiency syndrome. *Annals of Internal Medicine.* 101:421.

Kolter, D.P., Wang, J., and Pierson, R.N. (1985). Body composition studies in patients with the acquired immunodeficiency syndrome. *American Journal of Clinical Nutrition.* 42:1255.

LaPerriere, A., O'Hearn, P., Ironson, G., et al. (1988). Exercise and immune function in healthy HIV antibody negative and positive gay males. Paper presented at the ninth annual scientific meetings of the Society of Behavioral Medicine, Boston.

LaPerriere, A., Schneiderman, H., Antoni, M.H., et al. (1989a). Aerobic exercise training and psychoneuroimmunology in Aids research. In Baum, A., and Temoshok, L. (Eds.): *Psychological Perspectives on AIDS.* Hillsdale, NJ: Lawrence Erlbaum Associates, Inc., pp. 259-286.

LaPerriere, A., Ironson, G., Antoni, M.H., et al. (1989b). Aerobic exercise training as a buffer of anxiety and depression in HIV-1 infected individuals. *Proceedings of the Tenth Annual Scientific Meetings of the Society of Behavioral Medicine,* San Francisco.

LaPerriere, A., Fletcher, M.A., Klimas, N., et al. (1989c). Aerobic exercise training attenuates the stress of a positive test for anti-HIV-1. *Proceedings of the 5th International Conference on AIDS,* Montreal, Canada.

LaPerriere, A., et al. (in press). Aerobic Training in an AIDS

Risk Group. *International Journal of Sports Medicine.*

LaPerriere, A., et al. (1990). Exercise intervention attenuates emotional distress and natural killer cell decrements following notification of a positive serologic status for HIV-1. *Biofeedback and Self-Regulation.* 15(3):229.

Levy, S., Herberman, R., Lippman, M., et al. (1987). Correlation of stress factors with sustained depression of natural killer cell activity and predicted prognosis in patients with breast cancer. *Journal of Clinical Oncology.* 5:348.

Livnat, S., Felten, S., Carlson, S., et al. (1985). Involvement of peripheral and central catecholamine systems in neural immune interactions. *Journal of Neuroimmunology.* 10:5.

Markham, P., Salahuddain, S., Veren, K., et al. (1986). Hydrocortisone and some other hormones enhance the expression of HTLV-III. *International Journal of Cancer.* 37:67.

Matarazzo, J.D., Weiss, S., Herd, Jr., et al. (1984). *Behavioral Health: A Handbook of Health Enhancement and Disease Prevention.* New York: Wiley.

Mathews, P.M., Froelich, C.J., Sibbitt, W.L., et al. (1983). Enhancement of natural cytotoxicity by B-endorphin. *Journal of Immunology.* 130:1658.

McCabe, P.M., and Schneiderman, N. (1985). Psychophysiologic reactions to stress. In Schneiderman, N., and Tapp, J.T. (Eds.): *Behavioral Medicine: The Biopsychosocial Approach*, (pp. 99-131). Hillsdale, NJ: Lawrence Erlbaum Associates, Inc.

McCartney, N., Moroz, P., Garner, S.H., et al. (1988). The effects of strength training in patients with selected neuromuscular disorders. *Medicine and Science in Sports and Exercise.* 20:362.

McNair, D., Lorr, M., and Droppleman, L. (1981). *EITS Manual for the Profile of Mood States..* San Diego: Educational and Industrial Testing Service.

Miller, G.C., Murgo, A.J., and Plotnikoff, N.P. (1983). Enkephalins: Enhancement of active T-cell rosettes from lymphoma patients. *Clinical Immunology and Immunopathology.* 26:446.

Miller, G.C., Murgo, A.J., and Plotnikoff, N.P. (1984). Enkephalins: Enhancement of active T-cell rosettes from normal volunteers. *Clinical Immunology and Immunopathology.* 31:132.

Monjan, A. (1981). Immunologic competence in animals. In Ader, R. (Ed.): *Psychoneuroimmunology*, (pp. 185-228). New York: Academic Press.

Morgan, W.P. (1985). Affective beneficence of vigorous physical activity. *Medicine and Science in Sports and Exercise.* 17:94.

Morgan, W.P. (1979). Anxiety reductions following acute physical activity. *Psychiatric Annals.* 9:36.

Morin, S., Charles, K., and Maylon, A. (1984). The psychological impact of AIDS on gay men. *American Psychologist.* 39:1288.

Munoz, A., Wang, M.G., Good, D., et al. (1988). Estimation of the AIDS-free times after HIV-1 seroconversion. Paper presented at the meeting of the International Conference on AIDS, Stockholm, Sweden.

Ockene, J.K., Sorensen, G., Kabar-Zinn, J., et al. (1988). Clinical perspectives: Benefits and costs of lifestyle change to reduce risk of chronic disease. *Preventive Medicine.* 17:224.

Painter, P., and Zimmerman, S.W. (1986). Exercise in end-stage renal disease. *Journal of Kidney Diseases.* 7:386.

Painter, P., and Blackburn, G. (1988). Exercise for patients with chronic disease. *Postgraduate Medicine.* 83:185.

Pargman, D., and Baker, M.C. (1980). Running high: Enkephalin indicted. *Journal of Drug Issues.* 10:341.

Parmley, W.W. (1986). Recommendations of the American College of Cardiology on cardiovascular rehabilitation. *Cardiology.* 7:4.

Pawlikowski, M., Zelazowski, P., Dohler, K., et al. (1988). Effects of two neuropeptides, somatoliberin (GRF) and corticoliberin (CRF) on human lymphocyte natural killer activity. *Brain Behavior and Immunity.* 2:50.

Peterson, S.R., and Bell, G.J. (1987). *Training with Hydra Fitness.* Belton, TX: HydraFitness Industries, pp. 1- 51.

Plaut, M. (1987). Lymphocyte hormone receptors. *Annual Review of Immunology.* 5:621.

Protas, E.J., and Galantino, M.L. (1989). An exercise test for assessing endurance in AIDS patients. *Proceedings of the Annual APTA Conference*, Research Platform. 69:394.

Raglin, J.S., and Morgan, W.P. (1985). Influence of vigorous exercise on mood state. *Behavior Therapy.* 8:179.

Raise, E., Gritti, F.M., Sabbatini, S., et al. (1988). Reduction of T helper/inducers of B lymphocyte and increased of T suppressors as an early pattern of HIV infection. *Proceedings of the IV International AIDS Conference.* Stockholm, Sweden I, p 171.

Richman, D.D., Fischel, M., Grieco, M., et al. (1987). The toxicity of azidothymidine (AZT) in the treatment or patients with AIDS and AIDS-related complex. *New England Journal of Medicine.* 317:192.

Richter, E.A., Ruderman, N.B., and Schneider, S.H. (1981). Diabetes and exercise. *American Journal of Medicine.* 70:201.

Rigsby, L., Raven, P.B., Jackson, A.W., et al. (1989). The Effects of Exercise and Counseling on the Physiological, Psychological and Immunological Factors in HIV+ Individuals (abstract). Paper presented at the meeting of the American College of Sports Medicine.

Roth, D., and Holmes, D. (1985). Influence of physical fitness in determining impact of stressful life events in physical and psychological health. *Psychosomatic Medicine*. 47:164.

Sachs, M.J. (1984). The runner's high. In Sachs, M.L., and Buffone, G.W. (Eds.): *Running as Therapy: An Integrated Approach*. Lincoln: University of Nebraska Press.

Saltin, B., and Astrand, P. (1967). Maximal oxygen uptake in athletes. *Journal of Applied Physiology*. 23:353.

Saltin, B., and Golnick, P.D. (1983). Skeletal muscle adaptability: Significance for metabolism and performance. In Peachey L.D., Adrian R.N., and Geiger S.R. (Eds.): *Handbook of Physiology*. (pp. 555-631). Baltimore: Williams & Wilkins.

Simon, H. (1984). The immunology of exercise: A brief review. *Journal American Medicine Association*. 252:381.

Solomon, G.F., and Mead, C.W. (in press). Psychosocial and human considerations in the treatment of the gay patient with AIDS or ARC. *Journal of Human Medicine*.

Spence, D.W., and Galantino, M.L. (1990). Effect of Progressive Resistance Exercise on Muscle Function and Anthropometry of a Select AIDS Population. *Archives of Physical Medicine and Rehabilitation*. 71:644.

Sutton, J.R., Brown, G.M., Keane, P., et al. (1982). The role of endorphins in the hormonal and psychological responses to exercise. *International Journal of Sports Medicine*. 2:19.

Targan, S., Britvan L., and Dorey, F. (1981). Activation of human NKCC by moderate exercise: Increased frequency of NK cells with enhanced capability of effector-target lytic interactions. *Clinical Experimental Immunology*. 45:352.

Temoshok, L., Zich, M., Solomon, G.F., et al. (1987a). An intensive psychoimmunologic study of men with AIDS.

Paper presented at the III International Conference on AIDS, Washington, D.C.

Tross, S., Hirsh, D.A., Rabkin, B., et al. (1987b). Determinants of current psychiatric disorders in AIDS spectrum patients. *Proceedings of the III International Conference on AIDS*. Washington, D.C.

Tross, S. (1987). Psychological response to AIDS and HIV disease. *Proceedings of conference on Current Concepts in Psycho-oncology and AIDS*. New York: Memorial Sloan- Kettering Cancer Center. Unger, K.M., Moler, K.M., and Hansen, P. (1980). Selection of an exercise program for patients with chronic obstructive pulmonary disease. *Heart and Lung*. 9:68.

U.S. Department of Health, Education and Welfare. (1979). *Healthy People: The Surgeon General's Report on Health Promotion and Disease Prevention*. Washington, DC: United States Government Printing Office.

Vranic, M., and Berger, M. (1979). Exercise and diabetes mellitus. *Diabetes*. 28:147.

Watson, R.R., Moriguchi, S., Jackson, J.C., et al. (1986). Modification of cellular immune functions in humans by endurance exercise training during B-adrenergic blockade with atenolol or propranolol. *Medicine and Science in Sports and Exercise*. 18:95.

Wybran, J.T., Appelbloob, J.P., Famary, A., et al. (1979). Suggestive evidence for morphine and methionine-enkephalin receptors on normal blood T lymphocytes. *Journal of Immunology*. 123:1068.

Wybran, J.T. (1985). Enkephalins and endorphines: Activation molecules for the immune system and natural killer activity *Neuropeptides*. 5:371.

Wybran, J.T., Schandene, L., Van Vooren, J., et al. (1987). Immunologic properties of methionine-enkephalin, and therapeutic implications in AIDS, ARC, and cancer. *Annals New York Academy of Sciences*. 496:108.

8

Respiratory and Cardiac Complications

Mary Lou Galantino, MS, PT

It is only with the heart that one can see rightly; what is essential is invisible to the eye.

—Antoin De Saint-Exupery

INTRODUCTION

Cardiopulmonary complications of the patient with HIV disease originate from opportunistic infections, which, when diagnosed, are responsive to appropriate management. Categories of infectious agents of the pulmonary system include parasites, bacteria, fungi and viruses. Malignancies and non-Hodgkin's lymphoma may also cause pulmonary dysfunction. Lymphocytic interstitial pneumonitis (LIP) is frequently encountered in the pediatric population.

Patient management begins with knowledge of the pathophysiology of the pulmonary opportunistic infections in order to:

1. distinguish between acute infection and other systemic disorders
2. determine appropriateness of pulmonary physical therapy
3. establish exercise prescription in light of pulmonary and other systemic dysfunction.

Pulmonary infectious agents can be grouped into categories (Table 8-1). This chapter discusses the most common pulmonary pathogens and their infectious processes. HIV-related pulmonary disease is similar to other primary pulmonary diseases in that functional problems can be directly related to problems of inadequate ventilation. Ventilatory dysfunction may upset the delicate balance of arterial blood gases and pH, leading to inadequate tissue oxygenation. Although ventilation problems seen in HIV are similar to those of primary pulmonary disorders, coincidental infections of the nervous, gastrointestinal, renal and endocrine systems may at times confound management strategies.

PNEUMOCYSTIS CARINII PNEUMONIA

Pneumocystis carinii pneumonia (PCP) is the most common threatening opportunistic infection in the United States. The infection is also the most common cause of death in AIDS patients (Douglas, 1988), with more than 60 percent of AIDS patients developing PCP (Kovacs & Masur, 1989). Of these, anywhere from 30 to 85 percent experience a relapse of PCP within a period of one year (Hollander et al., 1986; Centers for Disease Control, 1986; Small et al., 1985). *Pneumocystis carnii* is a parasitic protozoan that is part of the normal flora of most adults and rarely causes disease unless the immune system is compromised. The clinical manifestations of PCP are progressive dyspnea; tachypnea; a persistent, non-productive dry cough; fever; hypoxemia and increased alveolar-capillary-oxygen gradient, respiratory acidosis and bilateral diffuse alveolar disease. Diffuse lymphadenopathy may appear in patients with severe pulmonary involvement. Auscultatory signs, other than dry

Table 8-1
INFECTIOUS AGENTS CAUSING PULMONARY COMPLICATIONS

PARASITES
Crytosporidia
Pneumocystis carinii
Toxoplasma gondii
Strongyloidosis

BACTERIA
Mycobacterium avium intracellulare
Mycobacterium tuberculosis
Pyogenic organisms

FUNGI
Aspergillus species
Cryptococcus neoformans
Candida species
Histoplasmosis

VIRUSES
Cytomegalovirus
Herpes simplex virus
Varicella — zoster virus

MALIGNANCIES
Kaposi's sarcoma
Non-Hodgkin's lymphoma

OTHER
Lymphoid interstitial pneumonitis—pediatric population

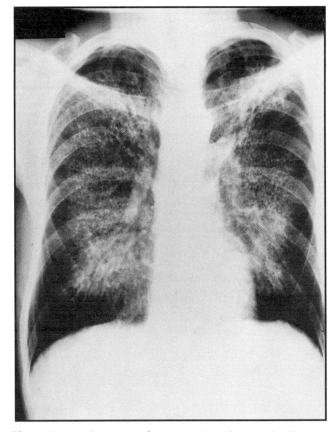

Figure 8-1. A chest x-ray of an HIV patient diagnosed with PCP.

rales, are minimal.

To definitively diagnose PCP, the causative agent must be demonstrated in material from lung aspirates or in smears of tracheobronchial mucus. No useful culture or serologic tests are in routine use to date. Chest x-rays show diffuse, symmetric, bilateral interstitial infiltrates (Figure 8-1). These changes extend peripherally from the hilar regions and have a solid, granular appearance. Pulmonary function tests reveal reduced total lung capacity, vital capacity and single breath diffusing capacity for carbon monoxide and increased expiratory flow rates. Gallium lung scans may also aid in diagnosis.

Treatment for the patient with PCP includes drug intervention, pulmonary/respiratory therapy and endurance retraining. Drug therapy consists of the following: intravenous pentamidine, trimethoprim-sulfamethoxazole (TMP/SMX), trimetrexate, clindamycin- primaquin, dapsone, difluoromethylornithine (DFMO), bactrim, septra, and co-trimoxalzole. Neither of the first two drugs has been proven clinically superior; both appear to be at least 75 percent

effective (Pedersen et al., 1989). The use of these drugs has also been shown to have severe toxic effects in 50 percent of cases and have failed in 25 percent (Haverkos, 1984; Wharton et al., 1984; Leoung et al., 1986).

Investigational studies of aerosolized pentamidine indicate that inhaled pentamidine might have increased effectiveness and decreased toxicity in mild cases of PCP (Conte et al., 1987). The dosage of IV pentamidine for 24 hours, should be dissolved in 250 ml of 5 percent dextrose in water and administered at a constant infusion rate for 1 hour. The minimum duration for treatment has not been established, but in most trials the drug was given for 14 to 21 days (Haverkos, 1984). The current daily dose recommendation for TMP-SMX is four doses at 6-hour intervals. If there is a suggestion that the drug will not be completely absorbed, it can be given orally (TMP-160 mg and SMX-800 mg) (Sattler et al., 1988). In 1989, aerosolized pentamidine was approved by the FDA for use in prophylaxis against PCP in high-risk individuals infected with HIV (Young et al., 1989). More clinical studies are necessary to judge safety and efficacy, although preliminary reports appear to be positive.

When using the aerosolized pentamidine, the patient

should inhale and exhale through the mouth, and, approximately every minute, the patient should exhale to residual volume and then maximally inhale (Montgomery, 1989). The proper breathing pattern should be used regardless of the patient's position; however, it is best if the patient is sitting, reclining or semireclining. These positions aid in achieving maximum apical alveolar deposition of pentamidine (Montgomery, 1989) because PCP has a tendency to recur in the upper lobes of the lung (Lowery et al., 1988). Extra precaution is warranted when administering aerosolized pentamidine due to the increased incidence of tuberculosis in patients with HIV disease. Patients should be evaluated for TB before treatment and, if appropriate, anti-TB therapy should be initiated (Centers for Disease Control, 1989).

Pulmonary rehabilitation has been shown to be an effective tool for patients with respiratory problems. Patients that are initially diagnosed with PCP or that only have PCP and no other opportunistic infections are living approximately 8 months longer then previously noted. This longevity appears to be linked with the use of azidothymidine (AZT, Retrovir) therapy (Lemp et al., 1990).

According to Gaskell (1975), treatment for the patient with general pneumonia depends on the severity of lobar involvement. Diaphragmatic breathing and localized basal expansion, holding the breath on full inspiration, should be initiated. The patient may be encouraged to cough, but if the lung is still consolidated coughing may not be productive. In this case, vigorous coughing should be discouraged; intermittent positive pressure breathing (IPPB) may be helpful in aiding removal of secretion in severe cases.

Patients with a nonproductive cough may not necessitate chest physical therapy unless other infectious agents coexist with copious production of tenacious secretions. Chest physical therapy has been demonstrated to cause a decreased PaO^2 in acutely ill patients with no sputum or thin mucoid-type sputum (Boudin, 1988); therefore, chest physical therapy (percussion and drainage) may not be indicated. Regimented and vigorous coughing sessions may be as effective as the much more elaborate regimen of postural drainage, deep breathing, vibration and percussion (Boudin, 1988).

The effects of bed rest deconditioning have been well documented (Saltin & Mitchell, 1968). As with other pulmonary disorders, mobility exercises, including bed exercises, may be used to gradually improve endurance of the patient with PCP. More specifically, pulmonary physical therapy may be indicated (Small et al., 1985). During all exercise activities, the importance of diaphragmatic breathing needs to be stressed. More than likely the clinician will have to teach the patient the techniques of proper diaphragmatic breathing before initiating an exercise regimen. Because arterial blood gases are helpful in determining the severity of pulmonary involvement, the therapist should review the patient's medical chart for laboratory results. An increase in alveolar-to-arterial oxygen difference, especially with exercise, is common in patients with PCP (Stover et al., 1985; Stover & Meduri, 1988).

TUBERCULOSIS

Chest radiographs of HIV patients who have pulmonary TB are similar to those of patients with primary TB with hilar or mediastinal adenopathy with or without noncavitating pulmonary infiltrates, located with approximately equal frequency in upper and lower lung fields (Weber et al., 1987). Thus, it is hard to distinguish pulmonary TB from other opportunistic infections, especially PCP, strictly on the basis of radiographs. Clinical symptoms are also similar (Cupples et al., 1989).

A presumptive diagnosis can be made by demonstrating of acid- fast bacilli in stained smears from sputum or other body fluids. On the basis of a positive smear, chemotherapy is justifiably initiated. Standard anti-TB drug regimens, including isoniazid, rifampin, ethambutol hydrochloride, and pyrazinamide, are effective in the treatment of HIV patients with TB (Suderam et al., 1986), although drug therapy may need to be extended beyond the normal nine months (American Thoracic Society, 1983). Within months after initiating drug therapy, the chest radiographs begin to return to normal in these patients despite their immunosuppressed state.

MYCOBACTERIUM AVIUM-INTRACELLULARE

Studies show that the infection *Mycobacterium avium-intracellulare* (MAI), is common in HIV disease (Cohen et al., 1983; Chan et al., 1984; Wong et al., 1985). *Mycobacterium avium* complex is the most common isolated cause of infection among all AIDS patients; however, *Mycobacterium* tuberculosis is more frequent among intravenous drug users and Haitians (Suderam et al., 1986). Noncavitary, nonapical tuberculosis and extrapulmonary disease are commonly cited as well (Centers for Disease Control, 1987).

Sputum cultures for MAI, in contrast to those of primary pulmonary TB, are usually positive, whereas pleural effusions are relatively small and infrequent (Fraser et al., 1979). Patients may have a coexisting pulmonary infection,

Table 8-2
PULMONARY COMPLICATIONS OF HIV

PULMONARY DISEASE	DIAGNOSIS	CLINICAL MANIFESTATION	TREATMENT

Mycobacterium Tuberculosis	—isolation of *M. tuberculosis* by culture
	—acid-fast bacilli
	—chest x-ray: hilar or mediastinal adenopathy
	—extrapulmonary
		—fever
		—lymphadenitis
			Drugs include:
			  isoniazid
			  rifampin
			  pyrazinamide
			  ethambutol
			Breathing exercises

Mycobacterium avium intracellulare (MAI)	—isolation of MAI from sputum or bronchoalveolar lavage —mycobacteremia —neutropenia	Associated with: —wasting syndrome consisting of fever, weight loss and cachexia —chronic diarrhea —progressive anemia —chronic malabsorption syndrome	No drug treatment regimen found ideal to ⇓ mycobacteremia or ⇑ survival (new Rx: clorythromycin) Additional drugs have been used: —ciprofloxacin —rifampin —ethambutol —amikacin —ansamycin Breathing exercises

Cytomegalovirus (CMV)	—(+) CMV culture
	—exudative alveolar inflammatory response that includes:
	  (1) cytotoxic suppressor T-lymphocytes
	  (2) focal to diffuse pneumonitis
	—chest x-ray: similar to PCP
		—similar to interstitial pneumonia
		—shortness of breath
		—dyspnea on exertion
		—dry, nonproductive cough
		—⇑ HR, ⇑ RR
		—hypoxemia
			Drugs:
			  DHPG–gancidozia
			  CPT–same as PCP

Pneumocystis carinii pneumonia	—⇑ alveolar-capillary oxygen gradient
	—respiratory acidosis
	—bilateral diffuse alveolar disease
	—diffuse lymphadenopathy
	—auscultation: dry rates
	—chest x-ray: bilateral interstitial infiltrates in the hilar region
	—Pulmonary Functon Tests:
	⇓ total lung capacity
	⇓ vital capacity
	⇓ single breath diffusing capacity for CO
	⇑ expiratory flow rates
		—progressive dyspnea
		—tachypnea
		—persistent, nonproductive cough
		—fatigue
			Prophylaxis:
			—aerosolized pentamidine
			—AZT
			Regimented and vigorous coughing sessions
			Diaphragmatic Breathing Exercises
			Drugs:
			  pentamidine
			  trimethoprim-sulfa-methoxazole
			  bactrim
			  dapsone
			  septra
			  co-trimoxazole
			
			Under investigation:
			  DFMO
			  trimetrexate
			  clindamycin-primaquin

and extrathoracic TB is commonly presented (Stead et al., 1968). Several experimental drugs are used in treating disseminated disease resulting from MAI and include ansamycin and clofazimine. Patients should be monitored closely after therapy, and, if clinically indicated, mycobacteriologic examinations should be repeated.

Although chest physical therapy is not indicated in the treatment of TB, it may be used in the treatment of associated complications (Gaskell, 1975). Occasionally patients may be diagnosed as having bronchiopneumonia and chest physical therapy (CPT) will have started before the diagnosis of tuberculosis has been made. In this case, CPT should be discontinued once the diagnosis is confirmed. After medical treatment has been initiated with antituberculous drugs, CPT will not spread the disease and it has an important part to play in preventing chest deformity and the loss of respiratory function due to thickening of the pleura and calcification. (Gaskell, 1975). In the case of tuberculous pleural effusion, administration of localized expansion exercises to all areas of involvement and belt exercises are indicated. If severe chest deformity occurs, the patient should lie on the unaffected side with pillows under the thorax in order to expand the ribs on the affected side. This position should be assumed for one half hour four times per day with intermittent expansion exercises reinforced.

PNEUMONIA AND CYTOMEGALOVIRUS

Cytomegalovirus (CMV) may be present as severe pneumonia in the patient infected with HIV. In these patients, CMV infection is second only to PCP as the most common cause of pneumonitis (Farthing et al., 1986). CMV is also associated with hemorrhagic, exudative, alveolar inflammatory response that includes cytotoxic suppressor T lymphocytes (American Thoracic Society, 1983). CMV lesions of the lungs range from focal to diffuse pneumonitis with numerous characteristic intranuclear and intracytoplasmic inclusion cells (Benyesh-Melnick, 1969).

The antiviral drug gancidozia (DHPG) is the drug of choice in the treatment of CMV, although DHPG is only capable of suppressing the progress of the disease (Broder, 1987). At present the disease is incurable. Rehabilitation intervention is similar to that of PCP. Breathing exercises are indicated and postural drainage necessary only if secretions are present.

In summary, the many pulmonary complications in the HIV seropositive patient warrant careful evaluation by the clinician, including analysis of laboratory results, chest x-rays and drug interventions. Compilation of this information will allow the rehabilitation specialist to design appropriate CPT intervention and exercise protocols. Table 8-2 presents an overview of pulmonary complications while Table 8-3 includes a procedure and precaution checklist for use in the rehabilitation setting.

CARDIAC COMPLICATIONS

Cardiac disease is common in patients with AIDS, having been described in 29 to 41 percent of some studies (Lafont et al., 1989; Monsuez et al., 1988). The types of cardiac abnormalities that have been seen in such patients include pericarditis, cardiac tamponade, marantic (thrombotic) endocarditis (Fink et al., 1984), dilated cardiomyopathy (Cohen et al., 1986), *Mycobacterium avium intercellulare* and cryptococcal endocarditis (Lewis et al., 1985)

Focal metastatic involvement of the heart due to KS is a reported clinical manifestation of cardiac involvement in AIDS (Silver et al., 1984; Autran et al., 1986), and other cardiac complications have been associated with other disease processes. In a study by Suderam et al. (1986), uncommon manifestations of TB involving the pericardium were noted. In one patient, these manifestations caused acute cardiac tamponade and, despite several months of anti-TB chemotherapy, subsequent chronic TB draining sinus. Another study (Cohen et al., 1986) reported three cases that demonstrated myocardial compromise secondary to dilated cardiomyopathy resulting from advanced HIV disease. Two studies (Craddock et al., 1987; Miller & Semple, 1987) reported autonomic neuropathy associated with the HIV virus. Miller and Semple's patient presented with an autonomic dysfunction similar to Shy Drager syndrome with orthostatic hypotension, anhidrosis and sphincteric disturbance. Cardiovascular function tests indicated severe sympathetic and parasympathetic nervous system damage.

No studies as yet have defined optimal guidelines for the evaluation and treatment of AIDS-related endocarditis. The roles of myocardial biopsy, immunosuppressive therapy and antiviral therapy remain undefined (Stansell, 1990). Clinical presentations of AIDS-associated dilated cardiomyopathy is similar to that of dilated cardiomyopathy of any cause. The therapy includes afterload reduction and diuretics. As the incidence of KS declines, the incidence of lymphoma rises (high-grade B-cell lymphoma, which may present as stage IV disease). Because most patients with pericarditis have myocardial inflammation, clinicians should become familiar with this AIDS complication and early pericardiocentesis.

To properly evaluate and treat the patient with HIV infection, therapists need to be conscious of pathogenic processes. Therapists should be aware that cardiopulmonary disease due to various opportunistic infections can compli-

Table 8-3
PROCEDURE AND PRECAUTION CHECKLIST

PROCEDURES:

1. Review chart for orders, clinical data, and chest radiograph report and identify opportunistic infection of patient.

2. Wash hands and explain procedure to patient. If a face mask is used, consider discussing this with the patient.

3. Perform breath sounds assessment to identify area to be drained.

4. Properly position patient and proceed with percussion and vibration.

5. Patient should be instructed to relax and take slow deep breaths using diaphragmatic, pursed-lip breathing.

6. Do a series of procedures, including postural drainage, clapping, and vibration of each area to be drained.

7. At the end of each procedure, encourage deep breathing and coughing exercises. Dispose of used tissues in blood and body secretions labeled bag.

8. Assess the effectiveness of these procedures with chest auscultations.

9. Incorporate incentive spirometry into the program and post-treatment breathing regimen.

10. For postural drainage, repositioning the patient several times throughout the day will provide continued efficacy of chest physical therapy.

11. Ongoing consultation with respiratory therapy about appropriate function tests (arterial blood gases, oxygen saturation) facilitates continued monitoring of the patient.

PRECAUTIONS

1. Use proper body mechanics.

2. Avoid chest physical therapy one to two hours after meals. Stop continuous enteral feeding 30 minutes to one hour before treatment.

3. If not contraindicated, encourage a high-fluid intake program for these patients; however, patients should be discouraged from taking large quantities of fluid just before and during treatment.

4. Be overly cautious on the cachectic, debilitated patient. Deviation from proper techniques can cause fractures of the ribs or hemoptysis to occur.

5. Use of masks and gloves is indicated for the therapist when working with patients on respiratory or reverse isolation, including patients with untreated TB or MAI.

cate the clinical course of these patients. Emphasis should be placed on the importance of thorough cardiac evaluation, especially submaximal testing, until more precise studies are completed on the incidence of myocardial disease (see chapter 7).

Fatigue due to lack of cardiac endurance is a common clinical complaint and is used to assess a patient's condition, yet few objective methods have been applied to measuring fatigue. An example for documenting subjective fatigue is described in the Fatigue Survey (Appendix D).

In a study by Johnson et al., (1990), HIV seropositive patients without pulmonary opportunistic infection underwent cardiopulmonary exercise testing, pulmonary function testing, bronchoalveolar lavage, chest roentgenography and gallium scanning. These patients demonstrated a mild tachypnea throughout exercise relative to the controls and had a significant increase in the slope of the heart rate/VO^2 relationship. They concluded that there is a limitation of oxygen delivery to exercising muscles, which may represent occult cardiac disease. Patients in this study did not participate in a regular program to observe effects of conditioning on the cardiovascular system.

The rehabilitation of these patients with occult disease requires consideration for adherence to cardiac rehabilitation protocols. Despite the many diagnosed cases of AIDS, cardiac complications have rarely played a major role in AIDS patient management, but autopsy results demonstrate a high incidence of cardiac disease (Stansell, 1990). Therefore, the clinically silent nature of cardiac complications is an important consideration in the design of an exercise protocol with the symptomatic patient with HIV disease.

INTENSIVE CARE PATIENTS

For the patient with pulmonary complications requiring intensive care, the therapist should be aware of a number of infection control procedures. Due to the potential for considerable environmental contamination from oral and blood secretions, patients with AIDS who are placed on mechanical support ventilators need specific attention. The air expired from the ventilator might disseminate airborne pathogens. The ventilator exhaust needs to be either filtered or vented outside. Patients with HIV disease in an ICU should ideally be placed in a private room with a private nurse. Gowns, masks and protective eyewear are recommended for all health care professionals who come into contact with these patients to prevent conjunctival contamination (Appendix B).

In one study conducted at San Francisco General Hos-

Table 8-4
CASE STUDY

PULMONARY COMPLICATIONS OF A HIV SEROPOSITIVE PATIENT: NP is a 39-year-old patient with HIV infection who was admitted with a history of alcoholism, diarrhea, and progressive dementia (central nervous system encephalopathy). Patient had been on ribavirin and azidothymidine (ZDV or Retrovir). NP also has had recurring episodes of severe herpes zoster that had been controlled by acyclovir.

HOSPITAL COURSE
Patient was admitted February 21, 1989, with a temperature of 102.6 degrees Fahrenheit and blood pressure of 115/85. Blood cultures were obtained, and intravenous fluids were administered. Do Not Resuscitate (DNR) status was explained to the patient's family at the request of the patient.

2-21-89   Chest radiograph showed atelectasis of the left lower lobe and complete collapse of the medial basal segment of the left lower lobe. The right lung was clear. Antibiotics were started (flagyl, or metronidazole, and primaxin). Respiratory therapy consult ordered. Chest physical therapy initiated. Minimal dilation of the intracerebral ventricular system was noted on CT scan of the brain; however, the dilation was increased since the last CT scan on March 17, 1988. Minimal cerebral atrophy was noted.

2-24-89   A cardiology consult and echocardiogram were requested, and a diagnosis of congestive heart failure with pulmonary edema was given. The electrocardiogram demonstrated sinus tachycardia. Intravenous hyperalimentation was halted, and support hose was placed on the patient.

REVIEW OF PULMONARY PHYSICAL THERAPY

2-21-89   Orders were received and evaluation was performed. Respiratory rate (RR) was regular with no shortness of breath, at rest. Pulmonary physical therapy was administered in right side-lying position. The physical therapist taught breathing exercises to NP, which included deep diaphragmatic, pursed-lip breathing and focus on expansion of the left rib cage. The patient was introduced to incentive spirometry.
Functional Status: NP was able to ambulate approximately 50 feet before complaints of shortness of breath (SOB). RHR = 100; post ambulation HR = 152. Bed mobility and transfers were independent.

2-22-89   Bilateral breath sounds were auscultated, and very slight shortness of breath was noted. Pulmonary physical therapy was continued every 3-4 hours.
Functional Status: Continued gait and endurance training with limitation of 50 feet.

2-23-89   Bilateral breath sounds were the same. Pulmonary therapy continued.
Functional Status: Decline in ambulation distance to 20 feet. RHR = 108; postambulation HR = 160. SOB with ADLs transfers if pacing techniques were not used.

2-24-89   Bilateral breath sounds decreased. Pulmonary therapy continued.
Functional Status: SOB with supine -> sit and sit -> stand activites. Ambulation distance ceased. RHR = 118 -> post-bedside commode transfer HR = 174. Energy conservation techniques employed.

2-25-89   Auscultation of the lungs revealed continuous audible rales. The chest radiograph worsened, showing mild cardiomegaly. NP expressed minimal subjective relief from breathing difficulty despite increased urine output from Lasix. Supplemental oxygen at 3 liters was added to the regimen, and physical therapy was continued with focus on a supine bedside regimen.
Functional Status: Focus on pulmonary rehabilitation to meet short-term goal of relieving respiratory distress.

2-26-89   Bilateral breath sounds were decreased throughout the chest. Pulmonary physical therapy resulted in decreased auscultation of rales in the left lower lobe.
Functional Status: Improvement in pulmonary status warranted reestablishment of transfer training with vs monitoring at the bedside.

2-27-89   Chest radiograph now improved. Effusion diminished. Pulmonary physical therapy continued.
Functional Status: As ventilatory status improved, RHR decreased and SOB diminished, a gradual graded exercise program, (initially in supine then sitting) was performed by the patient with therapist carefully monitoring HR and BP. Over the course of one week, NP achieved increased ambulation distance of 100 feet with no SOB.

3-01-89   Atelectasis resolved. NP's overall status improved. Breathing exercises reinforced.
Functional Status: Independent in all transfers, ambulation and ADLs. No respiratory complications noted. NP was instructed in self-monitoring of HR for continuance of endurance retraining.

This case study demonstrates the medical and physical therapy management of an HIV seropositive patient whose functional capacity rapidly deteriorated due to cardiorespiratory complications. Decreased ventilatory capacity was caused in part by congestive heart failure as well as atelectasis. The patient was initially stabilized by medical management and acute care pulmonary physical therapy. Once ventilatory problems were resolved, the patient's functional status continued to improve while in a structured program of pulmonary rehabilitation.

pital, 82 patients with AIDS were admitted to the ICU between March, 1981, and December, 1985. Of these patients, 69 percent died in the hospital; the death rate for patients who required mechanical ventilation because of PCP and respiratory failure was 87 percent (Wachter et al., 1986). In another study conducted at the Clinical Center at the National Institutes of Health (NIH), 216 patients were admitted to the medical ICU between July, 1981, and March, 1987 (Rogers et al., 1989). Of these patients, 77 percent returned to the ward in less that 24 hours. Of the remainder, 85 percent of the patients who required venti-latory support died, as did 67 percent of the patients with respiratory failure who did not require ventilatory support. Only 33 percent of the patients admitted to the ICU for cardiovascular disorders died.

Patients with PCP and respiratory failure continue to have a complicated process. The number of ICU admissions has declined since the time of the San Francisco General Hospital study despite the growing number of cases of AIDS. A survey of physicians at San Francisco General Hospital reports that physicians are aware of this decline and believe that mechanical ventilation is not often indicated under these circumstances. There also has been more discussion of resuscitation between the physicians and patients with AIDS. Recent reports indicate a better survival rate for patients with severe respiratory failure, which suggests that a reevaluation of previous recommendations concerning patients with advanced disease, PCP and acute respiratory failure is necessary (Friedman et al., 1989; Efferen et al., 1989). Table 8-4 is a case study that depicts respiratory decline and medical management for return to function.

SUMMARY

Good pulmonary hygiene is imperative for the HIV patient encountering pulmonary complications. Additional-ly, appropriate breathing exercises can enhance the administration of prophylaxis pentamidine. Given the in-creased survival rate of the patient with PCP, the therapist can assist in enhancing cardiopulmonary status. Problems of ventilation occur in both HIV and non-HIV cardiopulmon-ary disorders and methodology of pulmonary rehabilitation remains the same. Distinctions must be made between simultaneous opportunistic infections listed in Tables 8-1 and 8-2 and others. Guidelines for evaluation and mo-bilization of the patient with cardiorespiratory complica-tions warrant further research. (Chapter 7 further delineates the need for submaximal testing of the symptomatic patient undergoing a rehabilitation program.)

Acknowledgment

The author wishes to acknowledge Bess Kathrins, MS, PT, and Rick Dellagatta, MEd, PT, of Stockton State College for technical assistance in the development of this chapter.

References

American Thoracic Society. (1983). Treatment of tuber-culosis and other mycobacterial Diseases. *American Review of Respiratory Diseases.* 127:790.

Autran, B., Gorin, T., Leibowitch, M., et al. (1986). AIDS in Haitian women with cardiac Kaposi's sarcoma and Whipple's disease. *Lancet.* 1:767.

Benyesh-Melnick, M. (1969). Cytomegaloviruses. In Len-nette, E.H., & Schmidt, N.J. (Eds.): *Diagnostic Proce-dures for Viral and Rickettsial Infections.* New York: Public Health Association.

Boudin, K. (1988). Respiratory implications of AIDS *Cardi-opulmonary Record.* 3:12.

Broder, S. (1987). *AIDS Modern Concepts and Therapeutic Challenges.* New York: Marcel Dekker, Inc.

Cammarosano, C., and Lewis, W. (1985). Cardiac lesions in acquired immune deficiency syndrome. *Journal of Amer-ican College Cardiology.* 5:703.

Centers for Disease Control. (1986). Update: Acquired immunodeficiency syndrome, United States. *Morbidity and Mortality Weekly Report.* 35:757.

Centers for Disease Control. (1987). Diagnosis and man-agement of the mycobacterium infection and disease in persons with human immunodeficiency virus infection. *Annals of Internal Medicine.* 106:254.

Centers for Disease Control. (1989). Tuberculosis and human immunodeficiency virus infection: Recommen-dations of the advisory committee for the elimination of tuberculosis. *Morbidity and Mortality Weekly Report.* 38:236.

Chan, J., McKitrick, J.C., and Klein, R.S. (1984). *Myco-bacterium gordonae* in the acquired immunodeficiency syndrome. *Annals of Internal Medicine.* 100:400.

Cohen, I., Anderson, D., Virmani, R., et al. (1986). Con-gestive cardiomyopathy in association with the acquired immunodeficiency syndrome. *New England Journal of Medicine.* 315:628.

Cohen, R.J., Samoszuk, M.K., Busch, D., et al. (1983). Occult infections with *M. intracellulare* in bone-marrow biopsy specimens from patients with AIDS. *New Eng-land Journal of Medicine.* 308:1475.

Conte, J., Hollander, H., and Golden, J. (1987). Inhaled or reduced-dose intravenous pentamidine for *Pneumocystis carinii* pneumonia. *Annals of Internal Medicine.* 107:495.

Cupples, J.B., Blackie, S.P., and Road, J.D. (1989). Granulomatous *Pneumocystis carinii* pneumonia mimicking tuberculosis. *Archives of Pathological Medicine.* 113:1281.

Craddock, C., Bull, R., Pasvil, G., et al. (1987). Cardiorespiratory arrest and autonomic neuropathy in AIDS. *Lancet.* 2:16.

Douglas, S. (1988). Respiratory care and AIDS: Opportunistic infections of the AIDS patient. *AARC Times.* 12:21.

Efferen, L.S., Nadarajah, D., and Palat, D.S. (1989). Survival following mechanical ventilation for *Pneumocystis carinii* pneumonia in patients with the acquired immunodeficiency syndrome: A different perspective. *The American Journal of Medicine.* 87:401.

Farthing, C.E., Brown, S., Staughton, S., et al. (1986). *A Colour Atlas of AIDS.* London: Wolfe Medical Publications, Ltd.

Fink, L., Reichek, N., and St John-Suttion, M.G. (1984). Cardiac abnormalities in acquired immune deficiency syndrome. *American Journal of Cardiology.* 54:1161.

Fraser, R.G., and Pare, J.A.P. (1979). *Diagnosis of Diseases of the Chest,* vol. 2. Philadelphia: W.B. Saunders.

Friedman, Y., Franklin, C., Rackow, E.C., and Weil, M.H. (1989). Improved survival in patients with AIDS, *Pneumocystis carinii* pneumonia, and severe respiratory failure. *Chest,* 96:862.

Gaskell, D.V. (1975). Pulmonary infection. In Cash, J.E. (Ed.): *Chest, Heart and Vascular Disorders for Physiotherapists..* London: J.B. Lippincott, pp. 134-140.

Haverkos, H.W. (1984). Assessment of therapy of *Pneumocystis carinii* pneumonia. *American Journal of Medicine.* 76:501.

Hollander, H., Golden, J., and Stulberg, M. (1986). Recurrent AIDS-. related *Pneumocystis carinii* pneumonia (PCP); frequency, outcome and prevention. In *Program and Abstracts of the International Conference on AIDS. Paris: L'Association pour la Recherche sur les fedicits Immunitares Viro-Induits.* 51:7.

Johnson, J.E., Anders, G.T., Blanton, H.M., et al. (1990). Exercise dysfunction in patients seropositive for the human immunodeficiency virus. *American Review of Respiratory Disorder.* 141:618.

Kovacs, J.A., and Masur, H. (1989). Prophylaxis of *Pneumocystis carinii* pneumonia: An update. *The Journal of Infectious Diseases.* 160(5):882.

Lafont, A., Marche, C., Wolff, M., et al. (1989). Myocarditis in acquired immunodeficiency syndrome (AIDS): Etiology and prognosis (abstract). *Journal of American College of Cardiology.* 11:196A.

Lemp, G.F., Payne, S.F., Neal, D., et al. (1990). Survival trend for patients with AIDS. *Journal of the American Medical Association.* 263:402.

Leoung, G.S., Mills, J., Hopewell, P.C., et al. (1986). Dapsone trimethoprim for *Pneumocystis carinii* pneumonia in the acquired immunodeficiency syndrome. *Annals of Internal Medicine.* 107:45.

Lewis, W., Lipsick, J., and Cammarosano, C. (1985). Cryptococcal myocarditis in acquired immune deficiency syndrome. *American Journal of Cardiology.* 55:1240.

Lowery, S., Fallat, R., Feigal, D.W., et al. (1988). Changing patterns of pneumocystis carinii pneumonia on pentamidine aerosol prophylaxis. Presented at the Fourth International Conference on AIDS. Stockholm, Sweden.

Miller, R.F., and Semple, S.J.G. (1987). Autonomic neuropathy in AIDS. *Lancet.* 2:343.

Monsuez, J.J., Kinney, E.L., Vittecog, D., et al. (1988). AIDS heart disease: Results in 85 patients (Abstract). *Journal of American College of Cardiology.* 11:195A.

Montgomery, A.B. (1989). *Pneumocystis carinii* pneumonia in patients with the acquired immunodeficiency syndrome: Pathophysiology, therapy and prevention. *Seminars in Respiratory Infection.* 4:102.

Pedersen, C., Lundgren, J.D., Nielsen, T., and Andersen, W.H. (1989). The outcome of *Pneumocystis carinii* pneumonia in Danish patients with AIDS. *Scandinavian Journal of Infectious Diseases.* 21:375.

Rogers, P.L., Lane, H.C., Henderson, D.K., et al. (1989). Admission of AIDS patients to a medical intensive care unit: Causes and outcomes. *Critical Care Medicine.* 17:113.

Saltin, S., and Mitchell, J. (1968). Response to exercise after bedrest and after training. *Circulation.* 38 (Supplement VII).

Sattler, F.R., Cowan, R., Nielson, D.M., et al. (1988). Trimethoprim-sulfamethoxazole compared with pentamidine for treatment of *Pneumocystis carinii* pneumonia in the acquired immunodeficiency syndrome. *Annals of Internal Medicine.* 109:280.

Silver, M.A., Macher, A.M., Reichert, C.M., et al. (1984). Cardiac involvement by Kaposi's sarcoma in acquired immune deficiency syndrome (AIDS). *American Journal of Cardiology.* 53:983.

Small, C., Harris, C., Friedland G., and Klein, R. (1985). The treatment of *Pneumocystis carinii* pneumonia in the acquired immunodeficiency syndrome. *Archives of Internal Medicine.* 145:837.

Stansell, J.D. (1990). Cardiac, endocrine and renal complications of HIV infection. In Sande, M.A. and Voiberding, P.A. (Eds.): *Medical Management of AIDS* (pp. 195-206). Philadelphia: W.B. Saunders.

Stead, W.W., Kerby, G.R., Schleuter, D.P., and Jordahl, C.W. (1968). The clinical spectrum of primary tuberculosis in adults: Confusion with reinfection in the patho-genesis of chronic tuberculosis. *Annals of Internal Medicine.* 68:731.

Stover, D.E., White, D.A., Romano, P.A., et al. (1985). Spectrum of pulmonary disease associated with acquired immune deficiency syndrome. *American Journal of Medicine.* 78:429.

Stover, D.E., and Meduri, G.U. (1988). Pulmonary function tests. In White, D.A., and Stover, D.E. (Eds.): *Clinics in Chest Medicine.* 9:473.

Suderam, G., McDonald, R., Maniatis, T., et al. (1986). Tuberculosis as a manifestation of the acquired immu-nodeficiency syndrome (AIDS). *Journal of the American Medical Association.* 256:362.

Wachter, R., Luce, J., Turner, J., et al. (1986). Intensive care of patients with the acquired immunodeficiency syn-drome. *American Review of Respiratory Diseases.* 134:189.

Weber, A.L., Bird, K.T., and Janower, M.L. (1987). Primary tuberculosis in childhood with particular emphasis on the changes affecting tracheobronchial tree. *American Journal of Respiration.* 103:123.

Wharton, M., Coleman, D.L., Fitz, G., et al. (1984). Prospective randomized trial of trimethoprim-sulfamethoxazole versus pentamidine for *Pneumocystis carinii* pneumonia in the acquired immunodeficiency syndrome. *American Review of Respiratory Diseases.* 129:188A.

Wong, B., Edwards, F.F., Kiehn, T.E., et al. (1985). Continuous high-grade *Mycobacterium avium-intracellu-lare* bacteremia in patients with the acquired immunode-ficiency syndrome. *American Journal of Medicine.* 78:35.

Young, F.E., Nightingale, S.L., Cooper, E.C., and Trapnell, C.B. (1989). Aerosolized pentamidine approved for HIV-infected individuals at high risk for *Pneumocystis carinii* pneumonia. *Archives of Internal Medicine.* 149:2412.

9

Rehabilitation Perspectives for Neurologic Complications of HIV

Eugenie A.M.T. Obbens, MD, PhD
Mary Lou Galantino, MS, PT

To be poised against fatality, to meet adverse condition gracefully is more than simply endurance, it is an act of aggression, a positive triumph.
—Thomas Mann

INTRODUCTION

Neurologic dysfunction occurs frequently in patients with HIV infection. In adult patients with AIDS, the incidence ranges from 23 to 65 percent (Snider et al., 1983; Levy et al., 1985) and as high as 80 percent in some autopsy studies (Anders, et al., 1984; Petito, et al., 1986). In children with AIDS, neurologic dysfunction, including developmental delay, is reported to be as high as 90 percent (Belman et al., 1988). Neurologic dysfunction may be the presenting symptom of AIDS, as was seen in 10 percent of all AIDS cases reviewed retrospectively at the University of California at San Francisco (Levy et al., 1985). Damage of nervous tissue may be caused by HIV itself, by opportunistic infections in the nervous system, by autoimmune reactions or by specific tumors such as cerebral lymphoma. Signs and symptoms are varied and range from a mild sensory polyneuropathy to seizures, hemiparesis, paraplegia and dementia and may thus contribute to major disability for the patient.

OPPORTUNISTIC INFECTIONS

The impaired cellular immunity caused by HIV infection makes patients prone to opportunistic infections, including infections of the CNS. Most of these CNS infections are either fungal or viral, and bacterial infections in the CNS are much less common in these patients. The diagnosis of the offending pathogen is not always easy to make, especially in debilitated patients in whom a brain biopsy is contraindicated. A complicating factor is the occurrence of more than one pathogen, either in the same or in different lesions, in some patients with intracranial infections.

Cerebral Toxoplasmosis

Caused by *Toxoplasma gondii*, toxoplasmosis is the most common intracranial infection, with an incidence of 13 to 28 percent in all patients with AIDS (Navia et al., 1986a; Levy et al., 1988). The infection is thought to be caused by reactivation of dormant *Toxoplasma* cysts, which then produce inflammatory and necrotic abscesses. Signs and symptoms depend on the location and the mass effect of the abscesses. Focal deficits such as hemiparesis, ataxia, aphasia or seizures are very common, and are present in 73 to 89 percent of patients diagnosed with cerebral toxoplasmosis (Navia et al., 1986b; Levy et al., 1988). Other symptoms include severe headache and changes in mental status, such as confusion and lethargy. Meningeal signs are absent, but patients may have a fever. On computed tomography (CT) scans the lesions are best visualized with contrast enhancement. The most common appearance is of multiple ring-enhancing lesions in the cerebral hemispheres, although occasionally the lesions do not enhance or are not visualized at all. Magnetic resonance imaging (MRI) scans appear to be more sensitive in identifying disseminated abscesses. A more definitive diagnosis is made through an open brain biopsy, especially with immunoperoxidase tissue staining. This test is often not performed, however, because of the potential morbidity in these already ill and immunocompromised patients. Cerebrospinal fluid (CSF) abnormalities are usually nonspecific, often with a mild to moderate increase in CSF protein and a mild pleocytosis. In the serum, IgG or IgM antibodies may be detected against *T. gondii*, as are complement fixation titers, but they are not always helpful (Navia et al., 1986c).

Cerebral toxoplasmosis is a potentially curable infection, especially when treatment is started early, and occasionally treatment is warranted when the diagnosis is highly suspected but not proven. The recommended treatment is a combination of pyrimethamine and sulfonamides, which in one review resulted in a response rate of 82 percent (Levy et al., 1988). As relapses are not uncommon, patients are often continued on pyrimethamine after an initial response. With adequate treatment, death directly attributed to toxoplasmosis is rare.

Cerebral Lymphoma

Second to toxoplasmosis, cerebral lymphoma is the most common cause of intracranial mass lesions, accounting for five percent of all neurologic complications and 20 percent of mass lesions in AIDS patients (Marks et al., 1989). This is in contrast to the normal population, where cerebral lymphoma is quite uncommon, and seen mainly in older patients. Although patients usually have overwhelming systemic disease at the time of diagnosis, it is not unusual to develop neurologic symptoms before the diagnosis of AIDS is made.

The systemic illness may mask the initial neurologic symptoms of memory loss, confusion and lethargy. Other symptoms include headache, hemiparesis and seizures (Gill et al., 1985; So et al., 1986).

The intracranial tumor is best visualized on CT scan or MRI. One or more contrast-enhancing mass lesions are the usual CT picture, and MRI may show a few additional lesions not detected by CT scanning. If there is no evidence of increased intracranial pressure clinically or radiographically, a lumbar puncture can be performed. CSF often shows nonspecific abnormalities and occasionally some malignant or atypical cells. If the diagnosis is in doubt, a brain biopsy will almost certainly yield the diagnosis of a large B-cell lymphoma (Marks et al., 1989). At autopsy the diagnosis is always multifocal, sometimes with diffuse infiltration throughout the brain (So et al., 1986).

Patients succumb either from progressive neurologic disease or from coexisting systemic infections. Whole brain irradiation may cause tumor regression but may not increase survival time.

Cryptococcal Meningitis

Cryptococcus neoformans is the most common cause of fungal infection in the central nervous system, occurring in about five percent of all AIDS patients according to data reported to the Centers for Disease Control. As this infection is usually limited to the meninges, the presenting symptoms are those of a subacute meningitis, including headache, nausea, neck stiffness and altered level of consciousness (Kovacs et al., 1985). The diagnosis is made by demonstrating the presence of *C. neoformans* in the CSF. Blood cultures are often positive for *C. neoformans*, but CT and MRI scans are usually normal. The meningitis is treated with antifungal medication, either intravenous amphotericin B alone or in combination with oral flucytosine. This six week treatment regimen, followed by maintenance therapy, is often poorly tolerated. If the patient responds to treatment, the relapse rate is high, and complete resolution of the disease is unusual.

Progressive Multifocal Leukoencephalopathy (PML)

PML is an unusual demyelinating disease in the brain caused by papovavirus. This virus is present in a dormant state in most normal people and may become reactivated in patients with a depressed immune status. Reactivation occurs in less than one percent of all patients with AIDS. The illness presents with gradually progressive signs and symptoms of mental dysfunction, hemiparesis, aphasia, ataxia, cortical blindness and other focal deficits, leading to death within a few months. The diagnosis is suggested by CT scan, which may show nonenhancing areas of low density in the white matter, most often that of the cerebral hemispheres. These lesions do not appear to cause edema or mass effect (Krupp et al., 1985). The definitive diagnosis is usually made at autopsy, where areas of myelin loss are surrounded by large oligodendrocytes with intranuclear inclusion bodies. Treatment for PML includes ARA-C and antiviral drugs, and occasional spontaneous clinical improvement has been reported (Berger & Mucke, 1988).

Viral Encephalitis

The most common viruses causing CNS infection in this patient population are herpes simplex, herpes zoster and CMV. They have all been implicated as the causative agent of a viral encephalitis. Focal findings include aphasia, seizures, hemiparesis, diffuse evidence of infection and an intracranial mass, with fever and headache as the prominent symptoms. Herpes simplex virus type I (HSV) usually leads to a hemorrhagic encephalitis, with the medial temporal lobes and inferior frontal lobes most often involved. A bloody spinal fluid in these patients is highly suspicious for HSV encephalitis, as is a hemorrhagic lesion on CT scan. A biopsy of the hemorrhagic lesion is needed for a definitive diagnosis. Herpes simplex encephalitis used to carry a high morbidity and mortality, but both have lessened considerably with the introduction of antiviral drugs such as Ara-A and acyclovir. A more mild and diffuse form of HSV encephalitis has been seen in AIDS patients as well (Levy et al., 1985). HZV occurs in 5 to 10 percent of all patients with HIV infection. Manifesting as either dermatomal or disseminated skin lesions, HZV may develop early on in the asymptomatic stage of the disease, long before other opportunistic infections start to occur. Ten percent of these patients with HZV infection will develop a CNS infection, notably a meningoencephalitis. Other complications caused by HZV include transverse myelitis; herpes zoster ophthalmicus with vasculitis and contralateral hemiparesis; and blindness (Graham & Bredesen, 1988). Encephalitis caused by CMV appears to be less specific and uniform in presentation and may even be clinically asymptomatic, as suggested at autopsy (Morgello et al., 1987). CMV may give rise to a retinitis, a cerebral vasculitis or a radiculomyelitis. The diagnosis is not easy to make, as viral cultures of CSF are often negative. A clinical and radiographic response to acyclovir or analog medication has been reported (Grafe & Wiley, 1989).

AIDS DEMENTIA COMPLEX

Of all the neurologic complications of AIDS, dementia presumably caused by HIV infection of the brain is the most common one and is a major clinical problem. It has been reported under several names, including HIV encephalitis and subacute encephalopathy. The term AIDS dementia complex (ADC) has remained in vogue because it describes a syndrome of progressive cognitive loss in combination with motor and behavioral dysfunction in HIV-infected patients. Up to 25 percent of HIV patients will be diagnosed with this progressive dementia during life (Navia, Cho et al., 1986; McArthur, 1987). The first symptoms are often subtle, with apathy, social withdrawal, and some difficulty in concentration and in solving complex mental tasks. On examination there is a slowness in verbal and motor responses, especially in repetitive movements, with a deterioration in handwriting, and an unsteady gait. Over several weeks to months there is a steady progression of symptoms until the patient is bedridden and mute, often with para-

paresis and urinary and fecal incontinence (see Chapter 11). It is as yet unclear what exactly causes the extensive neurologic dysfunction, as the pathology is often limited to focal areas of macrophages and multinucleated cells (Petito et al., 1986; Navia, Jordan et al., 1986). It is well known that HIV especially interacts with T-helper lymphocytes by binding to the CD4 molecules on these cells. CD4 expression is also found on neurons and glial cells, the supportive cells in the nervous system, which suggest that these cells also serve as HIV receptors. Macrophages are large phagocytic or "scavenger" cells, aimed at clearing up debris. Multinucleated giant cells are HIV-infected macrophages fused together, probably through action of HIV, and are specific for HIV infection of the brain. It is unlikely that the HIV infection, restricted to these multinucleated cells, is directly responsible for the neurologic abnormalities. A physiologic alteration brought about by a secreted substance altered by HIV and responsible for disturbing normal brain function has been considered (Price et al., 1988).

An aseptic meningitis at the time of seroconversion, with HIV identified in the CSF, points to an early infection of the leptomeninges, if not the CNS in general (Ho et al., 1985). Even in the early stages of the dementia, cerebral atrophy and ventricular enlargement can be seen on a CT scan, indicating a degenerative process already ongoing for at least several weeks. An MRI scan occasionally will reveal abnormalities in the cerebral white matter, either diffuse or patchy. The dementia may be the first sign of HIV infection, and progression of this syndrome always seems to be associated with severe immunosuppression (Price et al., 1988).

Treatment has been directed toward attacking the virus with antiviral drugs that penetrate the blood-brain barrier and toward restoring the immune system with drugs such as AZT. Some improvement of cognition has been reported with AZT, but more studies are needed to evaluate its efficacy (Schmitt et al., 1988).

VACUOLAR MYELOPATHY

In the spinal cord, a pathologic abnormality specific to AIDS patients has been encountered in association with a subacute paraparesis. The presenting symptoms are weakness, spasticity and ataxia, which are steadily progressive over several weeks to months. Other findings are sensory and reflex changes, urinary and fecal incontinence, and often dementia. Such a myelopathy appears to occur often, and in autopsy studies has been encountered in 22 to 31 percent of AIDS cases (Grafe & Wiley, 1989; Petito et al., 1985). However, not all patients will have been symptomatic during life, especially when autopsy findings are mild. Microscopically, the most striking feature is a spongy vacuolization of the white matter, especially in the lateral and posterior columns of the thoracic spinal cord. The vacuolization is due to the presence of lipid-laden macrophages (Petito et al., 1985). The myelopathy does not appear to be caused by HIV, CMV or any other infectious agent. An autoimmune reaction has been suggested as a possible etiology. No treatment has been reported to halt or reverse the disease progression.

PERIPHERAL NEUROPATHY

The peripheral nerves may be affected in different ways and in different stages of the disease. (see Table 10-1, Chapter 10) The most common peripheral neuropathy, distal symmetric polyneuropathy (DSPN), occurs in 10 to 30 percent of patients with full-blown AIDS (Cornblath & McArthur, 1988). The neuropathy is characterized by a symmetric distal sensory loss and often painful dysesthesias and is usually associated with weight loss and with a higher incidence of dementia. In a prospective study involving 40 patients with AIDS, 13 (35 percent) had clinical evidence of a peripheral neuropathy (So et al., 1988). Most cases were mild, with findings limited to distal numbness and tingling, decreased ankle jerks and vibratory sensation in the toes. Three of the 13 patients had burning pain distally. Neuropathy also does not seem to respond to any specific drug treatment, although tricyclic antidepressants can alleviate the pain (Cornblath et al., 1988) (see Chapter 10).

In asymptomatic patients with HIV infection, an inflammatory demyelinating polyneuropathy (IDP) has been encountered on occasion. Here, the more striking neurologic feature is progressive weakness. Loss of deep tendon reflexes is a uniform finding, whereas sensory loss, when present, is usually mild. Patients eventually all improve, either spontaneously or with treatment, but they may relapse in between. In one study, where 118 patients were diagnosed with IDP over four years, nine patients (8 percent) were HIV positive, a diagnosis made in every instance after the neuropathy was manifested (Cornblath et al., 1987). As this neuropathy appears to have an underlying autoimmune cause, patients may benefit from treatment with corticosteroids or plasmapheresis.

Another disorder causing a lower motor neuron weakness in AIDS patients is an inflammatory polyradiculopathy. Here, the nerve roots of the cauda equina are inflamed, presumably due to CMV infection, resulting in distal weakness, numbness and tingling, and incontinence. These symptoms can progress to paraplegia and areflexia and may involve the upper extremities as well. No treatment has been known to affect the course of the disease. (Eidelberg et al., 1986; Miller et al., 1988).

Isolated cranial neuropathies may develop in patients with polyneuropathy, especially the trigeminal and the facial nerve, resulting in facial numbness or weakness. A mononeuropathy, such as a peroneal nerve palsy leading to footdrop or other compression neuropathies, are not uncommon in patients with a marked weight loss.

Recently there have been several reports of autonomic dysfunction in patients with HIV infection. This dysfunction is often not clinically manifested, especially in the early stages of infection, and only brought about by specific testing of sympathetic and parasympathetic functions, such as measuring orthostatic blood pressure, heart rate, respiration and skin responses. The relationship between autonomic and peripheral neuropathy is controversial (Cohen & Laudenslager, 1989; Zuckerman & Halperin, 1989), although patients with severe autonomic neuropathy usually exhibit other neurologic manifestations as well (Freeman et al., 1989).

HIV-ASSOCIATED MYOPATHY

A less common cause of weakness, HIV-associated myopathy presents with a progressive painless weakness in the proximal limb muscles. The weakness is symmetric, and often involve the muscles of the face and neck. Some patients also have signs and symptoms of peripheral neuropathy. The myopathy may occur in HIV-infected patients in every stage of illness (Simpson & Bender, 1988). The diagnosis can be made electrophysiologically with features of abnormal spontaneous activity and small polyphasic motor units on needle electromyography (EMG) (Gonzales et al., 1988). Muscle biopsies have shown necrosis of muscle fibers with and without inflammatory infiltrates. No evidence has been found of direct HIV infection of the muscle, and the underlying etiology has not been determined. The fact that patients improve on corticosteroids or plasmapheresis, however, points to an underlying autoimmune defect.

Recently, myopathy characterized by proximal muscle weakness and tenderness with mild elevation of creatine phosphokinase has been described in association with AZT therapy muscle biopsy showed widespread focal necrosis with little inflammation and recovery after discontinuation of AZT (Besser et al., 1988). A necrotizing myopathy has also been reported seemingly related to AZT (Gorard et al., 1988). Although it appears that AZT-induced myopathy is

Table 9-1a
SUMMARY OF NERVOUS SYSTEM DISORDERS
ASSOCIATED WITH HIV

OPPORTUNISTIC INFECTION	SIGNS AND SYMPTOMS	DIAGNOSIS	TREATMENT
1. Cerebral lymphoma	Memory loss Confusion Lethargy Headache Hemiparesis Seizures	CT/MRI: —contrast enhancing lesions CSF: —nonspecific abnormalities —some malignant or atypical cells	Drug: —whole brain XRT —chemotherapy Rehabilitation: —assistive device —stroke rehabilitation —transfer/gait training —cognitive retraining —ADL
2. Cerebral toxoplasmosis	Focal deficits: hemiparesis ataxia aphasia seizures severe headaches confusion lethargy fever	CT: —multiple ring enhancing lesions MRI: —disseminated abscesses CSF: —mild increase in CSF protein —mild pleocytosis Serum: —IgG or IgM —antibodies against *T. gondii* —meningeal signs are absent	Drug: —pyrimethamine sulfonamides Rehabilitation: 1. Management of headaches —modalities —manual therapies 2. Implementation of assistive devices; eg. —MAFO —glenohumeral support to prevent subluxation 3. Neurologic retraining 4. Transfer/gait training 5. Cognitive retraining
3. Cryptococcal meningitis	Headache Nausea Neck Stiffness Altered level of consciousness	CSF: —Presence of *c. neoformans* SERUM: —(+) for *c. neoformans* CT: —normal	Drug: 1. Antifungal medication —amphotericin B —oral flucytosine Rehabilitation: —pain management —appropriate neurologic and cognitive retaining

continued...

rare, the impact of this complication awaits further experience with long-term therapy.

REHABILITATION OF THE HIV PATIENT

As reviewed, HIV presents clinical problems, which may lend to an eclectic blend of neurorehabilitation strategies. The clinician may find it appropriate to incorporate various techniques from several strategies for treatment purposes.

Neuromuscular disturbances may first appear as movement disorders. Subtleties of altered movement can be detected early in assessment and during subsequent treatment phases. The HIV Evaluation Form (Appendix C) includes a neurologic evaluation and should be performed to delineate:
1. level of lesion
2. neuromuscular deficits
3. need for assistive devices
4. ADL
5. functional abilities.
A team approach is indicated with each allied health

Table 9-1a (continued)
SUMMARY OF NERVOUS SYSTEM DISORDERS
ASSOCIATED WITH HIV

OPPORTUNISTIC INFECTION	SIGNS AND SYMPTOMS	DIAGNOSIS	TREATMENT
4. Cytomegalovirus CMV	Retinitis cerebral vasculitis radiculo myelitis	CSF: (-) viral cultures	Drug: DHPG Rehabilitation: ADL NDT
5. Herpes Simplex Virus type I (HSV)	Hemorrhagic encephalitis Focal findings: —aphasia —seizures —hemiparesis	CT scan: Hemorrhagic lesion medical temporal lobes and inferior frontal lobes most often involved CSF: bloody	Drug: ARA-A Acyclovir rehabilitation: NDT
6. Herpes Zoster Infection (HZV)	Dermatomal or disseminated skin lesions Occasionally CNS: meningoencephalitis transverse myelitis herpes zoster ophthalmicus with vasculitis and contralateral hemiparesis blindness	Skin lesions	Drug: Acyclovir Rehabilitation: pain management spinal cord/stroke rehabilitation
7. Progressive Multifocal Leukoencephalopathy (PML)	Mental dysfunction Hemiparesis Aphasia Ataxia Cortical blindness	CT: —Nonenhancing areas of low density in the white matter (ie. cerebral hemispheres) —Areas of myelin loss surrounded by large oligodendrocytes with intranuclear inclusion bodies	Drug: —Nonspecific Rehabilitation: —Neurologic retraining —Retraining using visual stimulation focused at the edges of the field deficit

profession lending expertise in assessment, which provides the framework for the development of appropriate treatment programs. The importance of assessment tools is to assist the clinician in establishing goals that are achieved by quality, cost effective treatment. The establishment of goals should be realistic for the long and short term. Time frames for the potential actualization of the goals should be stated (Hopp & Rogers, 1989).

Evaluation of appropriate assistive devices should take into consideration the following:

1. immediate need to prevent subluxation of a joint

2. use of practical lower extremity orthoses to achieve functional ambulation (Chapter 18)

3. utilization of assistive device to compensate for balance

and coordination problems to facilitate more efficient and safe movement

4. appropriate positioning to maintain skin integrity

5. energy conservation techniques, particularly for progressive disease

6. family training (Chapter 18).

Given the ravages of CNS/PNS complications throughout HIV infection, the therapist may note vacillation in tone, muscle strength and functional abilities. Therefore, prudent use of extensive equipment throughout rehabilitation is warranted (Galantino et al., 1990).

Generally, treatment for the aforementioned nervous system disorders associated with HIV can include drug intervention and neuromuscular retraining (Table 9-1a,b).

Table 9-1b
SUMMARY OF NERVOUS SYSTEM DISORDERS
ASSOCIATED WITH HIV

PATHOLOGY	SIGNS AND SYMPTOMS	DIAGNOSIS	TREATMENT
1. AIDS Dementia Complex (ADC) HIV encephalitis Subacute encephalopathy	Progressive cognitive loss Motor and behavioral dysfunction Apathy Social withdrawal Deterioration in handwriting Unsteady gait	Pathology: focal areas of macrophages and multi-nucleated cells —CD4 expression is found on neurons and glial cells —Multinucleated giant cells are HIV infected macrophages fused together —Aseptic meningitis at time of seroconversion early infection of leptomeninges CT: cerebral atrophy ventricular enlargement MRI: abnormalities in cerebral white matter (diffuse or patchy)	Rehabilitation: —Neurobehavioral retraining —Cognitive retraining —Speech Therapy
2. Myopathy	Proximal muscle weakness	—Polymyositis —Elevated creatine kinase —Inflammatory infiltrates on muscle biopsy —Cause (a) direct HIV invasion in the muscle fibers (b) immune mediated mechanisms	Drug: Corticosteroids Rehabilitation

continued. . .

As in other disorders requiring rehabilitation, the goal of functional restoration remains paramount. Function may be assessed globally by ADL and focally by analysis of sequential developmental movement patterns. Problems of function are subdivided into problems of sensation, strength, muscle tone, posture and coordination as they contribute to the loss of functional movements (see Chapter 5). Problems such as perception of fatigue, pain, depression and anxiety are assessed in and of themselves as problems and as they effect the global problem of dysfunction (see Chapters 8, 10 and 11, respectively).

Swallowing disorders are common among patients with various CNS infections. A CNS lymphoma may produce right-sided hemiparesis and difficulty with speech formulation (ie. aphasia, facial weakness). Furthermore, hypopharyngeal and laryngeal problems may be due to KS and/or viral infections in the oral cavity. These infections may progress to airway obstruction (Flower & Sooy, 1987). Hoarseness can occur secondary to chronic cough and inflammation from candidiasis. Recurrent nerve paralysis may also be observed (Patow et al., 1984). A qualified physical therapist, occupational therapist or speech pathologist can evaluate through an oral motor examination, establish the basis of a communication disorder and implement therapeutic techniques (Table 9-2). Various tools can assess an individual's speech to identify needs in order to enhance communication.

Lesions of the visual cortex secondary to PML may cause cortical blindness and require ADL retraining. Opportunistic infections (ie. CMV retinitis) can produce field deficits. Thus visual stimulation programs may also be incorporated into the rehabilitation regimen. When cognitive deficits are

Table 9-1b (continued)
SUMMARY OF NERVOUS SYSTEM DISORDERS
ASSOCIATED WITH HIV

PATHOLOGY	SIGNS AND SYMPTOMS	DIAGNOSIS	TREATMENT
3. Peripheral neuropathy	6 types of PN (see Table 10-1)	—Acute demyelinating inflammatory sensorimotor polyradiculopathy —Chronic demyelinating polyneuropathy —Mononeuritis multiplex —Distal axonopathy —Progressive inflammatory polyradiculopathy —Sensory ataxic neuropathy	Drug: Tricyclic antidepressant Anticonvulsant Non-narcotic and narcotic analgesics Rehabilitation: —use of orthoses/braces and assistive devices when appropriate —pain management —PT/OT
4. Polymyositis	Subacute proximal weakness	—Increased creatine kinase —Abnormal EMG —Membrane irritability —Biopsy: fiber necrosis, variable degrees of inflammatory cell infiltration —May be no evidence of virus in muscle	Drug: Immunosuppressants Rehabilitation: Therapeutic exercise with proximal focus
5. Vacuolar myelopathy	—Weakness —Spasticity ataxia —Urinary and fecal incontinence —may be accompanied by dementia	Sensory changes reflex changes Pathology: vacuolization of the white matter (esp. the lateral and posterior columns of the thoracic spinal cord) Lipid-laden macrophages cause: autoimmune process	Drugs: Antivirals Rehabilitaion: —PT/OT —bowel/bladder program —functional activities/ADL

apparent, further neuropsychiatric testing may be helpful in achieving established goals (see Chapter 11). However, practical application in cognitive retraining requires consistency within the entire rehabilitation team. Additionally, care givers need to be instructed in safe and effective management of the neurologically impaired individual in the home (see Chapter 18). Although HIV presents the patient with a plethora of clinical and functional problems, the therapist has numerous management techniques to achieve therapeutic goals. Neurophysiologic techniques using sensory input, facilitation, inhibition and reflexic movement patterns have been used for decades in the rehabilitation of hemiparesis, spinal cord trauma and other degenerative neurologic diseases. The treatment principles of Bobath, Brunnstrom, Knott and Voss, and Rood supplement the earlier works of Sherrington, Hellebrandt, McGraw and Gessell, Fay, and others. These authors offer the clinician a variety of methods for the delivery of therapeutic exercise (NUSTEP, 1967). More recently, advances in the studies of motor control have led to the Motor Relearning Program (Carr and Shepherd) as well as other motor learning based concepts.

As with other exercise protocols, these neurophysiologic methods can be modified to accomplish goals such as increasing tone, increasing proprioceptive awareness, increasing coordination and endurance, and improving move-

Table 9-2
THERAPY TECHNIQUES FOR SWALLOWING PROBLEMS

SWALLOWING DISTURBANCE	THERAPY
PHYSIOLOGIC	
Oral Stage of the Swallow	
Reduction in lip closure	Lip exercise
Reduction in cheek tesion	Posture (tilt toward stronger side)
	Pressure on weaker side
Reduction in tongue elevation	Tongue exercise
	Position food posteriorly
	Prosthesis
	Posture (tilt head backward)
Reduced tongue lateralization, anterior to posterior movement	Prosthesis
	Tongue exercises
	Position food posteriorly
	Posture (tilt head backward)
Reflex	
Delayed or absent reflex	Thermal stimulation
	Posture (tilt head forward)
Pharyngeal Stage of the Swallow	
Reduced pharyngeal peristalsis	Alternate liquid/solid swallows
Pharyngeal hemiparesis	Posture (tilt toward stronger side, turn toward weaker side)
Reduced laryngeal elevation	Supraglottic swallow
Reduced laryngeal closure	Adduction exercise
	Supraglottic swallow
Cricopharyngeal hypertonicity	Myotomy
ANATOMIC	
Tongue scarring	Surgical release
	Position of food
Cervical osteophyte	Surgical removal
	Diet change
Scar tissue on pharyngeal wall	Posture
Scar tissue at base of tongue	Surgical removal
Tracheoesophageal fistula	Surgical closure
Zenker's diverticulum	Surgical removal

Printed with permission. Logemann, T.A. (1983) Therapy techniques of swallowing disorders. In Mathews (Ed.): Evaluation and Treatment of Swallowing Disorders (pp. 140) Austin, TX: Austin Pro-Ed.

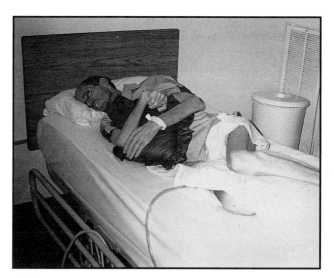

Figure 9-1a. Proprioceptive stimulation. David is placed in side-lying position to prevent contractures, with weight bearing on involved side. This maintains functional active and passive mobility.

ment efficiency. These techniques allow the clinician to accomplish any or all of the preceding goals by varying the parameters of frequency, intensity, and duration of training. An optimal level of input and feedback from therapist to patient stems from the manual contact required by these techniques. In treating a multitude of neurologic disorders caused by HIV opportunistic infections, a diverse selection of exercises, drills and techniques may be well founded. Proprioceptive neuromuscular facilitation (PNF) rhythmic stabilization, when used to train for pelvic stability and coordination, may foster better balance and transfer skills (Knott & Voss, 1986). The flexor/extensor synergies of Brunnstrom (1970) may be used to encourage reach and pull activities. The pivot-prone position denoted by Rood (NUSTEP,1967) can be used to encourage rolling and bed mobility. When choosing a technique, the concept of specificity of training should be viewed as the "thread" that ties the program together.

The following discussion describes the cohesiveness of therapy. David is a 34-year-old hospice patient diagnosed with ADC and acute HIV-related encephalitis. His past medical history is significant for cerebral palsy; however, this condition did not compromise his functional abilities before the diagnosis of infection. Slight right upper extremity involvement at the wrist and hand were noted with excessive activities, but David was independent in all ADL and ambulation. As the ADC and HIV disease advanced, increased tone was noted with exacerbation of right upper extremity flexion synergy. Difficulty with swallowing, transfers and ADL were also observed. Focus on rehabilitation to maintain patient independence

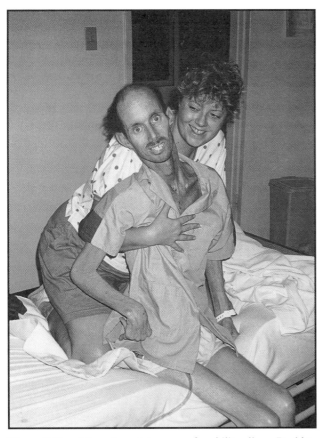

Figure 9-1b. Adequate maintenance of mobility allows David to assist the care-giver in assuming sitting position from supine or side-lying. Manual proprioceptive input at key points of control, as well as David's labrynthine righting reactions, facilitate erect sitting.

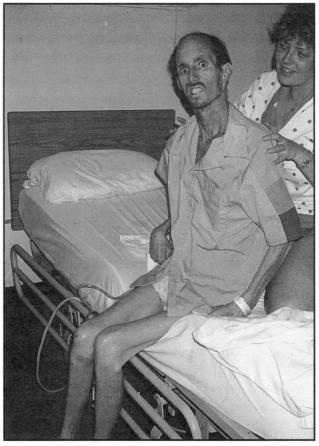

Figure 9-1c. With the head and trunk balanced, weight bearing through the pelvis and lower extremities facilitates his tonic lumbar reflex to create a readiness for sit to stand.

became David's major request. Aware of his physical decline and eventual loss of speech, David learned to communicate through speech therapy with various manual signals and a word association board and was determined to participate in occupational and physical therapy. Figure 9-1a-e demonstrates David's neurologic complications and therapeutic intervention.

The effects of prolonged systemic disease may lead to further debilitation. Autonomic neuropathy has been reported in patients with advanced disease with clinical features that range from postural hypotension to cardiovascular collapse in the setting of invasive procedures (Craddock et al., 1987). To counter these effects, therapeutic exercise should be carefully monitored. In cases of multisystem atrophy, monitoring vital signs and measuring cardiovascular endurance is the primary requirement during rehabilitation designed to improve functional capacity (Galantino & Levy, 1988). Improvement of such capacity offers the neurologically impaired

patient less restriction in activities and improvement in quality of life.

Once exercise training has begun, the effects of training on motor learning, strength, endurance and coordination should be reassessed. The parameters of training can then be adjusted to facilitate goal attainment. The therapist should remain acutely aware of the cognitive status of the patient and changes of perceptual motor skills. Visual and auditory cues are additional forms of sensory input and feedback. Training of functional skills is often initiated in environments free of noxious external stimuli. As the patient increases his skill level, the environment is subtly changed to challenge the patient. Variation in temporal and spatial requirements of the criterion skill is desirable to allow for greater versatility in the learning or relearning of the skill(s) (Fitts, 1967; Gentile, 1972). The therapist must use prudent judgment to challenge the patient without exacerbating frustration. A decision whether to use mass versus distributed practice sessions is

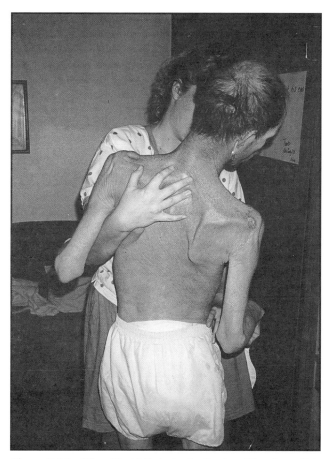

Figure 9-1d. When David first stands, the transition from sit to stand may once again facilitate abnormal postures, synergies and associated movements.

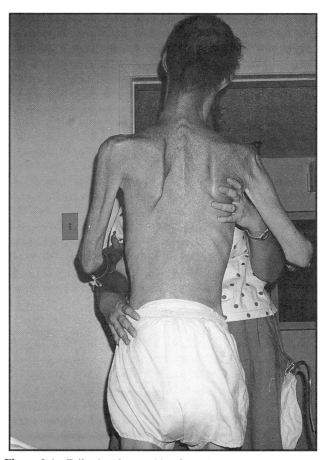

Figure 9-1e. Following the transition form sit to stand, input at key point of control assists internal mechanisms in assuming appropriate postures. Weight bearing creates a readiness for functional ambulation.

made by reviewing the goals of the exercise session. Component skills may be best learned through frequent, short sessions with practice and testing of the criterion skill encouraged (Schmidt, 1975; Singer, 1980; Magill, 1981). Above all, family training and home programs should be designed to enhance safe, functional activity for the neurologically impaired HIV patient. Creativity on the part of the therapist can be a great contribution to the quality of life.

SUMMARY

Neuromuscular complications may occur during all stages of HIV infection. This chapter reviewed multiple opportunistic infections, their multisystem and functional deficits and possibilities for rehabilitation intervention. Neurologic complications can affect 1) the muscular system, 2) peripheral nerve and root, 3) meninges, 4) spinal cord, and 5) brain.

References

Anders, K., Verity, M.A., Cancilla, P.A., and Vinters, H.V. (1984). Acquired immune deficiency syndrome (AIDS): Neuropathologic studies. *Journal of Neuropathology and Experimental Neurology*. 43:315.

Belman, A.L., Diamond, G., Dickson, D., et al. (1988). Pediatric acquired immunodeficiency syndrome: Neurologic syndromes. *American Journal of Diseases in Children*. 142:29.

Berger, J.R., and Mucke, L. (1988). Prolonged survival and partial recovery in AIDS-associated progressive multifocal leukoencephalopathy. *Neurology*. 38:1060.

Besser L.J., and Green J.B. (1988). Severe polymyositis-like syndrome associated with zidovudine therapy of AIDS and ARC (letter to the editor). *New England Journal of Medicine*. 318:708.

Brunnstrom, S. (1970). *New England Journal of Medicine*. 318:708.

Cohen, J.A., and Laudenslager, M. (1989). Autonomic nervous system involvement in patients with human immunodeficiency virus infection. *Neurology*. 39:1111.

Cornblath, D.R., and McArthur, J.C. (1988). Predominantly sensory neuropathy in patients with AIDS and AIDS-related complex. *Neurology*. 38:794.

Cornblath, D.R., McArthur, J.C., Kennedy, P.G.E., et al. (1987). Inflammatory demyelinating peripheral neuropathies associated with human T-cell lymphotropic virus type III infection. *Annals of Neurology*. 21:32.

Craddock C., Pasvok G., Bull R., et al. (1987). Cardiorespiratory arrest and autonomic neuropathy in AIDS. *Lancet*. 11:16.

Eidelberg, D., Sotrel, A., Vogel, H., et al. (1986). Progressive polyradiculopathy in acquired immune deficiency syndrome. *Neurology*. 36:912.

Flower, W. M., and Sooy, C.D. (1987,November). AIDS: An introduction for speech-language pathologists and audiologists. *American Speech and Hearing Association*. 29:25.

Fitts, P.M., and Posner, M. (1967). Human performance. Belmont, CA: Brooks/Cole.

Freeman, R.L., Roberts, M., Friedman, L., and Broadbridge, C. (1989). Autonomic function and HIV infection. *Neurology*. 39(supplement 1):238.

Galantino, M.L., and Levy J.K. (1988). HIV infection: Neurological implications for rehabilitation. *Clinical Management in Physical Therapy*. 8:6.

Galantino, M.L., Fried J., and Munkind J. (1990). Physical therapy management of patient with HIV infection. In Munkind, J. (Ed.): *AIDS and Rehabilitations*. New York: McGraw-y Hill.

Gentile, A.M. (1972). A working model of skill acquisition with application to teaching. *Quest*. 17:3.

Gill, P.S., Levine, A.M., Meyer, P.R., et al. (1985). Primary central nervous system lymphoma in homosexual men. *American Journal of Medicine*. 78:742.

Gonzales, M.F., Olney, R.K., So, Y.T., et al. (1988). Subacute structural myopathy associated with human immunodeficiency virus infection. *Archives of Neurology*. 45:585.

Gorard, D.A., Henry, K., Guiloff, R.J. (1988) Necrotizing myelopathy on zidovudine (letter to the editor). *Lancet*. 1:1050.

Grafe, M.R., and Wiley, C.A. (1989). Spinal cord and peripheral nerve pathology in AIDS: The roles of cytomegalovirus and human immunodeficiency virus. *Annals of Neurology*. 25:561.

Graham, S.H., and Bredesen, D.E. (1988). Neurologic complications of herpes zoster in patients with HIV infection. *Neurology*. 38(supplement 1):120.

Ho, D.D., Rota, T.R., Schooley, R.T., et al. (1985). Isolation of HTLV III from cerebrospinal fluid and neural tissues of patients with neurologic syndromes related to the acquired immunodeficiency syndrome. *New England Journal of Medicine*. 313:1493.

Hopp J.W., and Rogers E.A. (1989). *AIDS and the Allied Health Professions*. Philadelphia: F.A. Davis Co. Knott, M., and Voss, D.E. (1986). *Proprioceptive Neuromuscular Facilitation*, 2nd ed. New York: Harper and Row.

Knott, M., and Voss, D. (1968). Proprioceptive neuromuscular facilitation. 2d ed. New York: Harper and Row. Kovacs, J.A.,

Kovacs, A.A., Polis, M., et al. (1985). Cryptococcosis in the acquired immunodeficiency syndrome. *Annals of Internal Medicine*. 103:533538.

Krupp, L.B., Lipton, R.B., Swerdlow, M.L., et al. (1985). Progressive multifocal leukoencephalopathy: Clinical and radiographic features. *Annals of Neurology*. 17:344.

Levy, R.M., Bredesen, D.E., and Rosenblum, M.L. (1985). Neurological manifestations of the acquired immunodeficiency syndrome (AIDS): Experience at UCSF and review of the literature. *Journal of Neurosurgery*. 62:475.

Levy, R.M., Bredesen, D.E., and Rosenblum, M.L. (1988). Opportunistic central nervous system pathology in patients with AIDS. *Annals of Neurology*. 23:S7.

Logeman, J.A. (1983). Therapy techniques for swallowing disorders. In Mathews. *Evaluation and Treatment of Swallowing Disorders*. TX: Pro-Ed.

Magill, R.A. (1980). Motor learning: Concepts and applications. Dubuque, IA: William C. Brown Co.

Marks, W.J., McArthur, J.C., Royal, W., et al. (1989). Intracranial mass lesions in AIDS: Diagnosis and response to therapy. *Neurology*. (supplement 1):380.

McArthur, J.C. (1987). Neurologic manifestations of AIDS. *Medicine*. 66:407.

Miller, R., Storey, J., Greco, C., et al. (1988). Subacute radiculomyelopathy caused by cytomegalovirus in patients with AIDS. *Neurology*. 38:242.

Morgello, S., Cho, E.S., Nielsen, S., et al. (1987). Cytomegalovirus encephalitis in patients with acquired immunodeficiency syndrome. *Human Pathology*. 18:289.

Navia, B.A., Cho, E.S., Petito, C.K., and Price, R.W. (1986). The AIDS dementia complex. II. Neuropathology. *Annals of Neurology*. 19:525.

Navia, B.A., Jordan, B.D., and Price, R.W. (1986). The AIDS dementia complex. I. Clinical features. *Annals of Neurology*. 19:517.

Navia, B.A., Petito, C.K., Gold, J.W.M., et al. (1986). Cerebral toxoplasmosis complicating the acquired immune deficiency syndrome: Clinical and neuropathological findings in 27 patients. *Annals of Neurology*. 19:224.

Northwestern University Special Therapeutic Exercise Project. (1967). *American Journal of Physical Medicine.* 46:379.

Northwestern University Special Therapeutic Exercise Project: An exploratory and analytical survey of therapeutic exercise. (1967). *American Journal of Physical Medicine.* 46:1.

Patow, C.A., Stark, T.W., Findlay, P.A., et al. (1984). Pharyngeal obstruction by Kaposi's sarcoma in a homosexual male with acquired immune deficiency syndrome. *Otolaryngology and Head and Neck Surgery.* 92:713.

Petito, C.K., Cho, E.S., Lemann, W., et al. Neuropathology of acquired immunodeficiency syndrome (AIDS): An autopsy review. *Journal of Neuropathology and Experimental Neurology.* 45:635.

Petito, C.K., Navia, B.A., Cho, E.S., et al. (1985). Vacuolar myelopathy pathologically resembling subacute combined degeneration in patients with the acquired immunodeficiency syndrome. *New England Journal of Medicine.* 312:874.

Price, R.W., Sidtis, J., and Rosenblum, M. (1988). The AIDS dementia complex: Some current questions. *Annals of Neurology.* 23(supplement):27.

Schmidt, R.A. (1975). A schema theory of discrete of motor skill learning. *Psychological Review.* 82:225.

Schmitt, F.A., Bigley, J.W., and McKinnis, R. (1988). Neuropsychological outcome of zidovudine (AZT) treatment of patients with AIDS and AIDS-related complex. *New England Journal of Medicine.* 319:1573.

Simpson, D.M., and Bender, A.N. (1988). Human immunodeficiency virus-associated myopathy: Analysis of 11 patients. *Annals of Neurology.* 24:79.

Singer, R.N. (1980). *Motor Learning and Human Performance*, 3d ed. New York: MacMillan Publishing Co., Inc.

Snider, W.D., Simpson, D.M., Nielsen, S., et al. (1983). Neurological complications of acquired immune deficiency syndrome: Analysis of 50 patients. *Annals of Neurology.* 14:403.

So, Y.T., Beckstead, J.H., and Davis, R.L. (1986). Primary central nervous system lymphoma in acquired immune deficiency syndrome: A clinical and pathological study. *Annals of Neurology.* 20:566.

So, Y.T., Holtzman, D.M., Abrams, D.I., and Olney, R.K. (1988). Peripheral neuropathy associated with acquired immunodeficiency syndrome. *Archives of Neurology.* 45:945.

Zuckerman, M.J., and Halperin, J.J. (1989). Autonomic dysfunction in patients with HIV infection. *Neurology.* 39(supplement 1):410.

10

Pain Management

Mary Lou Galantino, MS, PT
Guy L. McCormack, MS, OT

The best way to dim one's pain is to cast it in the shadow of one's sympathy.

—John Andrew Holmes

INTRODUCTION

Although the number of patients with HIV disease has increased dramatically, few studies have been written about the prevalence of pain or descriptions of different pain syndromes in these patients. The symptom of pain may be overshadowed by a constellation of other overwhelming problems, which may include opportunistic infections, diarrhea, dyspnea, anorexia, weight loss and neuropsychologic symptoms. The development of specific disease-oriented treatment for AIDS, which increases survival but is not curative, creates a critical need to evaluate pain prevalence and its current management techniques.

The typical description of pain syndromes associated with HIV portrays a disorder producing a multitude of pathologic changes and deficiencies of the immune system. The possible causes of most of the pain syndromes or sites are complex. The high incidence of chest pain is presumed to be secondary to the prevalence of PCP. Abdominal pain, on the other hand, can have many causes: lymphadenopathy from the HIV infection or lymphoma, KS, infectious diarrhea, organomegaly, ileus and nonspecific gastritis. Common causes of headache are toxoplasmosis, central nervous system lymphoma, cryptococcus meningitis, or nonspecific headaches. Midsternal burning or dysphagia from esophagitis is usually caused by infection with herpes simplex, cytomegalovirus, or candidiasis. This type of infection is frequently resistant to antifungal treatment, and the pain associated with the esophagitis frequently requires opioids

for relief. Various types of peripheral neuropathy occur, most commonly the distal symmetric polyneuropathy, which causes painful, burning dysesthesia with minimal motor abnormalities (Table 10-1). A high incidence of neurologic symptoms has been documented in the AIDS population. One study estimated that about 40 percent of HIV patients present with neuropathologic symptomatology (Hilton, 1989). Levy et al. (1985) reported that 73 percent of patients affected with HIV have subtle neurological symptoms arising from peripheral and central nervous system involvement. One commonly overlooked neurologic aberration is pain. Laskin (1988) states that the patient with AIDS may experience pain from many sources, but is usually secondary to various opportunistic infections.

ADC is the most frequently documented neurologic manifestation of HIV. These patients exhibit apathy, withdrawal and depression; but their major complaint revolves around headaches, which are severe and persistent enough to cause sleep disturbances. These headaches respond poorly to analgesics. In addition to the headaches, these individuals experience dementia, which is manifested by cognitive, behavioral and sensory-motor dysfunctions (see Chapter 9, 11). Sensorimotor disturbances can include gait ataxia, loss of balance, paresthesia numbness and retinopathy (Hilton, 1989; Johnson & McArthur, 1986). There is little doubt that during the course of HIV disease, the patient will experience pain because of the detrimental effects on the nervous system. Pathology studies show that once HIV enters the bloodstream, multiple microglial nodules develop within the

Table 10-1
TYPES OF PERIPHERAL NEUROPATHY

TYPE	SIGNS AND SYMPTOMS	DIAGNOSIS	TREATMENT
Acute demyelinating inflammatory sensorimotor polyradiculoneuropathy	-Acute Guillain-Barre syndrome (GBS) -Usually occurs with asymptomatic seropositive individuals -Progressive weakness -Decreased DTR -Mild sensory loss	-HIV and hepatitis B antibodies -Polyclonal hypergamma globulinemia -CSF pleocytosis -Demyelination -Nerve biopsy: macrophage-mediated demyelination, lymphocytic infiltration	Plasmapheresis
Chronic Inflammatory demyelinating polyneuropathy (CIDP)	-Usually occurs with symptomatic and advanced HIV disease -Progressive weakness with motor symptoms developing over several months -Subacute onset soles of feet are numb	-Demyelinating polyneuropathy -Nerve biopsy: perivascular inflammmation with loss of myelinated fibers	-Nonsteroidal anti-inflammatory -Plasmapheresis (only for severe CIDP because the disorder can remit spontaneously) -Prednisone (careful administration as it is known to alter cell-mediated immunity, which may predispose patients to develop AIDS)
Mononeuritis multiplex *(a) Vasculitic Type	-Fever, weight loss -Anemia -Sensory or motor deficiency	-CSF pleocytosis Etiology: immune-complex deposition secondary to necrotizing vasculitis	-Prednisone -Cyclophosphamide
**(b) Multifocal Sensory Loss	-Sensory or motor deficiency	-CSF pleocytosis and increased protein -Nerve biopsy: axonal loss and demyelination -Perivascular inflammatory infiltrates	-Prednisone -Plasmapheresis
(c)Mononeuropathy	-Muscle weakness -Foot drop	-Peroneal nerve palsy	-Prevent compression neuropathies via optimal positioning
Progressive inflammatory polyradiculopathy	-Distal weakness with flaccid paraparesis -Numbness and tingling -Sphincter dysfunction -Hypoesthesias -Decreased DTR	-Nerve roots of cauda equina are inflamed, presumably due to CMV -Extensive loss of myelin and axons from both the dorsal/ventral roots	-Sympathetic nerve blocks

continued . . .

gray and white matter of the brain (Healy & Coleman, 1989). Scattered demyelination occurs in the spinal cord and the peripheral nervous system. Inflammatory abscesses are also scattered throughout the cerebral hemispheres (Hilton, 1989). HIV has been associated with malignant lymphomas, which have caused low back pain, muscular weakness and disturbance of orofacial musculature (Hilton, 1989; Johnson & McArthur, 1986; Healy & Coleman, 1989). Deafferentation

Table 10-1 (continued)
TYPES OF PERIPHERAL NEUROPATHY

TYPE	SIGNS AND SYMPTOMS	DIAGNOSIS	TREATMENT
Sensory ataxic neuropathy	-Seen primarily with symptomatic and advanced HIV disease -Paresthesia and dysesthesia confined initially to the soles of the feet, which may progress to the entire foot. -Contact-hypersensitivity and hyperpathia -Difficulty with ambulation, 2 intrinsic foot weakness -Decreased ankle jerk	-Dorsal root ganglion infection (ganglioneuritis) -Axonal neuropathy with secondary demyelination Electro-physiologically: (a) sural sensory response decreased (b) motor evoked amplitudes decreased (c) leg conduction velocities decreased (d) H reflexes - absent or prolonged	-Tricyclic antidepressants -Anticonvulsants -Salicylates -Narcotic analgesics -AZT
Distal symmetric polyneuropathy (DSPN) or distal axonopathy**	-Usually occurs in patients with AIDS -Associated with weight loss and higher incidence of dementia -Distal numbness and tingling -Decreased DTR -Decreased vibratory sense -Very painful and most disabling	-Loss of myelinated and unmyelinated fibers Etiology: -possibly metabolic, toxic or nutritional	-Tricyclic antidepressants -AZT -Interferon -Corticosteroids

* Rule out viral infection.
** Most difficult to treat.

pain, partial or complete damage to afferent nerve pathways, is rather common among individuals with HIV. The type of pain depends on the disease process that is secondary to HIV infection. The management of pain, therefore, depends on the origin, symptoms, and signs of pain.

Physical and occupational therapists are in an optimal position to conduct pain assessments, to address psychosocial issues, and to provide noninvasive interventions to improve the quality of life for the person with HIV disease.

PAIN ASSESSMENT

Pain is a puzzling phenomenon because it is neither purely physical nor psychologic in origin (McCormack, 1990). Although the pain may stem from an anatomic site on the body, the mind plays an important role in its perception. Therefore, the mind and body are an integrated circuit and what affects one will undoubtedly affect the other. Pain is also a personal and private sensation of discomfort. Thus, one can not truly measure the pain of another person. Yet, before therapeutic intervention can take place, the therapist must evaluate, formulate a baseline, and determine the individual needs of the patient. A Guide to Assessing the HIV Seropositive Patient can assist the therapist in discerning the etiology of pain patterns seen throughout HIV disease (see Appendix E).

Two studies that have reported on the prevalence of pain types in the HIV population are summarized here. Newshan et al. (1989) reviewed the pain experiences of 100 consecutive AIDS patients seen by the Pain Management Program at St Luke's/Roosevelt Hospital Center in New York City. The incidence of the pain location/syndrome was analyzed within each of two risk factor groups (44 homosexuals and 56 drug addicts). The most frequent type of pain was abdominal and the second most frequent; peripheral neuropathy in both groups. However, the third-ranked pain source was KS in the homosexual group and esophagitis in the drug addict group. Other prevalent types of pain found in both of these populations were mucositis, cellulitis, Stevens-Johnson syndrome, decubitus, corneal ulcers, and postoperative pain. Fifteen percent of all patients experienced a combination of different types of pain.

A study by Lebovits et al. (1989) at SUNY Health Center at Brooklyn describes a systematic evaluation of the prevalence of pain and pain management intervention in a general hospitalized AIDS population. The second most common presenting symptom was pain in 30 percent of the patients, second only to fever. The most prevalent pain location/syndrome was the chest (22 percent). Other pain types or locations were headache (13 percent), oral cavity (11 percent), abdomen (8 percent), peripheral neuropathy (6 percent), musculoskeletal system (6 percent), low back (3 percent), and thrombophlebitis (1 percent). In this study, there were no significant relationships between specific HIV syndromes and the incidence of pain, but this analysis was limited due to low incidence of some types of pain.

One of the first factors the therapist should evaluate is the origin of pain. Usually, the origin correlates with the intensity or type of unpleasant sensation the patient perceives. For example, pain can be classified as superficial somatic pain, which is caused by disturbance to the receptors in the superficial layers of the skin or from subcutaneous tissue just beneath the skin. Superficial cutaneous pain is usually very localized and corresponds to dermatomal boundaries (Johnson, 1977). The patient may describe the pain as sharp, bright tingling or stinging. Sometimes, but not usually, the pain intensity corresponds to the extent of tissue damage.

A second origin of pain may be called deep somatic pain because it arises from connective tissue such as muscles, joint capsules, tendons, ligaments and periosteum of bones. Deep somatic pain does not follow dermatomal patterns but is felt more in a three-dimensional pattern rather than in a linear plane. In other words, it is felt as a deep sensation projecting along nerve roots and produces a diffuse, dull aching pain. Thus it does not conform to a discrete two-dimensional configuration on the surface of the skin (Johnson, 1977; Lasagna, 1986; Empting-Koschorke et al., 1989).

Pain can also arise directly from peripheral neuropathies that produce another type of pain syndrome. Galantino and Brewer (1989) reported that in persons with HIV, peripheral neuropathies may involve sensory and/or motor fibers and be treated with various modalities. These peripheral neuropathies can be divided into subtypes based on the cell which is primarily affected (Parry, 1988; Cornblath, 1988) (Table 10-1).

In addition, side effects for patients with KS that result from chemotherapy, such as vincristine and bleomycin, can include peripheral neuropathies that are predominantly distal, symmetric sensory neuropathies. Peripheral neuropathies involving nerve fibers may manifest as causalgia, which is described as a lancinating paroxysmal pain. Causalgia produces a burning sensation and is particularly common with median and sciatic nerve involvement or with complications of autonomic fibers. Trophic skin changes may accompany causalgia, producing highly sensitive trigger point areas. The patient may be particularly guarded about touch to these sensitive areas because it may exacerbate the perception of pain. Paresthesia is another pain sensation associated with peripheral neuropathies. This may be felt as an abnormal electrical sensation producing shock-like sensations that tingle along the course of the nerve root.

Finally, pain may originate in viscera because of infection in tissues of internal organs located in the thorax or abdomen (lymphoma, KS and organomegaly). Because these organs are innervated by sympathetic nerve fibers, the pain may be projected to a region on the skin remote to the location of the internal organ. Referred pain, as it is called, is not well understood but is thought to occur because most of the internal organs of the body are supplied by pain fibers that pass along the visceral sympathetic nerves into the spinal cord by way of the lateral spinothalamic tract (Fields, 1987). For example, the heart pain fibers enter the spinal cord between C3 and T5. Pain arising from the heart muscle secondary to HIV cardiomyopathy may project to the left shoulder and neck region. Visceral pain may also conform to dermatomal patterns. KS of the gastrointestinal tract may be the cause of referred low back pain. Visceral pain is perceived as a cyclical, severe binding, gnawing or dull sensation. This cyclical sensation is probably produced by the automatic movements of organs such as peristalsis in the gastrointestinal tract (Guyton, 1987). By attending to the origins of pain, the therapist takes the first step to develop a therapeutic relationship and to identify words associated with the type of pain the patient is experiencing.

Many clinicians will objectify pain by measuring the dimensions of location, duration, intensity, quality and frequency (Johnson, 1977; Lasagna, 1986). The location of pain is best achieved by simply asking the patient to point to the area of discomfort. In addition, many clinicians use a pain chart, which is an anatomic line drawing showing anterior and posterior surfaces of the body. This chart provides a graphic representation so that the patient can color in the sites of discomfort. Once the pain locations are cited on the pain chart, the therapist can determine if any pattern exists in the locations of pain or if they correspond to common trigger points. The most common sites for trigger points are the upper trapezius, dorsum of the neck, subscapularis, gluteus medius and along the paralumbar muscles (Empting-Koschorke et al., 1989). By applying light manual finger pressure over the tender locations cited on the pain chart, the therapist can determine if there are smaller specific spots that evoke tenderness or sharp pain; these spots are usually the trigger points. Locating trigger points can lead to the evaluation of myofascial syndromes; therefore, it is important that the patient completes the pain chart to locate the general areas of pain. Second, the therapist should examine the sites by palpation to complete a collaborative examination. Cummings and Routan (1987) found only 43 percent accuracy rate in unassisted pain drawings completed by patients. The collaborative examination reveals pain locations not found on unassisted pain charts. The pain chart enables the therapist to detect changes in perceived pain when comparing subsequent assessments over time. The therapist should also ask questions about the duration of pain to try to determine if there are any rhythms or fluctuations in pain perception. It may also reveal aggravating or mitigating factors. For example, the therapist should inquire about which positions increase or decrease pain. What relieves or intensifies the pain? How much does it interfere with the activities of daily living? Do certain emotions influence the perception of pain?

Next, the therapist may choose to use a rating scale to quantify the intensity of pain. Pain intensity scales are easy to administer and score with relatively good sensitivity, reliability and validity (McCormack & Johnson, 1990). Some scales use a numeric scale in which a number from 0 (no pain) to 10 (worst pain imaginable) is used. The visual analog scale uses a straight line with "no pain" on one end and "pain as bad as it could be" on the other. The patient then marks the place along the continuum that signifies their intensity of pain. Another approach is to use a verbal scale, asking the patient to describe their pain in terms of minimal, moderate, severe or overwhelming. Unfortunately, verbal scales provide fewer choices and may be less sensitive (McCormack & Johnson, 1990).

The quality of pain represents the affective component of discomfort. It is also an indicator of the behavioral response to pain. One way to assess the quality of pain is to use scales, with a list of adjectives describing the sensations of pain. The McGill Pain Questionnaire developed in 1975 is such an instrument. This questionnaire contains a list of 102 words that patients have used to describe pain. The questionnaire is somewhat personal, but according to Wall (1987) pain is always subjective. The questionnaire also enables the therapist to develop a common language with the patient that enhances the communication process (Melzack, 1975;

Wall, 1987). This questionnaire may assist the therapist in developing metaphors that are unique to the patient's particular pain syndrome. The patient may say my "leg is on fire" when experiencing causalgia. Using the metaphor of "fire" the therapist can develop visualization scripts that are the antithesis to heat and burning sensations. For instance, the script might include the visualizations of cool blue colors bathing the painful extremity, putting "out the fire," and draining the ashes from proximal to distal out and away from the body.

The quality of pain appears to have cultural, social, and emotional implications. Psychologic stress factors may exaggerate the perception of pain and produce behaviors of anger, anxiety, depression, fear and irritability. It is not uncommon for persons who have endured pain for 2 to 3 months to demonstrate some personality changes (Lasagna, 1986; Empting-Koschorke et al., 1989). These changes might include inability to concentrate, hypochondriasis, depression, sleep disturbances and lack of appetite.

Psychologic stress has a physiologic basis for producing pain. Neurologically speaking, the older pain pathways have many collateral connections to the reticular formation in the brain stem hypothalamus and the limbic structures. Collectively, these structures can facilitate activity, which in turn diminishes microcirculation to pain receptors in the periphery, thereby changing their sensitivity levels. It is not unusual for a patient with chronic HIV infection to have stress and a heightened sensitivity to pain because of this "sympathetic overload." Thus, anytime the sympathetic branch of the autonomic nervous system prevails, it produces a physiologic overflow, creating increased muscle tone, changes in blood pressure, heart rate, respiration and gastrointestinal motility. Other physiologic signs of sympathetic overload are dilated pupil size, increased perspiration, blanching of the skin and nausea (Lasagna, 1986; Empting-Koschorke et al., 1989; Fields, 1987). The increased muscle tone associated with pain is only one of many cycles set into action. For instance, muscle tension related to anxiety can activate pain receptors in connective tissues, which in turn set off another continuous volley of pain transmissions that continues to activate the pain cycle. Studies show that too much sympathetic tone results from arousal of what is now called the hypothalamic-pituitary-adrenal axis (Green et al., 1981). If the therapist observes the previously mentioned physiologic signs or the behaviors (fear, anxiety, anger, irritability) associated with sympathetic overload, it is beneficial to halt the assessment to prevent exacerbation of pain. Instead, it has been found to be beneficial to use some inhibitory strategies to activate the parasympathetic branch of the nervous system to normalize physiologic processes. Deep breathing exercises, acupressure releases, visualizations, soft music and slow stroking over the primary rami or slow vestibular stimulation are effective for promoting parasympathetic dominance. Once the relaxation response is elicited, the therapist may resume testing and achieve better results in collecting the baseline data.

Fatigue is another variable that affects pain assessment reliability. Hidelman (1980) and Laskin (1988) postulated a cyclical relationship between pain and fatigue. According to Hidelman, fatigue brings on pain and pain brings on fatigue. This cycle becomes one more positive feedback loop in which pain and fatigue are constantly stimulating one or the other. Because fatigue is one of the primary symptoms experienced by patients with HIV infection, an understanding of this relationship is important to develop strategies for breaking this cycle.

Additional instruments for pain assessment are the Minnesota Multiphasic Personality Inventory (MMPI) (Empting-Koschorke et al., 1989), the Mensana Clinic Back Pain Test (Empting-Koschorke et al., 1989), the Pain Disability Index (PDI) (Tait, et al., 1987), and the Dallas Pain Questionnaire (DPG) (Lawlis, et al., 1989). These instruments have shown promise for assessing the qualitative aspects of the pain experience. For further review, McGuire (1984) has prepared a useful reference for use in clinical assessment of pain. The assessment of a patient's pain status is an ongoing process. The initial evaluation establishes the baseline (Appendix E), and subsequent assessments determine the effectiveness of interventions.

PAIN MANAGEMENT

To develop a comprehensive intervention program in the person with HIV, the therapist should understand the basics of pain theory. To begin, pain is a sensation that usually results from the stimulation of nociceptors. However, this definition by itself is too simplistic because it neglects the cognitive-emotional-affective components of pain. A better definition was generated by the International Association for the Study of Pain (1979), which states that "pain is an unpleasant sensory and emotional experience associated with actual or potential tissue damage or described in terms of such damage" (Laskin, 1988:38). This definition provides a theoretical basis from which to operate when developing strategies for intervention. First, pain usually results from stimulation to nociceptors found throughout the body. Physiologic studies have shown that nociceptors can be activated by chemical, thermal and mechanical stimuli. When these stimuli are converted into electrical-chemical impulses, the process is called transduction. Although specific nociceptors have been identified, other sensory receptors are known to carry pain impulses when the

magnitude and intensity of the stimulus is great enough (Fields, 1987). The term *transmission* refers to the process by which pain is carried to the thalamus and higher cortical centers where pain is realized. The transmission of pain is believed to be carried principally along neurons grouped into systems. Pain transmission consists of three neuronal components: the peripheral sensory nerves, which carry the impulse to its terminal in the spinal cord; the second order neuron, which can relay the impulse or inhibit it in the spinal cord; and the third order neuron whose cell body lies in the thalamus, which acts as a terminal for conveying the pain transmission to the cortex (Fields, 1987; Guyton, 1987).

Three tract systems are known to transmit pain. The older, paleospinothalamic pathways send many collaterals to the reticular formation, limbic structures, midbrain, hypothalamus, autonomic nervous system and widespread cortical areas (Lebovits et al., 1989; Empting-Koschorke et al., 1989). This system transmits pain messages that are diffuse and poorly localized and have been associated with behavioral reactions to nociception. The neospinothalamic tract consists of more recently evolved pathways that provide precise or discriminative sensory information about pain. The third tract system is the lemniscal system, which has classically been associated with conscious proprioception, vibration, pressure and tactile discrimination. However, this tract system may provide discriminative pain sensations and is involved in interpretation of pain stimuli (Lasagna, 1986; Fields, 1987).

Modulation is the third component of pain. Modulation refers to descending tracts that arise from central nervous system structures, such as raphe nuclei, reticulomagnus cellularis periaqueductal gray matter, and cortical assemblies of neurons that can inhibit pain transmission in the dorsal horn of the spinal cord.

Perception represents the least understood aspect of pain. It is not clear how the process takes place, but neurochemical connections in the cortex and most likely the limbic structures formulate psychologic, cognitive and emotional bonds to pain. Pain perception is a complex process because it involves sensory, emotional and cognitive affectors, which most likely subserve the connections of the hypothalamic-pituitary-adrenal axis. This description indicates that pain is indeed a multisystem phenomenon that requires a multifaceted approach. Such an approach is holistic because it involves the integration of the nervous, immune and the endocrine systems, which indicate that pain is indeed a multisystem phenomenon in needs of a multifaceted approach.

One of the most widely accepted pain theories is the gate control theory proposed by Melzack (1975, 1977, 1981) and Wall (1987) in 1965. This theory provides an excellent model because it incorporates the sensory and cognitive-emotional affective components that integrate to determine the person's perception of pain. Simply stated, the gate control theory proposes that pain impulses travel from the nerve endings (nociceptors) to the dorsal horn of the spinal cord in the substantia gelatinosa (lamina I and II), where synapses are made with the second order neurons or transmission cells (T-cells). These synapses are metaphorically referred to as gates that can close (inhibit) to keep the impulses from reaching higher centers where pain is realized. Whether the so-called gates are open or closed is contingent upon the size and type of nerve fiber that is stimulated. Small myelinated A delta and thinner unmyelinated C fibers are thought to carry pain signals to the gates, allowing the transmission to reach the brain. That stimulation of large-diameter sensory fibers from the peripheral tactile receptors activates the neurons that close the gates, thereby inhibiting transmission, has been a monumental discovery in developing of pain management techniques (Olsson & Parker, 1987; Melzack, 1981; Melzack, et al., 1977; McCormack, 1988). The depression of pain signals by stimulating the large diameter sensory fibers occurs when the stimulus is applied to the skin near the area of pain or along the dermatome (Guyton, 1987; Olsson & Parker, 1987; Melzack, 1981). Large fibers are best stimulated by cutaneous stimulation, such as finger-pressure, stretch, massage, vibration, acupuncture, mentholated rubs, the use of heat and cold or a variety of traditional dermal abrasive techniques (McCormack, 1988). Before applying cutaneous stimulation techniques, it is important to check with the nursing staff or the physician about pharmacologic analgesics.

A nonsteroidal anti-inflammatory drug and a narcotic may be prescribed for the person experiencing peripheral neuropathy (Nelson, 1986). Adjunctive drugs (ie. diuretics) may be used in conjunction with compression stockings to reduce swelling caused by internal pressure of lymphoma or KS. To provide consistency in pain relief, analgesics should be given on a routine basis and the cutaneous stimulation should complement the effects of the pharmacologic analgesics. In a study by Lebovits et al. (1989), the pharmacologic management of pain in the AIDS population showed frequent use of opioids, including acetaminophen and codeine. Suggestions from the investigators of some of the studies have included four principles adapted from the treatment for chronic pain from cancer, which may be useful in the HIV population: 1) use of nonsteroidal anti-inflammatory drugs (NSAIDs), 2) systematic approach to pain using the World Health Organization's guidelines for cancer pain treatment, 3) administration of analgesics on a fixed schedule rather than an as-needed schedule, and 4) use of tricyclic antidepressants as an adjuvant analgesic (World Health Organization, 1986).

These approaches to pain management, however, need to be examined in prospective studies of larger numbers of patients with HIV disease. The therapist may try a variety of cutaneous stimulation techniques so that the patient's nervous system does not habituate to the stimulus. Vibration and deep pressure will activate pacinian corpuscles and Ruffini's endings, which transmit along the thick (group II) fibers at velocities of 30 to 70 m/sec, whereas C fibers conducting pain only reach velocities of about 2 m/sec (Guyton, 1987). Therefore, deep manual pressure and vibration work well as beginning stimulus. Some patients do not like the feeling of the head of the vibrator when applied directly to the skin. Better results have been achieved by lying the palm of the hand over the painful site and then applying vibration through the therapist's hand. The feeling of vibration through the hand is less offensive. Pointed vibrators can be successfully applied over acupressure points to provide deep penetrating pressure over a small area. Pomeranz (1987) suggests that the acupressure points associated with analgesia are located in deep connective tissues near bones in muscle insertions. Trigger points may also be released for acute pain by applying deep finger pressure over the painful sites for seven seconds. Upon release, the patient is asked to move the extremity through range of motion. This movement further activates proprioceptors and low threshold afferents that synapse on the cells in the substantia gelatinosa in the dorsal horn of the spinal cord. For chronic pain lasting at least six months, lighter touch pressure is recommended. Acupressure releases that use several points to regulate a generalized balance and relaxation response will have a calming effect, and by eliciting a relaxation response, the immune system and self-healing processes are more activated (Kleinkort et al., 1981; Biederbach, 1987).

The mechanisms behind acupressure releases are not yet well understood, but there is growing evidence to suggest that the hypothalamus-pituitary-adrenal axis plays a major role in shifting the autonomic nervous system toward a parasympathetic response. Nevertheless, patients have been observed achieving states of deep relaxation and even sleep. During this phase, the patient's stress level drops and the natural physiologic healing processes predominate.

Some topical analgesics or mentholated rubs have been used to modulate the superficial pain sites. These agents may be applied in a circular motion over acupuncture points to bring temporary relief of pain. Ice has also been applied over the Ho-Ku point (Li-4) located in the web space of the hand between the first and second metacarpals to reduce pain in the head region (Klein, 1989).

Transcutaneous electrical nerve (TENS) stimulation to specific acupuncture and auricular points (external ear) has shown great promise as techniques for altering pain thresholds. Longobardi et al. (1989) used auricular TENS exclusively and reported a significant decrease in pain affecting distal extremities. TENS appears to work by activating the analgesia system in the brain and spinal cord. This system consists of the periaqueductal gray matter, raphe nucleus, and medullary and pontine reticular formation, which collectively compose a descending pain modulation system which acts on the cells in the dorsal horn of the spinal cord (Guyton, 1987; Wall, 1987).

TENS has been used with patients with HIV to control the pain associated with peripheral neuropathies (Galantino & Brewer, 1989). Electrodes were placed on various acupuncture points, and significant pain reduction enabled the patient to remain ambulatory longer. As mentioned earlier, six different peripheral neuropathies have been diagnosed in the HIV patient. It is important to carefully assess the use of TENS parameters, as clinical experience has noted muscle fasciculations with this pain syndrome. Rationale for these pain fasciculations are a matter of conjecture, and further clinical and diagnostic evaluation and research are warranted. A distinction needs to be made between the aspects of TENS versus low energy input (ie. microcurrent and laser). Another common problem in HIV patients is the pain associated with herpes zoster, which may persist long after open lesions subside. When this opportunistic infection is treated with an antiviral agent, such as acyclovir, in concert with TENS, there appears to be effective pain control. The placement of TENS electrodes for optimum pain attenuation in this condition is on synergistic or complementary points. An alternative electrode placement may be simply to bracket the shingles.

In summary, local and superficial pain of patients with HIV disease can be reduced with cutaneous stimulation or counter-irritation techniques. These techniques can be applied directly over the pain site, to areas around the pain, at acupuncture points, at trigger points and even at contralateral sites. Lasers, TENS, and microcurrent therapy have been promising modalities, especially when applied at specific acupuncture points. An excellent reference book for locating acupuncture points, which includes a comprehensive scientific literature review, is *Acupuncture Textbook and Atlas* (Stux & Pomeranz 1987).

Laser point stimulation and auriculotherapy in concert with other electrotherapeutic devices can be used for symptomatic relief and management of chronic, intractable pain or as an adjuvant for any pain treatment. With respect to wound healing (eg. decubiti), low energy laser can accelerate the healing process and is authorized for use with informed consent. Laser is a much more practical treatment for superficial wounds than hydrotherapy, especially in view of infection control. Recently, considerable attention has been paid to the Arndt-Schulz Law, which states that weak stimuli increase physiologic activity and very strong ones

retard, inhibit or abolish it. Thus, the use of low or subthreshold stimuli to relieve pain and heal wounds has become more prevalent. Two such modalities used in the treatment of HIV pain are microcurrent electrical neuromuscular stimulation and laser biostimulation. Both appear to be quite innocuous to the senses and produce significant results. Although the working mechanism of these devices is not fully known, they share a common pathway to pain relief via intervention in the cellular clean-up and repair cycles. Both modalities appear to stimulate the following:

1. membraneous exchange of intracellular and interstitial fluid
2. increased production of ATP
3. increased microcapillarization
4. increased collagen synthesis (Seitz & Kleinkort, 1986; Picker, 1989).

Microcurrent stimulation uses a current of less than 1000 microamps (ua) or one milliamp (ma). It is thought that the current will pass through the viscous protoplasm of an injured cell rather than follow the interstitial pathways such as currents of higher intensities. The direct pathway through the cell allows metabolites to move through the cell membrane, creating less intracellular impedance.

Virologic studies have demonstrated that the herpes virus can be reactivated by electrical stimulation of host nerve cells (Green et al., 1981, 1987). Therefore, the benefits of electrical stimulation must be weighed against the theoretical possibility of herpes simplex, herpes zoster, CMV or Epstein-Barr virus reactivation. No cases have been reported in which viral reactivation has occurred in conjunction with electrical stimulation.

COGNITIVE DISTRACTION

The patient with HIV may suffer from a variety of pain syndromes. As previously mentioned, severe headaches, referred pain and deep somatic pain are common among this population. Cognitive distraction involves a variety of techniques that manipulate the cognitive components of pain perception (Longobardi et al., 1989). By diverting the patient's attention and concentration away from the pain, a cascade of chemical, physiologic, and neuroendocrinologic events takes place to reestablish a sense of balance. Psychoneuroimmunology has begun to explore the chemical links between emotions and health. Neuropeptides, which are manufactured in the limbic system and other parts of the body, are transmitted through the bloodstream, providing the link between the body and mind (Pert et al., 1985). Therefore, behavioral approaches do indeed produce biochemical exchanges that occur along the hypothalamic-pituitary-adrenal axis, having far reaching results throughout the body (Antoni et al., 1989). The best documented influence of the body-mind link occurs along a biochemical pathway existing between the hypothalamus and the thymus gland where T-cells mature with the assistance of the adrenal pituitary glands. In stressful conditions such as pain, the hypothalamus produces a chemical called corticotropin-releasing factor, which causes the pituitary to secrete adrenocorticotropic hormone. This hormone causes the adrenal glands to release into the bloodstream steroid hormones called glucocorticoids. Elevated glucocorticoids can destroy T-cells, which provide a variety of immunologic tasks. Because HIV infection is an immunologic disorder, this finding is of enormous importance. Studies have shown that imagery, advanced meditation and visualization release neuropeptides into the bloodstream, which in turn direct the movement of the monocytes (macrophages) that are critical for tissue repair, elimination of antigens and stimulation T- and B-cells to fight diseases (Pomeranz, 1987; Lein et al., 1989; Longobardi et al., 1989). These findings provide new hope for managing HIV. Cognitive activities can perhaps fine-tune brain chemicals that act directly on free-roaming lymphocytes and rouse them to do battle with the antigens.

The power of the mind-body mechanism dates from approximately 5,000 years in India where the body was considered the projection of consciousness. One of the major goals of cognitive distraction is to affect the body by eliciting the "relaxation response," which is the opposite of the fight or flight reaction. Patients can learn to achieve this relaxed state through a number of procedures: progressive muscle relaxation, autogenics, and visualization. For instance, the therapist can teach the process of having the patient sit quietly with their eyes closed and concentrate on an object, short phrase, or even a relaxed muscle. Direct concentration can evoke the relaxation response once it is established as part of a daily routine. It tends to be a learned process that requires desire and repetition to achieve.

Deep breathing exercises are another useful technique to acquaint the patient with the relaxation response. Breathing is the basic rhythm of life. It is often forgotten as a preliminary exercise before therapy. The object is to have the patient concentrate on breathing. In doing so, the rate of breathing slows down automatically. As breathing slows, so do other physiologic mechanisms and the mind once again is diverted from pain. To augment the effects of deep breathing, the therapist instructs the patient to breath in through the nose and out through the mouth, with partly closed lips (a sighing sound may accompany the expirations). The rate of breathing can be set to a metronome so the expirations are calibrated to be twice as long as the inspirations. It is also beneficial to have the patient focus on an object while breathing, with the intent of producing a concentrated gaze.

Diaphragmatic breathing is another breathing technique. Here the patient is asked to place the palm of one hand over the abdomen and the other hand over the lower aspect of the sternum. In this way, the patient receives tactile feedback when the "belly" expands and contracts. The idea is to have the patient breathe in through the nose while expanding the abdomen. On exhalation the abdominal muscles contract, thus pushing out the air through the mouth. The combination of these maneuvers engage the mind in the steps of the processes, causing the cortical modulation system to suppress pain perception. Deep breathing also benefits the patients physiologically because inhalation through the nose activates parasympathetic fibers in the nasal mucosa (Guyton, 1987). Inhalation through the nose also draws in oxygen into the blood, forming oxyhemoglobin levels to increase and thus promote healing. In contrast, exhalation releases carbon dioxide and waste products. The patient in pain usually breathes in a shallow manner, using mostly the chest and intercostal muscles. Deep breathing opens up more alveoli in the lungs and oxygenates the bloodstream, allowing microcapillary beds to dilate and to supply tissues. Sympathetic nerve terminals have been found in lymph nodes and the spleen. These organs filter the blood and provide rich sources of antigens for lymphocytes (Hall & Goldstein, 1986). In addition, patients in pain have hypertonic muscles, which is a "splinting" reaction due to too much sympathetic tone. Simple breathing and stretch exercises also help to reduce the muscle tightness and relative status of the circulatory system. Muscle stretch exercises activate venous return and lymphatic drainage, which can become relatively stagnant in an immobilized state.

Music and imagery in combination produce significant changes in pain thresholds, heart rate, blood pressure and respiration (Taylor, 1987; Genden et al., 1989). Music can be personalized with ear phones so that the patient can select a range of sounds from easy listening to rock and roll. The volume dial can be used to simulate the intensity of pain. The greater the pain, the louder the volume. Therapists have used soft background music with "voice-overs," leading the listener through scenes at the ocean, beach or forest. Metaphors and the power of suggestion can have a type of hypnotic effect on the patient. Spiegel (1987) states that hypnosis is regaining respect in the medical community. Hypnosis may also be influenced by the patient's motivation and the intensity of pain being experienced. The patient should achieve deep relaxation before this technique is administered. The therapist should facilitate the process by

1. giving suggestions to the patient of sensations that the therapist has experienced in the past, for example, suggesting the feeling that novocaine has been injected or that the

arm has gone to sleep

2. focusing the sensation of muscle tension and pressure on another part of the body (eg. hand) to increase the response to suggestion. This way the patient can imagine to capture the pain in one hand. The tighter the fist is held, the more pain is in the hand, and when by throwing the pain away it will not return for several hours

3. suggesting the pain away through defining the pain outside of the body by stating that the involved part is floating down again. Once the patient experiences the arm back down, he or she will no longer feel the pain in that specific part of the body (which now does not seem to belong to him or her).

The first example is a form of hypnoanesthesia. The pain of secondary effects of HIV infection may have a clear organic basis, and hypnosis may help control this pain. HIV seropositive individuals with persistent pain need more than mere pain control. The psychologic and emotional consequences of the disease and the pain must also be considered. Deep relaxation and hypnotic suggestion are useful in pain management because they act as a facilitator and intensifier of physical and occupational therapy. It also heightens the patient's concentration by helping to integrate positive affirmations. Most people have learned intuitively how to reach a "trance state" of consciousness just by restructuring their thought processes. This is a "mind set" similar to daydreaming that uses metaphors to produce the physical feeling of anesthesia. Patients can learn to produce self-hypnotic states through disciplined control of their attention. The patient learns to put painful stimuli at the periphery of his awareness by focusing on a competing sensation in another part of the body. Some patients can imagine temperature changes or the painful area becoming numb with novocaine. Self-hypnosis or the power of suggestion as used by the therapist can enhance the patient's control over pain perception. Physiologically, hypnosis is not well understood. However, scientific evidence suggests a hypnotic trance produces distinct changes in physiologic function. In one study, the subject suppressed his brain's electrical response to a visual stimulus by imagining a cardboard box blocking his view of the stimulus (Kleinkort et al., 1981).

Relaxation techniques, such as progressive relaxation and EMG biofeedback, offer the patient another opportunity to take time out from the perception of pain. There are many professionally recorded scripts for progressive relaxation available. Patients' personal preferences vary considerably. Some patients prefer a male's voice, whereas others achieve a greater sense of relaxation from a female voice. The type of music is highly personal as well. Some patients find certain scores of music undesirable and prefer ocean sounds or Chinese gong sounds for relaxation. Once the script and the background sounds are selected by both the patient and therapist, it is important that they are used consistently. By hearing the same tape each treatment session the patient develops a "neuronal model" or mental program for the stimulus and can "fall into the relaxed state" more efficiently each time. The relaxation response should be elicited one to two times per day in the minimum amount of time for effective results. If the sounds or scripts are changed frequently, it produces a novel stimulus and the reticular activating system in the brain stem triggers the autonomic nervous system or cortex to cause states of arousal.

EMG biofeedback gives the patient direct visual and auditory awareness of subliminal or covert reactions in voluntary muscles. Biofeedback is used for muscle reeducation in this context to teach the patient how to relax hypertonic muscle groups. The EMG biofeedback machine measures microvolts that are caused by the depolarization of muscle fibers in response to a neural impulse. As an adjunct to more traditional therapy, biofeedback has produced neuromuscular changes not achieved by conventional methods (Lehninger, 1975). The frontalis muscle and the upper trapezius serve as excellent indicators of emotional stress related to pain intensity. As the patient learns to focus on certain target muscles and voluntarily causes them to be less tense, generalized relaxation ensues. The success of any relaxation technique may be related to fatigue levels. Kampfer (1982) concluded that reduction of muscle tension requires concentration of body functions and sustained mental and physical effort.

Stress management techniques may be best suited for the patient living with HIV who exhibits a great deal of physical fatigue (see Appendix D). Strangely enough, relaxation helps to relieve fatigue because it can break the pain-fatigue cycle and be especially energizing to the person with HIV.

Another useful adjunct to pain management is to provide an opportunity for emotional ventilation. Weeping, wailing, moaning, groaning and crying have produced favorable results. According to Frey, a researcher and biochemist, emotional stress and pain produce toxic substances in the body (Bricklin, 1987). The act of crying produces tears that contain by-products of stress and harmful substances produced by the central nervous system. In our society, when an adult cries it is perceived as weakness and is often suppressed. Some psychologists feel that crying is an instinctual act that has evolutionary significance for survival.

Groaning is thought to be a variation on crying. Savary recommends providing a safe environment where the patient can fully verbalize (Bricklin, 1987). According to Savary, groaning facilitates a relaxation response by involving the body in gentle, rhythmic activity. The act of groaning may produce strong vibrations within the internal tissues of the body, which effect a type of inner massage. Some patients report that groaning deeply helps them to relax and that they can feel the vibrations in the throat, chest and stomach. Unfortunately, groaning out loud is thought to be inappropriate in the hospital setting and may prompt the physician and nursing staff to increase pain medication. Yet rehabilitation clinics can, in most cases, provide a room where groaning, crying and other vocalizations can take place as part of therapy.

Humor is another therapeutic technique that has enjoyed popular support. Norman Cousins awakened the medical community to the importance of humor by describing how it assisted him in recovering from a collagen disease, ankylosing spondylitis, and later myocardial infarction. Humor can assist the HIV-infected patient living with HIV to cope with pain by providing cognitive and emotional distance between the person and the perception of pain. One premise behind humor is that it provides a stimulus for laughter, which is a method of venting nervous energy (Simon, 1988). It has also been suggested that humor operates as a defense mechanism to enable individuals to cope with daily problems and moderates the effects of stress (Klein, 1989). Patients often use humor as an emotion-focused coping strategy to change their perception of catastrophic illness. It is important for the therapist to allow the patient to verbalize in order to decrease anxiety. During intense pain, the use of humor may be inappropriate, but may be used as the level subsides. If the patient initiates humor, it should be supported and encouraged. Listen to what topics the patient finds to be amusing. It is sometimes useful to make jest of invasive hospital routines, hospital food, or "the world's most embarrassing situations." Just talking with patients about events that make them laugh, allows them to initiate humor therapy for themselves. To date, the correlation between physical health and the therapeutic use of humor is limited. Cousins (1983:1), however, stated that "laughter accomplishes one very essential purpose. It tends to block deep feelings of apprehension and even panic that all too frequently accompany serious illness. It helps free the body of the constricting effects of the negative emotions that in turn may impair the healing system."

MANUAL THERAPY APPROACH

Manual therapy techniques are beneficial adjuvants, particularly when the virus has invaded the central or peripheral nervous systems or when opportunistic infections have caused viral-related myelitis. Myofascial release and craniosacral therapy are specific techniques that relieve pain and restore function (Barnes, 1990; Upledger & Vredevoogd, 1983). These techniques are a noninvasive, gentle effective

addition to the therapists repertoire of techniques.

The importance of the role of the fascial system in pain and dysfunction has been documented (Upledger & Vredevoogd, 1983). Malfunction, or the binding down of the fascia, may be the reason for various pain syndromes. The fascia is a tough connective tissue that spreads throughout the body three dimensionally without interruption. The facia surrounds all of the somatic and visceral structures of the human body. Therefore, malfunction of the fascial system due to trauma, posture or inflammation can create a binding down of the fascia, resulting in abnormal pressure on nerves, muscles, bones or organs. This pressure can create pain or malfunction, sometimes with side effects and seemingly unrelated symptoms, which do not always follow a specific pain pattern. It is difficult to diagnose because the standard tests that a patient with HIV may undergo to determine the etiology of pain (CT, myelograms, x-rays) do not demonstrate the fascia.

The craniosacral concept is a potent therapeutic pattern grounded on certain anatomic, physiologic, and therapeutic observations that have proven to be effective in patients with fever. The normal rhythmic motion is quite stable. It does not fluctuate as do the rates of the cardiovascular and respiratory systems in response to exercise, emotion and rest. Therefore, it is a reliable criterion for the evaluation of pathologic conditions. It has been observed that patients suffering from acute illnesses with fever will exhibit abnormally rapid rates (Upledger & Vredevoogd, 1983). Incorporating craniosacral and myofascial release techniques is particularly effective throughout the spectrum of HIV diseases as the patient experiences multiple episodes of fever secondary to opportunistic infections.

Therapeutic Touch

Touch is a universal and basic component of therapy. A modern version of the laying on of hands in therapy is a technique called therapeutic touch. This technique is based on the concepts of using touch, centering and energy transfer. Dolores Krieger (1976) introduced Therapeutic Touch in 1974; since then it has become a standard intervention technique taught in many nursing programs. Quinn (1988) provided an excellent review of research conducted on therapeutic touch since 1974. To date, therapeutic touch has been shown to increase hemoglobin levels, influence certain enzyme activity, alter brain waves, induce relaxation and reduce pain (Keller & Bzed, 1986; and Quinn, 1988). The process involves centering, a conscious meditative act of clearing the mind; establishing the feeling of compassion with the intent to help or heal; and passing the hands over the patients' body first to assess or feel for differences in the bioelectric field (human energy field) that extends over the physical body. With practice, one can feel or sense differences in the field around the patient's body. Once the hands have scanned over the body of the patient, the hands are gently placed over the areas of accumulated tension. A growing body of research and several personal experiences have shown therapeutic touch to be a powerful technique for the relief of pain. Therapeutic touch appears to influence the electrical potential of the human body, which is basically composed of positive and negative ions. By passing the hands over the body energy is transferred and the polarity of the ions is reestablished to create a sense of balance. Touch is the essential key to the therapists role in the healing process.

SUMMARY

The need for touch continues throughout our lives. For the person living with chronic HIV disease, caring touch is an essential ingredient to the sense of well-being. The therapist may have personal concerns about the spread of the disease or struggle with the ethical and moral conflicts that surround HIV, but the essence of therapy and pain management is the non-judgmental act of compassion conveyed by the personal contact between therapist and patient. Because of the nature of HIV and its psychologic and social consequences, the patient is in dire need of touch and a holistic approach to pain management. The term *Haelen* is the root word of healing and it means to make whole. The term holistic derives from the philosophy that the whole is greater than the sum of its parts. Holistic approaches harness the patients' own recuperative and regenerative energies within the mind, body and spirit, enabling their natural physiologic processes to heal from within.

References

Antoni, M.H., Fletcher, M.A., Laperriere, A., and Schniederman, N. (1989). Center for the Biopsychosocial Study of AIDS: Aerobic exercise training and psychoneuroimmunology in AIDS research. In Baum, A., and Temoshok, L. (Eds.): *Psychosocial Perspectives on AIDS*, Hillsdale, NJ: Lawrence Elbaum Associates. Earlbaum Associates, Inc.

Barnes, J.F. (1990). Evaluation and Treatment Techniques In *Myofacial Release: The search for Excellence* (pp 33-1 191). Paoli, PA: John F. Barnes, P.T. and Rehabilitation Services, Incorporated.

Biederbach, M.C. (1987). *Effects of Electro- Acuscope/ Myopulse Therapy an Accelerated Tissue Repair.* Los Angeles: Institute of Bio-Molecular Education and Research.

Bricklin, M. (1987). *Prevention's Simple Healing Technique* (pp. 59-60). Emmaus, PA: Rodale Press Inc.

Centers for Disease Control. (1988, January). *AIDS Weekly Surveillance Report for the United States.* 3:27.

Cornblath, D.R. (1988). Treatment of the neuromuscular complications of human immunodeficiency virus infection. *Annals of Neurology.* 23 (supplement):88.

Cousins, N. (1981). *Anatomy of an Illness.* New York: W.W. Norton.

Cummings, G., and Routan, B. (1987). Accuracy of unassisted pain drawings by patients with chronic pain. *Journal of Orthopedic and Sports Physical Therapy.* 8:391.

Empting-Koschorke, L.D., Hendler, N., Kolodry, L.A., and Fraus, H. (1989, June). When pain is intractable. *Patient Care.* 23:107.

Fields, J.L. (1987). *Pain* (pp. 99-125, 171-198). New York: McGraw Hill Book Co.

Galantino, M.L., and Brewer, M. (1989, July). Peripheral neuropathies associated with AIDS-A case study in pain management for HIV. *Occupational Therapy Forum.* 11-1 13.

Galantino, M.L., and Spence, D. (1988). Physical medicine management of HIV patients. (pp 181-189). In *Nursing Care of the Person with AIDS/ARC.* Rockville, MD: Aspen Publications.

Genden, E., Lower, M., Beattie, S., and Beck, N. (1989). Effects of music and imagery on physiologic and self-report of analogued labor pain. *Nursing Research.* 38(1):37.

Green, M., Dunkel, E.C., and Pavan-Langston, D. (1987). Effect of immunization and immunosuppression on induced ocular shedding and recovery of herpes simplex virus in infected rabbits. *Experimental Eye Research.* 45:375.

Green, M.T., Rosborough, J.P., and Dunkel, E.C. (1981). In vivo reactivation of herpes simplex virus in rabbit trigeminal ganglia electrode model. *Infection and Immunity.* 34:69.

Guyton, A. (1987). *Basic Neuroscience-Anatomy and Physiology.* (pp 173-176). Philadelphia: W.B. Saunders Co.

Hall, N., and Goldstein, A. (1986). Thinking well: The chemical links between emotions and health. *The Sciences.* 26(2):34.

Hammer, S. (1984, April). The mind as healer. *Science Digest.* 47-50.

Healy R., and Coleman, T. (1989). A primer on AIDS for health professionals. *Health Education.* 19(6):4.

Hidelman, D. (1980). Fatigue: Towards an analysis and unified definition. *Medical Hypotheses.* 6:517.

Hilton, G. (1989). AIDS dementia. *Journal of Neuroscience Nursing.* 21(1):24.

Johnson, M. (1977). Assessment of clinical pain. In Jacux, A.K. (Ed): *Pain: A Source Book for Nurses and Other Health Professionals.* (pp. 139-166). Boston: Little Brown and Company.

Johnson, R., and McArthur, J. (1986). AIDS and the brain. *Trends in Neurosciences.* 9(30):91.

Kampfer, S.H. (1982). Relaxation training reconsidered. *Oncology Nursing Forum.* 9:15.

Keller, E., and Bzed, V.M. (1986). The effects of therapeutic touch on tension headache pain. *Nursing Research.* 35(2):101.

Klein, A. (1989). *The Healing Power of Humor..* Los Angeles: Jeremy P. Tarcher.

Kleinkort, J., Cook, M., and Webster, J., et al. (1981). *Therapeutic Medical Devices.* (p. 235). New York: Prentice Hall.

Krieger, D. (1976). Healing by the "laying on" of hands as a facilitator of bioenergetic change: The response of in vivo human hemoglobin. *Psychoenergetic System.* 1:121.

Lasagna, L. (1986, October). Pain and its management. *Hospital Practice.* 21:92.

Laskin, M.E. (1988). Pain management in the patient with AIDS. *Journal of Advanced Surgical Nursing.* 1(1):37.

Lawlis, F., Cuencas, R., Selby, D., and McCoy E. (1989). The development of the Dallas pain questionnaire. *Spine.* 14(5):511.

Lebovits, A.H., Lefkowitx, M., McCarthy, D., et al. (1989) The prevalence and management of pain in patients with AIDS: A review of 134 cases. *The Clinical Journal of Pain.* 5:245.

Lehninger, A.L. (1975). *Biochemistry.* (p. 995). New York: Worth Publishers.

Lein, D.H., Clelland, J., Knowles, C.J., and Jackson, J.R. (1989). Comparison of effects of transcutaneous electrical nerve stimulation of auricular, somatic and the combination of auricular and somatic points on experimental pain threshold. *Physical Therapy.* 69(8):671.

Levy, R., Bredesen, D., and Rosenblum, M. (1985). Neurological manifestations of the acquired immunodeficiency syndrome (AIDS). *Journal of Neurosurgery.* 62:475.

Longobardi, A.G., Clellund, J.A., and Knowles, C.J. (1989). Effects of auricular transcutaneous electrical nerve stimulation on distal extremity pain: A pilot study. *Physical Therapy.* 69:10.

Macek, C. (1983). Adjunctive role for biofeedback neuromuscular rehabilitation. *Medical News.* 12:1533.

McCormack, G. (1988). Pain management by occupational therapists. *American Journal of Occupational Therapy.* 42(9):582.

McCormack, G. (1990). Psychophysiological theories of pain and implication for treatment. *Occupational Therapy Practice.* 1(3):1.

McCormack, G.L., and Johnson, C. (1990). Systems of objectifying clinical pain. *Occupational Therapy Practice.* 1(3):17.

McGuire, D. (1984). The measurement of clinical pain. *Nursing Research.* 33:152.

Melzack, R. (1975). The McGill pain questionnaire: Major properties and scoring methods. *Pain.* 1:277.

Melzack, R. (1981). Myofascial trigger points: Relation to acupuncture and mechanisms of pain. *Archives of Physical Medicine and Rehabilitation.* 62:47.

Melzack, R., Stillwell, D., and Fox, E. (1977). Trigger points and acupuncture points for pain: Correlations and implications. *Pain.* 1:3.

Nelson, W. (1986). Clinical management of AIDS patients. *California Nurse.* 82 (4):10.

Newshan, G., Wainapel, S., and Schmitx, D. (1989). Pain related syndromes and their treatment in persons with AIDS. Paper presented at Eighth Annual Scientific Meeting of the American Pain Society, Phoenix, Arizona.

Olsson, G., and Parker, G. (1987). A model approach to pain assessment. *Nursing 87.* 17(5):52.

Parry, G.J. (1988). Peripheral neuropathies associated with human immunodeficiency virus infection. *Annals of Neurology.* 23:S49.

Pert, C.B., Ruff, M.R., and Weber, R.J. (1985). Neuropeptides and their receptors: A psychosomatic network. *Journal of Immunology.* 135 (2):820.

Picker, R.J. (1989). Current Trends, Parts I and II. *Clinical Management.* 9 (2):10.

Pomeranz, B., and Gabriel, S. (1987). Acupuncture Neurophysiology. In Adelman, G. (Ed.) Berlin, NY, Springer-Verlag 2:6-7.

Quinn, J.F. (1988). Building a body of knowledge: Research on therapeutic touch. 1974-1986. *Journal of Holistic Nursing.* 6(1):37.

Seitz, L., and Kleinkort, J. (1986). Low power laser: Its application in physical therapy. In Micholvitz (Ed.): *Thermal Agents In Rehabilitation.* Philadelphia: F.A. Davis.

Simon, J.M. (1988). Therapeutic humor: Who's fooling whom? *Journal of Psychosocial Nursing.* 26(4):9.

Spiegel, D. (1987, March-April). The healing trance. *The Sciences.* 35-39.

Stumf, K. (1989). Mechanisms to account for biofeedback's effect on motor control. *Occupational Therapy Forum.* 4(47):3.

Stux, G., and Pomeranz, B. (1987). *Acupuncture Textbook and Atlas.* New York: Springer-Verlag.

Tait, C., Pollard, C., and Margolis, B. (1987). The pain disability index: Psychometric and validity data. *Archives of Physical Medicine and Rehabilitation.* 68:438.

Taylor, A.F. (1987). Pain. *Annual Review of Nursing Research.* 5:23.

Upledger, J.E., and Vredevoogd, J.D. (1983). The craniosacral concept: Basic terminology. In *Craniosacral Therapy.* (pp. 5-25). Seattle: Eastland Press.

Wall, P.D. (1987). Pain: Neurophysiological mechanisms. In Adelman, G. (Ed.): *Encyclopedia of Neuroscience.* vol. II, (pp. 904-906). Boston: Birkhauser.

Weshsler, R. (1987, February). A new prescription: Mind over malady. *Discover.* vol. 23 (pp. 51-61).

World Health Organization. (1986). *Cancer pain relief.* Comprehensive Cancer Pain Management. Washington, D.C. (pp. 14-23).

11

Neurobehavioral Considerations

Joel K. Levy, PhD

Memory is not just the imprint of the past time upon us; it is the keeper of what is meaningful for our deepest hopes and fears.

—Andre Maurois

INTRODUCTION

As if the diseases that result from the decline of the immune response due to HIV were not catastrophic enough, HIV is neurotropic and causes CNS and PNS disorders, including dementia and organic psychiatric syndromes (Perry & Marotta, 1987), movement disorders (Nath et al., 1987) and neuropathies and myopathies (Cornblath & McArthur, 1988; Lange et al., 1988; So et al., 1988; Simpson & Bender, 1988; Gaut, et al., 1988). The psychosocial stresses associated with learning that one has a chronic disorder and coming to grips with the multitude of fears that accompany that realization were thought to precipitate major functional psychiatric disorders. However, it was also observed that the virus itself may bring about depression, resulting from brain dysfunction (Brew et al., 1988). Therefore, HIV has a perplexing quality: It causes extreme distress, in that the awareness that one has a catastrophic illness may precipitate anxiety, sadness and despondency to the point of losing touch with reality; it also attacks brain areas, which leads to impairment of cognitive function, depression, mania or psychosis (Perry & Marotta, 1987). It is thus extremely important not to label any psychiatric symptomatology as being reactive, especially after the first few months after diagnosis of seropositivity, when the possibility of organically based disturbances may be increasing and medical intervention may postpone profound disability. Thus, challenge exists to appropriately diagnose behavioral problems in HIV spectrum disorders. Those providing care for the HIV seropositive patient should be familiar with the most up-to-date knowledge on the virus' neurotropic effect in order to understand the processes going on within their patients. This investigation may include electrophysiologic, neuroimaging and neuropsychologic assessment and, perhaps, pharmacotherapeutic trials. Short-term discomfort may thus be minimized and long-term planning for the patient's care may be coordinated.

THE SEARCH FOR THE ETIOLOGY OF HIV ENCEPHALOPATHY

The complete mechanism of HIV encephalopathy is, as yet, undetermined. It is known that cells in the nervous system (Hill et al., 1987) possess the receptor for the virus. Theoretically, if the virus can gain entry into the substance of the nervous system, it may either attach to this receptor and replicate or go into dormancy. The cell may be destroyed in replicating the virus (Brew et al., 1988). The viral activity within the cell may also disrupt the cell's metabolism and dysregulate neurochemical functions (Brew et al., 1988).

Price and colleagues (Brew et al., 1988) have described the distribution of HIV in the brain and the distribution of infected macrophages, microglia and multinucleated giant-cells. They found that patients with dementia did not necessarily have productive infections (viral release) in the brain. They proposed that HIV-related central nervous system impairment comes from the production of some types of toxic substances. These toxic substances have not been totally characterized; however, the more demented the patients, the more frequently cellular changes are found. Thus, production or nonproduction of virus in CNS infection appears to be one index of the severity of the impact on the brain.

Another possibility for the neurologic problems is that the virus causes demyelination, as might be suspected of an agent that attacks the brain white matter. However, Marshall et al. (1989), in investigating the protein content of cerebral spinal fluid from HIV seropositive patients, found no significant increase in myelin basic protein in the CSF. Increase in myelin basic protein have been linked to an increase in demyelination. These co-workers failed to detect this protein in HIV disease in comparison to increases found in the demyelinating disorders such as multiple sclerosis. They concluded that demyelination may not be the most likely cause of HIV neurologic problems.

Using positron emission tomography (PET), regional metabolic abnormalities have been identified subcortically, and increased metabolism of glucose has been found in the basal ganglion and thalamus early in the course of HIV infection (Brunetti et al., 1989). This development is followed by a regional and then a generalized lowered metabolism of glucose as the involvement progresses. Such findings support the notion that the virus is interrupting, by toxic substance or by morphologic change, neurotransmission or metabolism, which may affect the passage of information from one cell to another. PET has also proved useful in reflecting the therapeutic response of the disease to antiviral treatment with AZT. Brunetti et al. (1989) described reversal of metabolic abnormalities in the brain cortex after treatment with AZT. They found increased glucose metabolism after treatment which they correlated in improved brain glucose utilization with improved neurologic function. This result may reflect the ability of AZT to diminish viral activity and the inflammation that accompanies it, therefore allowing metabolism and neurotransmission to normalize.

Regarding the specific neurotransmitters that may be the target of HIV interruptions, Hollander et al. (1986), in an early finding of CNS sensitivity to dopaminergic medication, proposed a dopamine dysregulation hypothesis for CNS involvement with HIV. They found that patients treated with dopaminergic agonists for Parkinsonian movement disorders became psychotic. Other studies have found that acutely psychotic HIV patients, treated with dopamine antagonists, developed severe Parkinsonian symptoms. From these two separate directions, HIV encephalopathic patients treated with dopaminergic drugs demonstrated extreme sensitivity to these types of medications. Additionally, from a localization perspective, Pert and colleagues (Hill et al., 1987) have found large numbers of cells with the CD4 receptor, the receptor for the virus, in areas of the brain usually associated with movement, affective and cognitive functions in the temporal limbic areas and in basal ganglia.

These areas are also known to have dopaminergic cells. In a series of studies, Fernandez et al. (1988) found that the use of the dopamine agonist methylphenidate improved mood and cognitive functioning in patients with HIV encephalopathy. In these cases, methylphenidate did not seem to drive the patients into a severe psychotic condition or thought disorder, but rather lifted mood and brought rate of information processing into an improved range. The selectivity of HIV in dysregulating dopaminergic cells appears to be a possible hypothesis in the encephalopathy, and more research is needed to determine whether manipulation of this neurotransmitter system can help with the effects of HIV-related affective, cognitive and behavioral deficits.

DIAGNOSIS OF HIV ENCEPHALOPATHY

CT and MRI have also been helpful in diagnosing involvement of the brain in HIV-seropositive patients (Kelly & Brandt-Zawadzki, 1983; Jarvik et al., 1988). These techniques have demonstrated brain substance changes by lucency or signal intensity, indicative of involvement of areas of white matter known to be the target of HIV effects. MRI has been especially useful in demonstrating areas of involvement in the white matter using the T2-weighted signals (Brew et al., 1988). T1-relaxation times have not demonstrated clear differences between a matched population of aged HIV-seropositive patients and controls (Freund-Levi et al., 1989).

As mentioned before, analysis of cerebral spinal fluid from lumbar puncture has been useful in delineating what happens cellularly as a result of HIV-CNS infection. Marshall et al. (1989) failed to find increase in myelin basic protein, which argued against a demyelinating process as the cause of HIV encephalopathy. However, it has been shown that HIV viral particles are present in CSF (Brew et al., 1988), implying that the virus may break through the brain-CSF barrier and circulate freely. Immunoglobulin (IgG) has been demonstrated in CSF in abnormally large quantities and has been an indication of HIV-CNS infection (Elovaara et al., 1988). The amount of virus and antibody, however, has not been helpful in reflecting the range and severity of neurologic involvement (Reboul et al., 1989). However, another constituent of CSF, beta-2-microglobulin, has recently been found to be more highly correlated with dementia severity (Brew et al., 1989; Elovaara et al., 1989). There was a high correlation between amount and both the severity of HIV dementia and the severity of constitutional disease.

Another useful diagnostic tool has been electrophysiologic investigation. Studies have shown that the electroencephalogram (EEG) becomes more abnormal and the percentage of patients showing abnormal EEG is in correlation with worsening constitutional illness (Gabuzda et al., 1988; Parisi et al., 1989). The latter determined that one fourth of asymptomatic patients had abnormal EEGs. In their sample of patients with persistent generalized lymphadenopathy, 30 percent showed a variety of abnormalities, from frontotemporal theta slowing to diffuse theta slowing to frontotemporal delta activity. These electrophysiologic disturbances occurred in patients even before the onset of AIDS (Parisi et al., 1989). The study be Gabuzda et al. (1985) demonstrated that 35 percent of patients with symptomatic HIV complex had mild to severe abnormal findings and about two thirds of patients with AIDS had mild to severe abnormal EEG; a common sign was intermittent or continuous theta or delta activity in both hemispheres.

Electrophysiologic evoked response studies are also helpful in screening for disorders in the central nervous system. Smith et al. (1988), using brain stem auditory potentials and somatosensory evoked potentials, found significant prolonging of response latency measures compared to responses in non-infected individuals. Such a delay of latency was deemed reflective of impaired neural transmission. These abnormalities may be an early indication of neurologic involvement.

PRESENTATIONS OF HIV ENCEPHALOPATHY

HIV spectrum disorders have been compared to syphilis, another formerly widespread illness that caused a multiplicity of problems including systemic and neurologic dysfunctions. Because of the variety of presentations, syphilis was called the "great imitator." Perry and Marotta (1987) have called HIV the "new great imitator" in its ability to simulate many types of systemic, neurologic and psychiatric diseases. It is important to have careful medical and neurobehavioral examinations to determine any organic contribution and to delay worsening of the disorder.

The disease has many neurobehavioral presentations. Frequently encountered neurobehavioral effects in HIV disease are organic mental disorders (OMDs), including delirium, dementia, and organic affective disorder and stress-distress disorders such as anxiety syndromes. Organic personality disorder and organic delusional disorder may also occur (Perry & Marotta, 1987).

Delirium

Delirium is seen in end stages of HIV disease and is characterized as a widespread brain metabolic disturbance (Lipowski, 1987). It may begin with difficulty in thinking, restlessness, and memory problems and may be confused with other OMDs such as dementia or amnestic syndrome. Irritability may be present. Misperceptions and other visual illusions may occur and sleep may be disturbed. A mental status examination focuses on the *Diagnostic and Statistical Manual of Mental Disorders* (American Psychiatric Association, 1987). Criteria such as arousal, attention, short-term memory and orientation may uncover characteristic deficits. Care givers should also be alert to patients' fluctuations in symptoms. Involuntary movements are also common. Aggressive and swift treatment with pharmacologic agents appears to offer the most hope of countering delirium (Fernandez et al., 1989).

Dementia

Dementia is a permanent intellectual impairment of often broad scope and may include problems in memory, language, cognition, visuospatial skills and personality. It is a frequent neurologic complication of HIV infection. The dementia of HIV disorders appears to involve a subcortical degenerative process. This subcortical type of impairment usually affects functions of alertness, arousal, memory and rate of information processing (Filley et al., 1989). HIV-related inflammation of brain white matter appears to cause degradation of the neural signal in this condition, as opposed to other primary degenerative dementias, such as that of the Alzheimer's type. This distinction between cortical and subcortical dementia, however, has been criticized (Whitehouse, 1986). Both areas are affected in HIV encephalopathy, but the characteristics of the disturbance make it more appropriate to term it primarily subcortical. Neuropsychologic tests that assess memory registration, storage and retrieval, psychomotor speed, information processing rate and fine motor function are most helpful to quantify cognitive disturbance (Fernandez & Levy, in press). Syndromes such as aphasia, agnosia, apraxia, motoric, visuospatial, and sensory-perceptual functions may also be encountered, usually later in the course of the disease. Focal opportunistic infection or neoplastic invasion of the CNS usually accounts for these specific cortical events.

Early signs and symptoms, both cognitive and psychiatric, of HIV dementia are detailed in Table 11-1 (Brew et al., 1988; Levy & Fernandez, 1989). These may be considered as effects of the systemic illness or sometimes as a psychologic reaction to learning about or living with HIV infection. Forgetfulness, attention and concentration deficits, slowing of mental processing and loss of interest in everyday activities fall into this category. Patients may be painfully aware of these deficits, which may engender further distress and cognitive problems.

Table 11-1
EARLY SIGNS AND SYMPTOMS OF HIV-RELATED
NEUROBEHAVIORAL IMPAIRMENT

COGNITIVE	AFFECTIVE/BEHAVIORAL
Memory difficulties (especially affecting verbal rote or episodic)	Apathy Depressed mood
Concentration/attention impairment	Anxiety
Comprehension impairment	Agitation Mild disinhibition
Visuospatial/manual constructional difficulties	Hallucinations
Psychomotor slowing or dyscoordination	
Mental tracking difficulties	
Mild frontal lobe dysfunction	
Handwriting and fine motor control difficulties	
Problem-solving difficulties	

Brew, B.J. Sidtis, J.J., Petito, C.K. and Price R.W. (1988). The neurologic complications of AIDS and Human immunodeficiency virus infection. In Plum, F. (Ed.): Advances in Contemporary Neurology. Used with permission.

Table 11-2
LATE SIGNS AND SYMPTOMS OF HIV-RELATED
NEUROBEHAVIORAL IMPAIRMENT

COGNITIVE	AFFECTIVE/BEHAVIORAL
Global dementia	Severe disinhibition
Mutism	Mania
Aphasia	Delusions
Severe frontal lobe dysfunction	Severe hallucinations
Severe psychomotor retardation	Agitation
Distractibility	Paranoia
Disorientation	Severe depression
	Suicidal ideation

Brew, B.J., Sidtis, J.J., Petitio, C.K. and Price, R.W. (1988). The neurological complications of AIDS and Human immunodeficiency virus infection. In Plum, F. (Ed.): Advances in Contemporary Neurology. Used with permission.

Symptoms of cognitive and psychiatric disorders seen late in the course of the disease (Brew et al., 1988; Fernandez & Levy, in press) are described in Table 11-2. The dementia may progress to moderate or severe cognitive deficits, motor involvement and seizures (Brew et al., 1988). Disinhibited behavior; psychosis; motor disturbances such as ataxia, spasticity and hyperreflexia; incontinence of bladder and bowel; muteness; and catatonia may be present.

The signs and symptoms of the AIDS dementia complex are not difficult to identify in the late stages of the immune decline, when severe wasting and frequent bouts of illness occur. In the early stages, however, controversy continued about what constitutes the early stages of cognitive involvement. Results of neuropsychologic evaluations revealed that asymptomatic infected subjects, carefully screened for prior drug and neuropsychiatric histories, did not differ from seronegative, matched controls on cognitive tasks (McArthur et al., 1989; Goethe et al., 1989). Other studies have shown differences between seropositive asymptomatic patients and seronegative patients on such direct physiologic measures as eye movements (Tervo et al., 1986; Currie et al., 1988) and evoked potentials (Goodin et al., 1990). If

cognitive impairments are to be detected in the early stages of HIV disorders, sensitive tasks requiring memory and retrieval, speed of information processing, problem solving and sometimes verbal fluency are helpful in making this assessment (Kovner et al., 1989; Van Gorp et al., 1989; Tross et al., 1988). Table 11-3 lists neuropsychologic tests that have been found useful in delineating the degree of the cognitive problems of HIV encephalopathy (Fernandez & Levy, in press). Also included are tasks that screen for focal opportunistic infections that may occur in the CNS.

If a tumor or focal infection in the brain develops as a result of immune decline, then neuropsychologic deficits can be as varied as the areas these opportunistic events may affect. Toxoplasmosis, fungal infections and lymphoma all may occur anywhere in the brain and thus may appear as symptoms resembling a stroke or tumor (Bredesen et al., 1988). Focal motor or sensory deficits may develop. Personality changes including mood alteration, inappropriate behaviors, loss of planning and goal-directed activities may occur with frontal involvement. Visual perceptual difficulties may occur with occipital lesions. Aphasia, anomia and verbal memory problems may occur with involvement of the dominant hemisphere's temporal lobes. Visuospatial difficulties may occur with nondominant hemisphere parietooccipital lesions. Any text on localization of lesions in neuropsychology (eg. Kertesz, 1983) describes the characteristic areas involved with these neurobehavioral symptoms. A comprehensive neurobehavioral examination must be undertaken to quantify these deficits in a person presenting with a history of HIV seropositivity and new cognitive, behavioral or mood complaints. This examination, along with a neuroimaging study, will characterize the location and behavioral impact of the lesion. Post-treatment testing can disclose residual cognitive deficits and help in planning for rehabilitation, both physical and cognitive, to attempt to restore the best possible function for continuing daily activities.

At this time, there is no definitive treatment for the dementia of HIV. Some of the cognitive/memory impairment may be helped with the psychostimulant methylphenidate (Fernandez et al., 1988). This medication has significantly improved mental tracking, information processing rate and long-term memory storage. AZT has also been shown to improve neuropsychologic functioning in severely ill patients as compared to placebo (Schmitt et al., 1988). This antiviral drug has also been shown to directly affect neurophysiologic function in the form of glucose utilization by the brain, a marker of brain metabolism. As previously described, after patients received AZT, PET scans showed improved brain metabolism (Brunetti et al., 1989).

The impact of this dementia on practical issues such as ADL is under study. One may document deficits in basic areas of cognitive functioning with neuropsychologic tests, which then relate to categories of difficulty in real life. However, a global index is needed to describe how this condition may affect a person's integrated behavioral functioning. The Global Deterioration Scale (Table 11-4), which was developed for use in geriatric patients to measure the impact of Alzheimer-type dementia (Reisberg et al., 1982), offers a sensitive measure of the impact of HIV encephalopathy and dementia. This scale can be used to quantify whether the impairment has reached a level that interferes with independent functioning. It may suggest the need for more skilled care than that which can be given by family or friends. The scale can also distinguish between levels of systemic disease; patients with the more severe immune decline as indicated by severe constitutional symptoms were more frequently in the upper ranges of the scale than those with only lymph gland involvement (Fernandez & Levy, in press). It was also found, however, that significant confusion or early dementia could occur in those with less systemic involvement. This fact should be kept in mind while working with this spectrum of disorders.

ORGANIC MOOD SYNDROMES

Because of its affinity for mood-related structures in the CNS, HIV causes organic mood syndromes frequently. Almost 85 percent of HIV-seropositive patients will develop

---

Table 11-3
HIV NEUROPSYCHOLOGICAL SCREENING BATTERY

General
Mini-Mental State Examination

Memory
Buschke-Fuld Verbal Selective Reminding Test
Wechsler Memory Scale Logical Memory Passages
Benton Visual Retention Test
Rey-Osterrieth Complex Figure (copy; 3 and 45 min. recall)

Language/Speech
Controlled Oral Word Association (from Benton Multilingual Aphasia Examination)
Visual Naming Test (from Benton Multilingual Aphasia Examination)

Orientation
Pfeiffer Short Portable Mental Status Questionnaire
Benton Temporal Orientation Test

Visuospatial
Bender-Gestalt Test
Raven Progressive Matrices

Intellectual/ Executive Psychomotor
Similarities, Digit Span, Arithmetic, Digit Symbol from the WAIS or WAIS-R
Trail Making Test, Parts A and B
Wisconsin Card Sorting
Finger Tapping Test
Grooved or Purdue Pegboard
Reaction time—simple auditory, simple visual, and four-choice visual
Shipley Institute of Living Scale
Stroop Color Word Test

HIV neuropsychological screening battery (From Fernandez F. and Levy J.K. (in press). Adjuvant treatment of HIV dementia with psychostimulant. In Ostrow, D. (Ed.): Behavioral Aspects of AIDS and Other Sexually Transmitted Disease. Used with permission.

some type of mood disorder at some time during the course of the illness (Perry & Tross, 1984). Differentiating these disorders is a complex task that requires more physical investigation than is usually appropriate for seronegative persons.

Mania

Mania has been observed in patients with HIV much less often than depression. In view of the fact that HIV encephalopathy usually involves psychomotor slowing, apathy and hypoattention, a presentation of mania is usually a result of

Table 11-4
GLOBAL DETERIORATION SCALE (GDS) FOR AGE-ASSOCIATED COGNITIVE DECLINE

GDS Stage	Clinical Phase	Clinical Characteristics
1. No cognitive decline	Normal	No subjective complaints of memory deficit. No memory deficit evident on clinical interview.
2. Very mild cognitive decline	Forgetfulness	Subjective complaints of memory mild deficit, most frequently in cognitive following areas: 1) forgetting where one has placed familiar objects, 2) forgetting names one formerly knew well. No objective evidence of memory deficit on clinical situations. Appropriate concern with respect to symptomatology.
3. Mild cognitive decline	Early confusional	Earliest clear-cut deficits. Manifestations in more than one of the following: 1) patient may have gotten lost when traveling to an unfamiliar location, 2) co-workers become aware of patient's relatively poor performance, 3) word and name finding deficits become evident to intimates, 4) patient may read a passage or a book and retain relatively little material, 5) patient may demonstrate decreased ability in remembering names upon introduction to new people, 6) patient may have lost or misplaced an object of value, 7) concentration deficit may be evident on clinical testing.
		Objective evidence of memory deficit obtained only with an intensive interview conducted by neuropsychiatrist or neuropsychologist. Decreased performance in demanding employment and social settings. Denial begins to become manifest in patient. Mild to moderate anxiety accompanies symptoms.
4. Moderate cognitive decline	Late confusional	Clear-cut deficit on careful clinical interview. Deficit manifest in following areas: 1) decreased knowledge of current and recent events, 2) may exhibit some deficit in memory of one's personal history, 3) concentration deficit elicited on serial subtractions, 4) decreased ability to travel, handle finances, etc.
		Frequently no deficit in following areas: 1) orientation to time and person, 2) recognition of familiar persons and faces, 3) ability to travel to familiar locations.
		Inability to perform complex tasks. Denial is dominant defense mechanism. Flattening of affect and withdrawal from challenging situations occur.
5. Moderately severe	Early dementia	Patient can no longer survive without some assistance. Patient is unable during interview to recall a major relevant aspect of their current lives, eg. their address or telephone number of many years, the name of close member of their family, the names of the high school or college from which they graduated.
		Frequently some disorientation to time (date, day of week, season, etc.) or to place. An educated person may have difficulty counting back from 40 by 4s or from 20 by 2s.
		Persons at this stage retain knowledge of many major facts about themselves and others. They invariably know the name of their significant others. They require no assistance with toileting or eating, but may have some difficulty choosing the proper clothing to wear.

continued . . .

Table 11-4 (continued)
GLOBAL DETERIORATION SCALE (GDS) FOR AGE-ASSOCIATED COGNITIVE DECLINE

GDS Stage	Clinical Phase	Clinical Characteristics
6. Severe cognitive decline	Middle dementia	May occasionally forget the name of significant others upon whom they are entirely dependent for survival. Will be largely unaware about recent events and experiences in their lives. Retain some knowledge of their lives, but this is very sketchy. Generally aware of their surroundings, the year, the season, etc. May have difficulty counting from 10, both backward and sometimes forward. Will require some assistance but occasionally will display ability to travel to familiar locations. Diurnal rhythm frequently disturbed. Almost always recall their own name. Frequently continue to be able to distinguish familiar from unfamiliar persons in their environment.
		Personality and emotional changes occur. These are quite variable and include: 1) delusional behavior, eg. patients may accuse their significant others of being an imposter, may talk to imaginary figures in the environment, or to their own reflection in the mirror, 2) obsessive symptoms, eg. person may continually repeat simple cleaning activities, 3) anxiety symptoms, agitation, and even previously nonexistent violent behavior may occur, 4) cognitive abulia, ie. loss of willpower because an individual cannot carry a thought long enough to determine a purposeful course of action.
7. Very severe cognitive decline	Late dementia	All verbal abilities are lost. Frequently there is no speech at all—only grunting. Incontinent of urine; requires assistance toileting and feeding. Lose basic psychomotor skills, eg. ability to walk. The brain appears to no longer be able to tell the body what to do.
		Generalized and cortical neurologic signs and symptoms.

From Reisberg, B., Ferris, S.H., deLeon, M.J., et al., (1984). Clinical assessment of cognition on the aged. In Shamoran, C.A. (ed.), Biology and treatment of Dementia in the Elderly. Clinical Insight Series. Washington, DC: American Psychiatric press, Inc. Used with permission.

focal infections or neoplasia in areas associated with this mood disorder. However, HIV and herpes may induce mania. A case associated with a right frontal lymphoma has been encountered. Mania may also result from neurotoxicity of medication used to treat other aspects of HIV disorder, and cases of AZT-induced mania have been reported (O'Dowd & McKegney, 1988). Lithium, which is effective in treating idiopathic bipolar disorder, may also be useful in managing this disorder.

Depression

Ascertaining the appropriate diagnosis of depression in HIV disease is difficult because of 1) the diverse etiologies of the same overt presentation, 2) the concomitant feelings of hopelessness that can accompany these diverse etiologies, and, 3) systemic symptoms of depression (such as appetite change, difficulty with concentration, and sleep disturbance) that overlap both HIV systemic disease and the diverse depressive syndromes (Fernandez, 1989). Thus, criteria used to diagnose depression in a standard way (eg. DSM-III-R) may not be applicable to the weighing of vegetative and psychological symptoms. Some investigators have proposed that in HIV-related depression, the psychological facets such as guilt, feelings of hopelessness and suicidality be weighted more in the differentiation of depression from the systemic disease (Cavanaugh et al., 1983; Clark et al., 1983). The DSM-III-R should be consulted for specific criteria and their time frames for making such a determination.

Depression in HIV may have many causes. Among them are medication side effects, viral or other infective involvement of mood control centers in the brain and reaction or adjustment difficulties to the illness itself. Viral etiologies include HIV itself, cytomegalovirus, Epstein-Barr virus and herpes simplex. Central nervous system tumors that are AIDS-related may also involve the mood centers. Likewise, vascular disorders (Vinters et al., 1988; Scaravelli et al., 1989; Frank et al., 1989; Engstrom et al., 1989), which sometimes stem from varicella-zoster vasculitis may also cause strokes that may be associated with organic depression. These involvements are usually lateralized to the left hemisphere. Neurotoxicity from some antimicrobial, antiviral and immunorestorative agents may also induce depression.

Treatment of depression of any type in the HIV seropositive patient requires caution. We have found that the HIV-involved nervous system is often more sensitive to drug effects than the CNS in some other systemic medical illnesses. Therefore, a trial of any antidepressive agent should begin cautiously with a low dose. When tricyclic antidepressants are used, the associated anticholinergic activity may cause side effects. Fernandez and co-workers (1988) have found that, in some more advanced patients, depression responds to treatment with a psychostimulant (Holmes et al., 1989). These compounds have some adverse effects and must be carefully administered and closely observed by a physician experienced with their use. (eg. Some patients have experienced a syndrome of abnormal movements or involuntary movements precipitated by these compounds.) Nevertheless, these drugs seem to improve mood, condition and even, paradoxically, appetite in many cases.

Anxiety

Obviously anxiety frequently accompanies HIV disease. Many stresses revolve around this set of disorders and the experiences that go along with them (Fernandez, 1989). Stress and distress develop from the beginning, with the notification of the results of antibody testing (Fernandez, 1989). The distress may recur with indicators of progression from one stage of HIV disease to another.

When supportive measures for caregivers and family fail to provide relief in cases of stress, pharmacotherapy with anxiolytic medication may provide for reduction of this distress. Under careful administration and supervision, these agents help without inducing dependency. One must also keep in mind, however, that anxiety disorders may also have an organic basis. There may be involvement of those centers of the brain mediating these responses by viral infective or neoplastic processes. In these cases, a search for this organic etiology must be done to abate the distress.

Other Organic Syndromes

In some cases, viral or neoplastic involvement may involve specific centers of the brain that control memory or personality function. Thus, one may get an amnestic disor-

der with involvement of the temporolimbic areas by herpes, which leaves other cognitive functions relatively intact. In addition, the virus, a vascular event or a circumscribed tumor, may involve only frontal areas, causing change in personality (the organic personality syndrome). Higher cognitive functioning of memory and other visuospatial perceptive functions may be spared, but there is a marked change in the person's personality, with either disinhibition and inappropriate actions or statements or an overwhelming behavioral inertia that causes loss of motivation and, even further, withdrawal from everyday activities.

Because intravenous substance use is one of the risk factors for HIV infection, one must also be sensitive to the fact that these individuals may continue to use these medications and suffer further cognitive impairment. There is an especially serious risk associated with the illicit use of stimulants, either intravenously administered or inhaled. Use of such agents as amphetamines and cocaine has been associated with cerebrovascular infarcts in non HIV-infected substance abuse patients (Nolte & Gelman, 1989; Nalls et al., 1989; Rothrock et al., 1988; Wojak & Flamm, 1987). If patients continue to use these stimulants, the risk for cerebrovascular problems and associated cognitive impairment resulting from this brain injury would seem to increase, especially in the presence of a weakened vasculature due to the viral vasculitis sometimes encountered in HIV spectrum disorders. Data are currently lacking on this problem, but studies are in progress. This example provides another instance of the way that functional behavioral problems may overlap with organic mental disturbances in this spectrum of disorders.

CASE STUDY

This case study illustrates the overlap of multiple neurobehavioral disabilities encountered in HIV spectrum disorders. A 55-year-old man with a history of substance abuse was referred for neuropsychologic evaluation after a suicide attempt. He had developed PCP two years earlier, at which time he was diagnosed with AIDS. He previously had a diagnosis of HIV encephalopathy, as well as painful peripheral neuropathic involvement of mainly the lower but also the upper extremities. He thus was given a diagnosis of organic affective disorder and treated, with some relief, with desipramine, haloperidol and methylphenidate. His neuropathy was treated with microcurrent stimulation and other physical therapeutic interventions.

Neuropsychologic testing disclosed a level of intellectual functioning below that which would be expected, given the patient's educational and vocational background, although it was in the average range. IQ testing is based on timed (as well as power) testing; therefore, the slowing of information processing associated with the encephalopathy and the painful neuropathy probably accounted for some of the problems with this area of functioning. He also demonstrated slowed speech, suggestive of central effects of the virus. Verbal rote memory was severely impaired, probably due to the encephalopathy but also perhaps associated with medication effects. He also showed severely impaired visuospatial problems, including poor nonverbal memory, nonverbal analysis and abstract reasoning, which was uncharacteristic of HIV dementia. These functions are usually spared until later in the encephalopathy. Thus, his performance on neurobehavioral testing was consistent with moderately advanced HIV-related dementia with affective complications. He was continued on antidepressants and stimulants, and suggestions were made to assist his failing memory with memory logs, alarm watches for reminding him of times for medications and restructuring of his environment to facilitate locating necessary items for ADL and to minimize demands that aggravate his neuropathic pain. He continued with physical therapy to maintain endurance and mobility as well as to receive analgesic relief. Although the patient's painful existential condition certainly would appear to contribute to a despondency that could lead to thoughts and acts of suicide, he also had demonstrable evidence of central and peripheral nervous system organic involvement and qualified for diagnoses of organic affective disorder and dementia.

SUMMARY

The many-faceted complications of HIV infection on neurologic and mental and behavioral functioning are a tremendous challenge for health care providers. With its effects on multiple systems in the body, the disease dictates a team approach for optimal care with specialties such as internal medicine, microbiology, physical medicine and rehabilitation, neurology, immunology and psychiatry. The specific neurobehavioral problems that may occur may be addressed by psychologists, neuropsychologists, speech/language/learning pathologists, physical therapists, occupational therapists and social service personnel. The patient's complex nutritional needs may be addressed by nutritionists. The depth of need in many cases of HIV spectrum disorder, especially as it advances, calls for the expertise of this diverse group of providers to optimize the patient's functioning.

Many gaps remain in our understanding of HIV-related neurobehavioral disorders. As yet undetermined are the point at which neurobehavioral problems begin and the recognition of cognitive impairment, especially subtle levels

that may occur early in the course of the disorder. More information is emerging about changes in the central nervous system caused by the virus and reflected by neurochemical markers in the cerebrospinal fluid. Correlation of these markers with behavioral test results, as well as electrophysiologic data, may help clarify when the early effects of HIV encephalopathy occur.

Since a large percentage of HIV-seropositive patients develop some type of nervous system involvement, this disease entity calls for a closer and more integrated approach to the understanding of HIV behavioral disturbances between biologically based psychological health care providers and those with a more psychosocial perspective. The disease causes tremendous upheaval in the patient's psychosocial framework and significant stress on the nervous system, both of which leave the patient with severely strained resources to deal with the medical, emotional, legal and practical issues that face the person with AIDS. As our knowledge of the complexities of this set of diseases increases, the utilization of many skills will be necessary to maintain as optimal a level of daily functioning as possible for as long as possible.

References

American Psychiatric Association. (1987). *Diagnostic and Statistical Manual of Mental Disorders,*. 3rd ed., revised. Washington, D.C.: author.

Bredesen, D. E., Levy, R. M., and Rosenblum, M. L. (1988). The neurology of human immunodeficiency virus infection. *Quarterly Journal of Medicine*. 68:665.

Brew, B. J., Bhalla, R. B., Fleisher, M., et al. (1989). Cerebrospinal fluid 2 microglobulin in patients infected with human immunodeficiency virus. *Neurology*. 39:830.

Brew, B. J., Sidtis, J. J., Petito, C. K., and Price, R. W. (1988). The neurologic complications of AIDS and human immunodeficiency virus infection. In Plum, F. (Ed.): *Advances in Contemporary Neurology*. Philadelphia: F. A. Davis.

Brunetti, A., Berg, G., DiChiro, G., et al. (1989). Reversal of brain metabolic abnormalities following treatment of AIDS dementia complex with 3'-azido-2'3'-dideoxythymidine (AZT, zidovudine): A PET-FDG study. *Journal of Nuclear Medicine*. 30:581.

Cavanaugh, S., Clark, D. C., and Gibbons, R. D. (1983). Diagnosing depression in the hospitalized medically ill. *Psychosomatics*. 24:809.

Clark, D., Cavanaugh, S. V., and Gibbons, R. D. (1983). The core symptoms of depression in medical and psychiatric patients. *Journal of Nervous and Mental Diseases*. 171:705.

Cornblath, D. R., and McArthur, J. C. (1988). Predominantly sensory neuropathy in patients with AIDS and AIDS-related complex. *Neurology.* 38:794.

Currie, J., Benson, E., Ramsden, B., et al. (1988). Eye movement abnormalities as a predictor of the acquired immunodeficiency syndrome dementia complex. *Archives of Neurology.* 45:949.

Elovaara, I., Sepälä, I., Poutiainen, E., et al. (1988). Intrathecal humoral immunologic response in neurologically symptomatic and asymptomatic patients with human immunodeficiency virus infection. *Neurology.* 38:1451.

Elovaara, I., Iivanainen, M., Poutiainen, E., et al. (1989). CSF and serum-2 microglobulin in HIV infection related to neurological dysfunction. *Acta Neurologica Scandinavica.* 79:81.

Engstrom, J. W., Lowenstein, D. H., and Bredesen, D. E. (1989). Cerebral infarctions and transient neurologic deficits associated with acquired immunodeficiency syndrome. *American Journal of Medicine.* 86:528.

Fernandez, F., Adams, F., Levy, J. K., et al. (1988). Cognitive impairment due to AIDS-related complex and its response to psychostimulants. *Psychosomatics.* 29:38.

Fernandez, F., Levy, J. K., and Galizzi, H. (1988). Response of HIV-related depression to psychostimulants: Case reports. *Hospital and Community Psychiatry.* 39:628.

Fernandez, F. (1989). Psychiatric complications in HIV-related illness. In *The American Psychiatric Association's Primer on AIDS.* (pp. 6-1--6-27). Washington, DC: American Psychiatric Press.

Fernandez, F., Levy, J. K., and Mansell, P. W. A. (1989). Management of delirium in terminally ill AIDS patients. *International Journal of Psychiatry in Medicine.* 19:165.

Fernandez, F., and Levy, J. K. (in press). Adjuvant treatment of HIV dementia with psychostimulants. In Ostrow, D. (Ed.): *Behavioral Aspects of AIDS and Other Sexually Transmitted Diseases.* New York: Plenum.

Filley, C. M., Franklin, G. M., Heaton, R. K., and Rosenberg, N. L. (1989). White matter dementia. Clinical disorders and implications. *Neuropsychiatry Neuropsychology and Behavioral Neurology.* 1:239.

Frank, Y., Lim, W., Kahn, E., et al. (1989). Multiple ischemic infarcts in a child with AIDS, varicella zoster infection, and cerebral vasculitis. *Pediatric Neurology.* 5:64.

Freund-Levi, Y., Saaf, J., Wahlund, L-O., and Wetterberg, L. (1989). Ultra low brain MRI in HIV transfusion infected patients. *Magnetic Resonance Imaging.* 7:225.

Gabuzda, D. A., Levy, S. R., and Chiappa, K. H. (1988). Electroencephalography in AIDS and AIDS-related complex. *Clinical Electroencephalography.* 19:1.

Gaut, P., Wong, P.K., and Meyer, R.D. (1988). Pyomyositis in a patient with the acquired immunodeficiency syndrome. *Archives of Internal Medicine.* 148:1608.

Goethe, K.E., Mitchell, J.E., Marshall, D.W., et al. (1989). Neuropsychological and neurological function of human immunodeficiency virus-seropositive asymptomatic individuals. *Archives of Neurology.* 46:129.

Goodin, D.S., Aminoff, M.J., Chernoff, D.N., and Hollander, H. (1990). Long latency event-related potentials in patients infected with human immunodeficiency virus. *Annals of Neurology.* 27:414.

Hill, J.M., Farrar, W.L., and Pert, C. B. (1987). Autoradiographic localization of T4 antigen, the HIV receptor, in human brain. *International Journal of Neuro-science.* 32:687.

Hollander, H., Golden, J., Mendelson, T., and Courtland, D. (1986). Extrapyramidal symptoms in AIDS patients given low- dose metoclopramide or chlorpromazine. *Lancet.* 2:1186.

Holmes, V.F., Fernandez, F., and Levy, J.K. (1989). Psychostimulant response in AIDS-related complex patients. *Journal of Clinical Psychiatry.* 50:5.

Jarvik, J.G., Hesselink, J.R., Kennedy, C., et al. (1988). Acquired immunodeficiency syndrome. Magnetic resonance patterns of brain involvement with pathologic correlation. *Archives of Neurology.* 45:731.

Kelly W.M., and Brandt-Zawadzki, M. (1983). The neurology of human immunodeficiency virus infection. *Radiology.* 149:486.

Kertesz, A. (Ed.). (1983). *Localization in Neuropsychology.* New York: Academic Press.

Kovner, R., Perecman, E., Lazar, W., et al. (1989). Relation of personality and attentional factors to cognitive deficits in human immunodeficiency virus-infected subjects. *Archives of Neurology.* 46:274.

Lange, D. J., Britton, C. B., Younger, D. S., and Hays, A. P. (1988). The neuromuscular manifestations of human immunodeficiency virus infections. *Archives of Neurology.* 45:1084.

Levy, J.K., and Fernandez, F. (1989). Neuropsychiatric care for critically ill AIDS patients. *Journal of Critical Illness.* 4:33.

Lipowski, Z. J. (1987). Delirium (acute confusional states). *Journal of the American Medical Association.* 258:1789.

Marshall, D.W., Brey, R.L., and Butzin, C.A. (1989). Lack of cerebrospinal fluid myelin basic protein in HIV-infected asymptomatic individuals with intrathecal synthesis of IgG. *Neurology.* 39:1127.

McArthur, J.C., Cohen, B.A., Selnes, O.A., et al. (1989). Low prevalence of neurological and neuropsychological abnormalities in otherwise healthy HIV-1-infected individuals: Results from the Multicenter AIDS Cohort Study. *Annals of Neurology.* 26:601.

Nalls, G., Disher, A., Daryabagi, J., et al. (1989). Subcortical cerebral hemorrhages associated with cocaine abuse: CT and MR findings. *Journal of Computer Assisted Tomography.* 13:1.

Nath, A., Jankovic, J., and Pettigrew, L.C. (1987). Movement disorders and AIDS. *Neurology.* 37:37.

Nolte, K.B., and Gelman, B.B. (1989). Intracerebral hemorrhage associated with cocaine abuse. *Archives of Pathology and Laboratory Medicine.* 113:812.

O'Dowd, M.A., and McKegney, F.P. (1988). Manic syndrome associated with zidovudine. *Journal of the American Medical Association.* 260:3587.

Parisi, A., Strosselli, M., Di Perri, G., et al. (1989). Electroencephalography in the early diagnosis of HIV-related subacute encephalitis: Analysis of 185 patients. *Clinical Electroencephalography.* 20:1.

Perry, S.W., and Marotta, R.F. (1987). AIDS dementia. A review of the literature. *Alzheimer Disease and Associated Disorders.* 1:221.

Perry, S.W., and Tross, S. (1984). Psychiatric problems of AIDS inpatients at the New York Hospital: Preliminary report. *Public Health Reports.* 99:200.

Reboul, J., Schiller, E., Pialoux, G., et al. (1989). Immunoglobulins and complement components in 37 patients infected by HIV-1 virus: Comparison of general (systemic) and intrathecal immunity. *Journal of the Neurological Sciences.* 89:243.

Reisberg, B., Ferris, S.H., de Leon, M.J., and Crook, T. (1982). The Global Deterioration Scale for assessment of primary degenerative dementia. *American Journal of Psychiatry.* 139:1136.

Rothrock, J.F., Rubenstein, R., and Lyden, P.D. (1988). Ischemic stroke associated with methamphetamine inhalation. *Neurology.* 38:589.

Scaravelli, F., Daniel, S. E., Harcourt-Webster, N., and Guiloff, R.J. (1989). Chronic basal meningitis and vasculitis in acquired immunodeficiency syndrome. A possible role for human immunodeficiency virus. *Archives of Pathology and Laboratory Medicine.* 113:192.

Schmitt, F.A., Bigley, J.W., McKinnis, R., et al. (1988) Neuropsychological outcome of zidovudine (AZT) treatment of patients with AIDS and AIDS-related complex. *New England Journal of Medicine.* 319:1573.

Simpson, D.M., and Bender, A.N. (1988). Human immunodeficiency virus associated with myopathy: Analysis of 11 patients. *Annals of Neurology.* 24:79.

Smith, T., Jakobsen, J., Gaub, J., et al. (1988). Clinical and electrophysiological studies of human immunodeficiency virus-. seropositive men without AIDS. *Annals of Neurology.* 23:295.

So, Y.T., Holtzman, D.M., Abrams, D.I., and Olney, R.K. (1988). Peripheral neuropathy associated with acquired immunodeficiency syndrome. Prevalence and clinical features from a population-based survey. *Archives of Neurology.* 45:945.

Tervo, T., Elovaara, I., Karli, H., et al. (1986). Abnormal ocular motility as early sign of CNS involvement in HIV infection (letter). *Lancet.* 2:512.

Tross, S., Price, R.W., Navia, B., et al. (1988). Neuropsychological characterization of the AIDS dementia complex: A preliminary report. *AIDS.* 2:81.

Van Gorp, W.G., Mitrushina, M., Cummings, J.L., et al. (1989). Normal aging and the subcortical encephalopathy of AIDS: A neuropsychological comparison. *Neuropsychiatry, Neuropsychology, and Behavioral Neurology.* 2:5.

Vinters, H.V., Guerra, W.G., Eppolito, L., and Keith, P.E. (1988). Necrotizing vasculitis of the nervous system in a patient with AIDS-related complex. *Neuropathology and Applied Neurobiology.* 14:417.

Whitehouse, P. J. (1986). The concept of subcortical and cortical dementia: Another look. *Annals of Neurology.* 19:1.

Wojak, J.C., and Flamm, E. S. (1987). Intracranial hemorrhage and cocaine use. *Stroke.* 18:712.

12

Rehabilitation of the Pediatric Population

Michael Pizzi, MS, OTR/L

Most people see what is and ask "Why?" I see what is and ask "Why not?"

—Bobby Kennedy

INTRODUCTION

HIV infection in children is not manifested in any one clinical picture. Detection of the infection in infants usually occurs as a result of opportunistic infections that indicate immune system compromise. Infants with HIV infection are then referred to therapists by a pediatrician or pediatric neurologist because of neurologic and developmental deficits. Often an undiagnosed infant is referred because of neurologic and developmental abnormalities secondary to HIV rather than directly because of HIV infection.

HIV infection used to be considered rapidly fatal. Early research indicated a survival rate of 6 to 12 months postdiagnosis. With vigorous medical intervention for HIV-related opportunistic infections in the United States, the advent of promising drugs such as AZT and dideoxyinosine (DdI), prognosis has improved for some children. We now are beginning to see the effects of interventions that unmask chronic neurologic and developmental deficits and for which therapy interventions can be effective in improving the quality of life for children with HIV and their families. Children acquire HIV through several routes of transmission. Falloon et al. (1988) describe blood-product-transfusion-related infection during treatment for hemophilia (or other coagulation disorders) and sexual

abuse as two routes of transmission. The primary mode of transmission is transplacentally or perinatally. This latter group comprises over 80 percent of the total number of infected infants and children (Institute of Medicine, 1986). In the United States, mothers of these infected children are HIV positive through blood transfusion or through IV drug use. Because such women are disproportionately black or Hispanic, poor and urban, most children living with HIV belong to such groups. Postpartum transmission via infected breast milk may also be possible, as suggested by the case of a breast-fed child who had been born to a woman infected by postpartum transfusion (Ziegler et al., 1985).

In the United States, current predictions estimate 10,000 to 20,000 HIV-seropositive children by 1991, the majority of whom are from African American and Hispanic cultures (Institute of Medicine, 1986). Many more thousands are expected worldwide. As the substance abuse problem escalates in the heterosexual community, the number of pediatric HIV cases will proliferate. Thus, when we care for children with HIV/AIDS, we must begin by caring for the adults. Our health care system must prepare for the growth of this population and begin to identify necessary support services, such as occupational therapy (OT) and physical therapy (PT), that facilitate adaptive functioning for children with HIV and their care givers.

Table 12-1
SYNDROMES AND NEUROLOGIC FINDINGS IN CHILDREN WITH HIV

Wasting syndrome

Lymhoid interstitial pneumonitis

Recurrent bacterial infection

Cardiomyopathy

Hepatitis

Renal disease

Developmental delay/loss of developmental milestones

Chronic encephalopathy

Seizure disorders

Motor dysfunction

Microcephaly

Abnormal CT scan findings - cortical atrophy, calcifications

Table 12-2
REFLEX DEVELOPMENT

REFLEX	APPROXIMATE AGE IN MONTHS (normal response)
Primary Reflexes	
Rooting	0 - 3
Sucking	0 - 3
Moro	0 - 5
Galant	0 - 3
Palmar grasp	0 - 3
Plantar grasp	0 - 10
Crossed extension	0 - 1
Primary standing/walking	0 - 2
Placing reaction	0 - 6
Tonal Reflexes	
Asymmetric tonic neck	0 - 6
Symmetric tonic neck	0 - 12
Righting Reaction	
Labrynthine righting on head (prone)	0 - life
Labrynthine righting on head (supine)	4 - life
Landau	3 - 24
Body righting	4 - life
Protective Balance Reaction	
Protective extension	6 - life
Equilibrium reactions	
prone/supine	5 - life
sitting	7 - life

CLINICAL MANIFESTATIONS

Children with HIV present a spectrum of clinical manifestations (see Appendix F). These children may range from being asymptomatic to critically/terminally ill. Scott (1987) and Oleske (1987) describe a range of clinical manifestations (Table 12-1).

The time from infection to overt AIDS is shorter in children than adults and shorter in children infected perinatally than in those infected through transfusion. Perinatally infected children have a median age at diagnosis of nine months, whereas children with transfusion acquired HIV have a median age at diagnosis of 17 months (Rogers et al., 1987).

Falloon and colleagues (1988) describe several nonspecific manifestations (eg. weight loss, low birth weight or failure to thrive, diarrhea, hepatosplenomegaly, dermatitis, fevers), bacterial infections (eg. sepsis, pneumonia, meningitis) and opportunistic infections (eg. PCP, disseminated cytomegalovirus, *Candida*, disseminated MAI). Four percent of HIV-infected children develop KS. Both KS and HIV-related lymphomas are more common in adults (Rogers et al., 1987).

The most common neurologic manifestation in children with HIV is encephalopathy, which can be the primary manifestation of HIV in children, resulting in developmental delay or in a deterioration of motor skills and cognitive functioning (Belman et al., 1985; Rubinstein, 1986; Epstein et al., 1986; Diamond, 1989). Neurologic abnormalities such as paresis, pyramidal tract signs, ataxia, abnormal tone

or pseudobulbar palsy have been noted (Rubinstein, 1986). Microcephaly has been described in younger children (Epstein et al., 1986). CT scans have shown cerebral atrophy, ventricular enlargement, and calcification in the basal ganglia and frontal white matter (Belman et al., 1985; Epstein et al., 1986).

The clinical manifestations, particularly encephalopathy of HIV in infants and children, have a profound impact on normal growth and development. The arenas of reflex, motor, cognitive, social-emotional and play development are areas where OT and PT can have a profound impact on facilitating adaptive responses.

NORMAL GROWTH AND DEVELOPMENT

A child's interactions with both the physical and social environments begin at birth and can be described as

Table 12-3
NORMAL GROWTH AND DEVELOPMENT (MOTOR)

TASK	DEVELOPMENTAL AGE
Body lying prone	birth
Body lying supine	birth
Rolling side to side	1 - 4 weeks
Rolling prone to supine	6 months
Rolling supine to prone	7 months
Propped sitting	6 months
Sitting with hands propped	7 months
Crawling all fours	7 - 8 months
Standing	7 - 8 months
Sitting unsupported	10 - 12 months
Walking holding onto furniture	10 months
Walking without support	10 - 12 months

Table 12-4
PIAGET'S COGNITIVE DEVELOPMENT

PHASE	STAGE	APPROXIMATE CHRONOLOGIC AGE
Sensorimotor	Reflexes, habits, circular reactions (primary, secondary, tertiary), deduction	0 - 2 years
Preoperational	Symbolism and imagery "magical thinking"	2 - 6 years
Concrete operational	Basic logic; inductive reasoning	6 - 12 years
Formal operational	Abstract thinking; deductive reasoning	12 years

From Piaget, J. (1959). The Construction of Reality in the Child. New York: Basic Books, Inc.

playful and exploratory (Reilly, 1974). The fundamental tool of children for occupational and physical skill development is play. Among the skills children develop through play are personal activities of daily living (PADL). Underlying sensorimotor and cognitive abilities facilitating development of play are ADL and occupational roles. It is important for therapists to have a basic knowledge in normal growth and development to identify abnormal growth and development in children with HIV infection.

Reflex and Motor Development

Several theorists and clinicians have identified a normal sequence of motor and reflex development (Gesell, 1940; Fiorentino, 1963; Bayley, 1965; Brazelton, 1973; Coley, 1987). Developmental charts and chronologic scales assist therapists in identifying skill levels of children and chronologic and developmental levels according to current functional levels (Tables 12-2 and 12-3).

Cognitive Development

Jean Piaget (1959) is most noted for his development of cognitive theory (Table 12-4). Piaget views human beings as alert, interactive with the environment, and able to process and interpret information, rather than passive recipients of information. He views people as adaptive through processes of assimilation, whereby new information is processed, and accommodation, which allows the integration of the new information into the person's view of life. Growth occurs through both of these processes.

Social-Emotional Development

Erikson (1975) focuses on psychosocial development via eight emotional stages or issues (Table 12-5). Each stage or issue in his theory must be resolved before proceeding adaptively to the next one. Erikson's developmental theory views human beings as interpersonal in nature, relating to the social and cultural environment through successful progression of the eight stages. How one achieves resolution of a particular issue hierarchically affects how one will deal with subsequent issues.

Play Development

Play is the most important activity in childhood. Play skill development and performance vary between children and between age groups. Motor and psychosocial/emotional development and competence and mastery in the environment are developed through play (Florey, 1971; Reilly, 1974; Robinson, 1977). Play function and dysfunction are examined through the domains of materials, action, people and settings (Takata, 1974) (Table 12-6). Goals and treatment are then designed around the need areas in each domain.

Table 12-5
SOCIAL-EMOTIONAL DEVELOPMENT
ERIKSON'S EIGHT STAGES

STAGE	AGE
Trust versus Mistrust	0 - 1
Autonomy versus Shame	1 - 3
Initiative versus Guilt	3 - 5
Industry versus Inferiority	5 - 11
Identity versus Role Diffusion	11 - 18
Intimacy versus Isolation	Young Adult
Generativity versus Stagnation	Middle Adult
Ego Integrity versus Despair	Later Adult

From Erikson, E.H. (1975). Eight Ages of Man: Life and Continuous Process. New York: Alfred A. Knopf, Inc.

EVALUATION OF THE INFANT/CHILD WITH HIV

A complete assessment of the child's functioning must be undertaken. Typical assessment strategies can include chart review, clinical observations, history taking, developmental play and ADL assessments, interviews of care givers and standardized testing (Pizzi, 1989b; Harris-Copp & Schlussel, 1989).

Neurodevelopmental evaluation is a major part of the overall assessment of children with HIV. It is most important in children 0 to 5 years of age. A holistic assessment includes the psychosocial and environmental (physical and social) domains of functioning. These domains, in concert with the domain of physical functioning, include the skills of play and self-care.

Pizzi (1989b) designed an assessment battery that (Table 12-7) can be incorporated to accommodate the preferences of individual therapists.

CLINICAL INTERVENTIONS

In the population of children with HIV infection, important and different issues arise regarding intervention. Noteworthy are the issues of regression in skill performance, cultural considerations, care givers who may also be coping with their own HIV disease, stigma, and environmental issues. (Most patients are poor urban dwellers with few economic or community resources; Pizzi, 1989b). Therefore, traditional treatment interventions must be examined with regard to these population-specific considerations.

Children with HIV may never achieve normal developmental milestones; they may develop slowly or experience loss of function. Therapists promote development of these milestones through neurodevelopmental treatment, positioning, adaptive equipment and play. Intervention with children with HIV should include the family system and care giver education (Pizzi, 1989b).

Self-Care

Self-care includes eating, bathing, grooming, hygiene, dressing, functional communication and mobility. Skills and established routines of daily living necessitate constant reassessment and adaptations due to the many complications and manifestations of HIV disease, such as motor and neurologic complications, frequent hospitalizations, psychosocial problems (eg. poor self-concept, self-esteem or body image), and influence of care givers on skill development. Treatment of self-care must also include treatment and recognition of underlying clinical problems. Environmental and cultural influences on development of self-care skills and routines must also be considered. For example, are family behaviors interfering with adaptive function and behaviors of the child? Are there cultural considerations regarding activity levels and self-care performance and routines? Is the physical environment able to support self-care, motor development and age-appropriate play? Does the family system value self-care or mobility independence for the child with HIV, or is it more important to develop other functional skills?

Adaptive Equipment and Strategies

Adaptive equipment and strategies to develop age-appropriate self-care and motor skills are often necessary. Children with HIV-related neurologic manifestations require a structured environment and few distractions to accomplish tasks. For example, using one command at a time (eg. put legs into pants, pull up pants, zip up pants), using the same environment to perform daily living skills (eg. child's room, bathroom), and having no one else around to distract the child can help him or her become more independent in dressing. Built up handles, plateguards, scoop dishes, and Velcro clothing are suggested for other self-care needs. Adapted wheelchairs, seating, and positioning can support care givers in fostering independent self-care function.

Self-Concept

Following the play taxonomy developed by Takata (1974), therapists can make play recommendations to facilitate adaptive motor responses, including reflex and sensory integration, facilitate and inhibit tone, and facilitate exploratory behaviors and competence in the environment. Care

Table 12-6
PLAY DEVELOPMENT

SENSORIMOTOR (0-2 YEARS)

Materials: Toys, objects for sensory experiences such as rattles, balls, blocks, straddle toys, chimes, simple pictures, color cones, large blocks using sight, smell, hearing, touching and mouthing.

Actions: Gross motor including stand/fall, walk, pull, sit on, climb, open/close. Fine motor including touch, mouth, hold, throw/pick up, bang, shake, carry, motoric imitation of domestic actions.

People: Parents and immediate family.

Setting: Home—crib, playpen, floor, yard, immediate surroundings.

* Emphasis is on independent play with exploration; habits expressed in trial and error.

SYMBOLIC AND SIMPLE CONSTRUCTIVE (2-4 YEARS)

Materials: Toys, objects, raw materials (water, sand, paints, clay, crayon) for fine motor manipulation and simple combining and taking apart; wheeled vehicles and adventure toys to practice gross motor actions.

Action: Gross motor including climb, run jump, balance, drag, dump, throw. Fine motor including empty/fill, scribble/draw, squeeze/pull, combine/take apart, arrange in spatial dimensions. Imagination with story telling; fantasy. Objects represent events and things.

People: Parents, peers, and other adults.

Setting: Outdoors—playground or play equipment in immediate neighborhood. Indoors—home, nursery.

* Emphasis is on parallel play and beginning to share. Symbolic play expressed in simple pretense and simple constructional use of materials.

DRAMATIC AND COMPLEX CONSTRUCTIVE AND PREGAME (4-7 YEARS)

Materials: Objects, toys, raw materials for fine motor actions and role playing; large adventure toys for refining gross actions for speed and coordination; pets; nonselective collections.

Action: Gross motor including "daredevil" feats of hopping, skipping, turning somersaults, dance. Fine motor including combining materials and making products to do well, to use tools, to copy reality. Dramatic role playing, including imitating reality in part/whole costumes, story telling.

People: Peer group (2-5 members), imaginary friends, parents, immediate family, other adults.

Setting: School, neighborhood and extended surroundings (excursions), upper space and off the ground.

* Emphasis is on cooperative play with purposeful use of materials for constructions; dramatization of reality and building habits of skill and tool use.

GAMES (7-12 YEARS)

Materials: Games played with rules (dominoes, checkers, table-card games, ping-pong); raw materials and tools for making complex products (weaving, woodwork, carving, needlework). Gross muscle sports, hopscotch, kite flying, skating, basketball. Books-puzzles, "things to do," biography, adventure, sports. Selective collection or hobby. Pet.

Action: Gross motor, including refined and combining skills of jumping, hopping and running. Fine motor including precision in using variety of tools, finer object manipulation and construction. Making, following and breaking rules; competitions and compromise with peers.

People: Peer group of same sex; organized group such as scouts; parents; other adults

Setting: Neighborhood, playground, school, home.

* Emphasis is on enhancement of constructional and sports skills as expressed in rule-bound behavior, competition and appreciation of process cooperative play.

RECREATION (12-16 YEARS)

Materials: Team games and sports and special interest groups for music, dancing, singing, discussing. Collections and hobbies; parties, books, table games.

Action: Gross motor including team sports and individual precision sports (tennis and golf). Fine motor including applying and practicing fine manipulative skills to develop craftsmanship, special talents. Organized group work.

People: Peer groups of same and opposite sex; parents and other adults.

Setting: School, neighborhood and extended community, home.

* Emphasis is on team participation and independent action, expressed in organized sports, interest groups and hobbies during leisure time.

Table 12-7
ASSESSMENT BATTERY FOR
CHILDREN/ADOLESCENTS
WITH HIV INFECTION

Developmental Assessments
Play Assessments
Activities of Daily Living Assessments
Adolescent Role Checklist
Adaptive Behavior Inventory for Children
Quick Neurologic Screening Test
Bruininks-Oseretsky Motor Proficiency Test
Piers-Harris Children's Self Concept Scale
Goodenough-Harris Drawing Test
Comprehensive Test of Adaptive Behaviors
Bayley Scales
Clinical Observations
Interiew with Child/Adolescent
Interview of Caregiver

From Pizzi, M. (1989, December). Occupational therapy: Creating possibilities for children with HIV infection, ARC, and AIDS. AIDS Patient Care. 31-36.

giver education on play and play development are crucial elements in treatment for HIV seropositive children. Play recommendations, presented at the level of understanding of the care giver, should be both written and oral to ensure that care givers understand the recommendations and their purpose (Pizzi, 1989b).

Often, self-concept affects play and self-care behaviors. Children with HIV, especially older children who have an understanding of the illness, can present clinically as withdrawn, anxious, and noncommunicative. Children are also very perceptive and observe adult behaviors. From these behaviors, they may sense that they are "different" or "special." Care givers often state that there is a noted change in the child's play and in family interactions. This psychosocial component can be addressed through interview with the care giver or child and through play observation. Intervention with a focus on activity produces successful outcomes and provides immediate positive feedback.

To help guide effective clinical interventions, therapists also need information about the child's level of understanding of HIV and whether the child has been told the diagnosis and by whom. This information and knowledge of the child's behaviors before the HIV diagnosis can yield significant clinical data and support the patient-therapist relationship. Psychosocial interventions include activities that are short term, interesting to the child, and easily completed. Children can be actively involved in projects

with subsequent task achievement that enhances self-esteem. An option is involvement in community projects, where the child makes a contribution to others and is acknowledged for that effort (eg. being a leader in developing a neighborhood carnival to raise money for charity, going to the store on a daily or weekly basis for an elder in the community) (Pizzi, 1989b).

Physical Environment

Adaptations to the physical environment are also needed when children experience physical symptoms of HIV. The physical environment includes the home, school and playground. Children with HIV often have difficulties negotiating environments due to motor problems, diminished visual acuity and endurance problems. Adaptations to the physical environment can facilitate the child's involvement in life activity and promote greater mobility. For example, a bed-bound child can use a lap tray to hold books or write a paper or for leisure tasks while lying down. An intercom or walkie-talkie can allow communication with others who may be in a different part of the house. Moving the child's bedroom to the most pleasant and active part of the house fosters ongoing communication and relationships within the family system. Ramps to accommodate wheelchairs can easily be built for the child at home and at school. Therapists can also be involved in adapting playgrounds in the child's community for the child with special needs.

Family System

The family system may consist of both parents, a single parent, a grandmother or even the pediatric unit of a hospital. The family system is often responsible for ongoing services that require their involvement in the rehabilitation process from the beginning of assessment through treatment. Families with HIV-seropositive children often demonstrate and experience guilt, fear, anxiety, shame and grief. Whether in denial, acceptance, or understanding of HIV disease, the care giver's reactions will affect the child and, hence, the child's functioning. It has been noted clinically that the level of communication about the disease from care giver to child affects function. For example, parents, who knew the diagnosis of their child, finally told their 10 year-old son and eventually shared the information with community members and their church. They encountered much support and outpouring of concern. The child began to experience a freedom from being "special," showed improvement psychosocially and played more interactively with friends (Pizzi, 1989a).

The varying functional levels of care givers, psychoemotionally and physically, can impede or enhance the child's current and future functioning, especially when care givers themselves are HIV seropositive or have AIDS. Care givers who are symptomatic often must cope with musculoskeletal, neurologic and cardiopulmonary difficulties, as well as the physical and psychosocial needs of the child with HIV. Therapists who provide services to infants with HIV, children and their families must be flexible and adaptable in scheduling therapy sessions to meet the needs of the family as well as the child. Identification of an HIV-seropositive child in a family is a window into a family system that is infected. Transmission from mother to infant prenatally or perinatally is often the first indication that the mother is seropositive.

The sadness experienced in helping either natural or foster parents cope with the grief associated with having a child with HIV is often addressed by therapists in occupational and physical therapy. Hopefulness is engendered by the positive effects from touching, adaptation, holding, and improving the child's quality of life. This may be noted through improving the quality of movement, feeding, breathing, playing and daily life skill management. By teaching care givers various ways to hold, move, sit and play with their neurologically impaired child, a more positive bond is established. Parents sometimes perceive these positive aspects as a welcome respite from coping with the bouts of illness and trips to emergency rooms that are an inherent part of coping with AIDS. Three occupational therapists are currently developing a Family Assessment of Occupational Functioning (FAOF) to address occupational needs and behaviors of family systems (Pizzi, 1989a).

A PEDIATRIC HIV CLASSIFICATION SYSTEM

Questions arise about when to intervene with OT or PT; how to best schedule the frequency and duration of therapy; and how to educate natural and foster families, other care givers, teachers, social workers, and social service agencies about the need and efficacy of therapy intervention. Intensive therapy is warranted at various times in the progression of HIV-associated disorders. At other times, periodic evaluation, monitoring, and parent or school education and training is more appropriate. Unfortunately, there are also times when parents and therapist decide that rehabilitation is a low priority because keeping appointments creates too much stress for the family or exceeds the child's energy levels.

Longitudinal follow-up of large numbers of children has permitted categorization of several neurologic courses in pediatric HIV infection (Belman et al., 1985), but the course of any one child is determined only with careful, consistent, standardized documentation and longitudinal follow-up. Information from diagnostic tests and clinical reports help identify the clinical course of the disease and understanding of the underlying pathology. Belman et al. (1985) reported six categories of neurologic progression based on a study of six children. These categories have been further expanded by Harris-Copp and Schlussel (1989) based on their clinical experiences. They are defined as follows:

1. rapidly progressive
2. subacute relentlessly progressive
3. subacute progressive with plateau
4. static encephalopathy
5. moderately impaired neurologic course
6. mildly impaired neurologic course
7. normal mental and motor neurologic course

Categories two through four are grouped together because it is difficult to determine whether changes are a result of the progressive disease process or whether the factors identifying them permit misclassification. Children in these groups may alternate between categories. For example, when first seen for evaluation, a child may present with what appears to be static encephalopathy, decline over the course of treatment, and then respond to treatment as deterioration decelerates. This course is marked by severe developmental, cognitive, and neurologic deficits with frequent increasingly severe acute illnesses.

Categories five through seven are now becoming apparent as a result of longitudinal follow-up. Children representative of these groups may not have been identified until preschool age or later and may have previously been asymptomatic. They later develop neurologic signs or opportunistic infections, which may require reclassification over time as neurologic deficits occur with disease progression. Some children in these groups previously may have been identified as static encephalopathy. They also may have had acute illnesses and other signs of HIV infection, such as lymphadenopathy, and may demonstrate slow, subtle deterioration in motor or mental status.

Depending on when the child is referred or identified as needing therapy services, the exact neurologic course is undetermined until HIV infection status is identified. The child is then followed with careful documentation of neurologic and developmental progress or regression.

The sometimes rapid onset of spasticity or rigidity, which quickly progress to contractures and subsequent loss of function and motor milestones, is frustrating for the therapist, child and care giver. The psychologic illness associated with deterioration precludes therapeutic intervention. At times, parents should endeavor to keep therapy appointments for the child to prevent contractures and rapid loss of function. Therapy includes facilitation of movement, prevention of contractures, facilitation of automatic reactions, and provision of adaptive equipment and positioning to continue function. The quality of life for the child and the family may be enhanced by intervention and by providing positive goals, even in periods of deterioration.

Therapists treating an undiagnosed child should be alert to indications of deterioration, including abrupt changes in tone, appearance of primitive reflexes not previously observed, loss of developmental milestones, developmental plateaus, chronic respiratory or other infections from opportunistic pathogens, loss of feeding skills, and a progressive generalized apathy. These symptoms are by no means conclusive indications of HIV infection or AIDS but may alert the therapist to refer the child for medical workup to rule out progressive neurologic disease. The importance of an accurate evaluation and clear documentation of therapy outcomes become critical in identifying changes that occur over time.

SUMMARY

This chapter has presented an overview of normal growth and development and the impact of HIV infection on infants, children and their families. Clinical interventions from the perspective of occupational and physical therapy have been described, noting that assessment and treatment must include the family system as the unit of care. A pediatric HIV classification system has been described to assist therapists in developing timely and appropriate clinical interventions.

Acknowledgment

This chapter was adapted and reprinted from the chapter, "Infants and Children with HIV infection: Perspectives in Occupational and Physical Therapy," written by Michael Pizzi, MS, OTR/L and Meredith Harris-Copp, EdD, RPT for the book *Productive Living Strategies For People with AIDS,*. Michael Pizzi, Guest Editor, with kind permission of Haworth Press, 10 Alice Street, Binghamton, New York, 13904-1580.

References

Bayley, N. (1965). Comparisons of mental and motor test scores for age 1-15 months by sex, birth order, race, geographic location and education of parents. *Child Development*. 36:379.

Belman, A., Ultmann, M.H., Horoupian, D., et al. (1985). Neurological complications in infants and children with acquired immunodeficiency syndrome. *Annals of Neurology*. 18:560.

Brazelton, T.B. (1973). *Neonatal Behavior Assessment Scale*. Philadelphia: J.B. Lippincott Co.

Coley, I.L. (1987). *Pediatric Assessment of Selfcare Activi-*

ties. St. Louis: C.V. Mosby.

Diamond, G.W. (1989). Developmental problems in children with HIV infection. *Mental Retardation*. 27(4):213.

Epstein, L.G., Sharer, L.R., and Oleske, J.M. (1986). Neurological manifestations of HIV infection in children. *Pediatrics*. 78:678.

Erikson, E.H., (1975). Eight ages of man. In *Life the Continuous Process.*, New York: Alfred A. Knopf, Inc.

Falloon, J., Eddy, J., Roper, M., and Pizzo, P. (1988). AIDS in the pediatric population. In DeVita, V. Hellman, S., and Rosenberg, T. (Eds.): *AIDS: Etiology, Diagnosis, Treatment and Prevention*. (pp. 339-351). Philadelphia: J.B. Lippincott Co.

Fiorentino, M. (1963). *Reflex Testing Methods for Evaluating CNS Development*, (2nd ed. 2nd printing). Springfield, IL: Charles C. Thomas.

Florey, L. (1971). An approach to play and play development. *American Journal of Occupational Therapy*. 25(6):275.

Gesell, A. (1940). *The First Five Years of Life*. New York: Harper and Row.

Harris-Copp, M. (1988). The HIV infected child: A critical need for physical therapy. *Clinical Management in Physical Therapy*. 8(1):16.

Harris-Copp, M., and Schlussel, S. (1989, June). Paper presented for the conference Children, AIDS and Developmental Disabilities: A Challenge for the 1990s. New York, NY.

Institute of Medicine. (1986). *Confronting AIDS: Directions for Public Health, Health Care and Research.*. Washington, DC: National Academy Press.

Michelman, S. (1971). The importance of creative play. *American Journal of Occupational Therapy*. 25(6):285.

Oleske, J.M. (1987). Natural history of HIV infection II. In *Report of the Surgeon General's Workshop on Children with HIV Infection and Their Families*. Washington, DC: United States Department of Health and Human Services.

Piaget, J. (1959). *The Construction of Reality in the Child.*. New York: Basic Books, Inc.

Pizzi, M. (1988a, April). Pediatric AIDS. Workshop presented at the Annual Conference of the American Occupational Therapy Association. Baltimore, MD.

Pizzi, M. (1988b, November 23). Pediatric AIDS: Occupational therapy assessment and treatment. *OT Week*, 6-7, 10.

Pizzi, M. (1989a, November). AIDS and Rehabilitation: The Care giver and Their Needs. Paper presented at the Annual Conference of the American Congress of Rehabilitation Medicine. San Antonio, TX.

Pizzi, M. (1989B, December). Occupational therapy: Creating possibilities for children with HIV infection, ARC, and AIDS. *AIDS Patient Care*. 31-36.

Reilly, M., (1974). *Play as Exploratory Learning.* Beverly Hills: Sage Publications.

Robinson, A.L. (1977). Play: The arena for acquisition of rules for competent behavior. *American Journal of Occupational Therapy.* 31(4):248.

Rogers, M.F., Thomas, P.A., and Starcher, E.T. (1987). Acquired immunodeficiency syndrome in children: Report of the Centers for Disease Control national surveillance, 1982-1985. *Pediatrics.* 79:1008.

Rubinstein, A. (1986). Pediatric AIDS. *Current Problems in Pediatrics.* 16:361.

Scott, G. (1987). Natural history of HIV infection in children. In *Report of the Surgeon General's Workshop on Children with HIV Infection and Their Families.* Washington, DC: United States Department of Health and Human Services.

Takata, N. (1974). Play as a prescription. In Reilly, M. (Ed.): *Play as Exploratory Learning,* pp. 209-246. Beverly Hills: Sage Publications.

Tower, G. (1983). Selected developmental reflexes and reactions: A literature search. In Hopkins, H.L., and Smith, H.D. (Eds.): *Willard and Spackman's Occupational Therapy,.* 6th ed. (pp. 175-187). Philadelphia: J.B. Lippincott.

Ziegler, J.B., Cooper, D.A., and Johnson, R.O. (1985). Postnatal transmission of AIDS associated retrovirus from mother to infant. *Lancet.* 1:896.

13

Disability in HIV Infection: Theory and Practice

Michael O'Dell, MD

Experience does not teach us that every enthusiasm is absurd. From it we learn simply to wait for results, not from high-sounding words, but from hard work and great courage.

—Andre Maurois

INTRODUCTION

As has been outlined in Chapter 2, the clinical management of AIDS has so far centered on control and prevention of further HIV infection. Treatment strategies have been devised for those already infected, both symptomatic and asymptomatic (Yarchoan, 1989; Bolognesi, 1989). Understandably, treatment of acute, life-threatening complications has received more attention than anticipation of future, chronic physical sequela. With improved prophylaxis and treatment of secondary infections, there has been a recent modest increase in AIDS survival time (Lemp et al., 1990) The introduction of AZT has probably contributed to this overall increase (Lemp et al., 1990; Fischl et al., 1989). This trend in increased life expectancy among person with AIDS is expected to continue with the introduction of new and less toxic treatments (Gill, 1988).

Increased survival has allowed enough time for development of chronic physical disability in some individuals with AIDS. Several authors have suggested that the future of AIDS is that of a chronic disease (Lewis, 1989; Arno et al., 1989; Cotton, 1989; Benjamin, 1989), leading others to cite the importance of AIDS in the future of rehabilitation medicine (Melvin, 1989; Opitz, 1990). More and more, AIDS will be viewed as only the end stage of a chronic infection with HIV (Benjamin, 1989). In the next several years, the time between onset of disability and death will increase dramatically. The relative attractiveness of rehabili-

tation intervention will be augmented by a longer time in which disability may adversely affect quality of life. The development of less toxic treatment approaches with less morbidity will also contribute to prolonged life spans of persons with HIV infection. The logical progression from improved medical and surgical management to lengthened survival to greater risk for physical disability can not be overemphasized. To this end, overall management of HIV illness will increasingly encompass rehabilitation assessment and intervention for physical disability.

The classification of human disablement has been formulated by the World Health Organization (1980) under the direction of Philip Wood. In the Wood classification, an impairment is "any loss or abnormality of psychological, physiological, or anatomical structure or function." The specific definition of a disability is "any restriction or lack (resulting from an impairment) of ability to perform an activity in the manner or within the range considered normal for a human being." Social dysfunction is termed handicap and is defined as a "disadvantage for a given individual, resulting from an impairment or disability, that limits or prevents the fulfillment of a role that is normal (depending on age, sex, social and cultural factors) for that individual." In general, disability implies an inability to perform ADL, functionally ambulate, or effectively communicate (Duckworth, 1984).

Impairments associated with HIV infection have been extensively described in virtually every organ system (Cornblath, 1988a; Kaye, 1989; Aronow, 1988; Rankin, 1988; Marcusen, 1985). Handicap has also been examined to some degree (O'Dowd, 1988; Tross & Hirsh, 1988; Francis, 1989). Until 1989, no information was available on disability in AIDS, and there remains little information on disability in HIV infection before an AIDS-defining event.

DISABILITY STUDIES IN AIDS

There is currently well-documented evidence of significant AIDS-related disability in the last year of life (Kapantais & Powell-Griner, 1989) and at the time of discharge from acute hospitalization (O'Dell, 1989). Other research indicates that persons with AIDS view themselves as more disabled than those with generalized lymphadenopathy or HIV-seronegative controls (Saykin et al., 1989). We know clinically that disability is wide-spread among the population. Concomitant HIV infection in those with non-AIDS-related disability has been reported (Meythaler, 1988) and discussed (Auerback & Jann, 1989), but will not be addressed here. To date, no research has been compiled examining the epidemiology or natural history of physical disability in the HIV population. This work, along with detailed rehabilitation need assessment, poses the most pressing current HIV disability research issues. With this background data, research can examine the need for efficacy and cost-effectiveness of wide scale rehabilitation intervention in HIV disease.

Kapantais and Powell-Griner (1989) published data from the National Mortality Followback Survey in August, 1989. Disability in the final year of life was examined in patients with AIDS from information obtained retrospectively from interviews with caretakers. Comparisons were made with data from a large sample of non-AIDS patients also in the final year of life. Between 40 and 60 percent of patients required assistance with bathing, eating, toileting, and dressing sometime in the year before death. Forty-seven percent required assistance with walking. No information was provided about communication. These percentages were actually similar in both the AIDS and non-AIDS groups. The age difference between groups was significant: 88 percent of the non-AIDS group was over 55 years old, whereas 87 percent of the AIDS group was under 55 years old. Another key difference between groups was the composition of the care givers. Among those with AIDS, a neighbor or friend provided assistance in 38 percent of cases. Ninety-one percent of non-AIDS patients had family assistance.

The only other study of disability in AIDS was conducted at The Graduate Hospital, Philadelphia (O'Dell, 1989).

Using the Functional Independence Measure (FIM) (See Appendix C-2) as a one-time, objective measure of disability, 37 patients with AIDS (CDC Group IV HIV disease) were evaluated at the time of discharge from acute hospitalization. Although one might expect significant disability in this setting, no data were available. Disability in this setting has impact on discharge planning, home services and caretakers. In addition, some disabilities documented may be amenable to readily available rehabilitation intervention. Sixty percent of the sample required human assistance in at least one of the 18 areas measured by the FIM. Nearly a third required assistance in five or more areas. Deficits in stair climbing and ambulation were the most frequent and most severe problems, occurring in 51 percent and 38 percent of the sample, respectively. ADL most frequently requiring assistance were bathing (29.3 percent) and feeding (27.6 percent) with a lesser frequency of upper and lower extremity dressing deficits (18.9 percent and 21.6 percent, respectively).

Using Analysis of Variance (ANOVA), significant relationships were observed between both duration of AIDS diagnosis ($P<0.01$) and length of hospital stay ($P<0.05$), and degree of disability (as measured by the number of FIM areas requiring at least some human assistance). Number of hospitalizations was taken as a gross measurement of overall (longitudinal) disease severity and demonstrated a trend toward, but not reaching, statistical significance. Patient age did not correlate with degree of disability.

When disability (measured by total FIM score) versus duration of AIDS diagnosis were plotted, it is clear that increasing disability occurs with longer disease duration. However, it is important to note the great variability of this relationship. Nine of 20 patients with a diagnosis over one year who had remained relatively functional, even at the resolution of an acute illness. This same trend has been observed in a nonselected population of outpatients using the Karnofsky Performance Status as the functional assessment tool (Riggs, in press). Both studies suggest that there is a subpopulation of individuals with HIV infection who remain relatively functional (ie. low disability) late into the disease process. Although also limited by a small sample size, Weinstein (1990) has noted a similar variability in self-assessed functional behavior.

It would be clinically useful to predict which individuals tend to do well functionally and which do not. The primary manifestation of HIV infection might appear to be a logical predictor of function. Nonetheless, this characteristic was not demonstrated in the sample of 37 patients. This failure may be due to the small size of the sample. (The FIM documents only disability and says nothing about the underlying impairment(s) that may be responsible for that disability.) The influence of generalized fatigue may have been great considering that most deficits were more in the endurance-type activities of ambulation and stair climbing. Disease manifestation does affect the overall survival rate in AIDS (Lemp, 1990; Overton, 1988; Anderson & Medley, 1988), but larger, longitudinal studies are needed to delineate the relationship, if any, between disease manifestation and physical disability.

DISABILITY IN AIDS—A FRAMEWORK OF REFERENCE

The medical and surgical management of AIDS is a dynamic process and so, too, are issues related to physical disability. As mentioned previously, the two are closely linked. Better control and treatment of specific medical complications continues to evolve. Examples include PCP prophylaxis (Golden et al., 1989; Fischl et al., 1988) and improved, less toxic treatments for cryptococcal meningitis (Tozzi et al., 1989) and MAI (Murray & Mill, 1990).

From a functional standpoint, each specific complication or combination of symptoms leads to different functional deficits. Hypothetically, as the relative incidence and mortality of PCP declines, CNS complications might gain significance. If relatively more treatable lesions (toxoplasmosis) predominate over less treatable lesions (progressive multifocal leukoencephalopathy), then intervention for disability may be more appropriate. On the other hand, if other severe pulmonary complications (eg. cytomegalovirus pneumonia) occur in conjunction with a relatively treatable CNS complication, intervention may be less appropriate. This fact demonstrates that not only will the incidence and prevalence of HIV-related disability be changing over the next several years but also the specific face of the disabilities seen. This poses a formidable challenge in the design and methodology used in HIV disability research. The combination of these factors determines the relative utility of rehabilitation professionals evaluating HIV patients to have some idea of the functional significance and prognosis of a wide variety of HIV complications.

Because of this constantly changing scenario, it may be helpful to discuss a rather theoretic framework of reference for physical disability in HIV disease. HIV disability and its measurement functional assessment (see Appendix C) will probably be influenced by two major factors: characteristics of the population affected and characteristics of the disease process itself.

POPULATION CHARACTERISTICS

The predominantly young age of the HIV-seropositive population significantly influences the approach to disability. The effect of physical disability on vocation will be more pronounced than in typical models of geriatric dysfunction (Spence & Brownwell, 1984). Rehabilitation interventions that maintain persons with HIV infection in an employable state may be the greatest challenge to the field. It would also be a contribution of tremendous economic impact (Carwein & Ray, 1989). As the demographics of the epidemic change over the next several years (toward the urban poor), return to employment may be less of a consideration. For those who are working, vocational status itself may be the most sensitive reflection of overall functional ability, depending on the intellectual and physical demands of the occupation. The amount of time a person is able to work and any additional assistance required will be important variables to consider in functional assessment and treatment and intervention outcome.

The extremely high baseline function in this young population also poses difficulties in the measurement of disability. Tools to quantify functional demise must be very sensitive. They will need to focus on much higher level problems than simple ambulation and ADL around which much of rehabilitation centers. It will be essential to develop and use the concept of instrumental-activities of daily living (I-ADL) within the HIV population. I-ADL are those activities that allow one to function in the immediate environment (Lawton, 1971). Activities such as house cleaning, cooking, laundry, using the telephone and public transportation and ambulating beyond household distances are examples. These activities are in contrast to ADL, which are self-care oriented and generally considered lower level-activities (Spector et al., 1987). I-ADL decline will probably closely follow or occur simultaneously with vocational demise, depending on the exact circumstance. It is not at all unusual to see I-ADL and vocational demise before an AIDS-defining event, that is in persons with symptomatic HIV infection. Overt ADL dysfunction has tended to occur primarily in those with AIDS (CDC Group IV), many of whom have progressed far into the disease process.

Compensation and treatment for physical disability require motivation by the patient. The psychologic status of the patient is critically important when considering function (Chapters 11 and 15). Depression may significantly influence physical performance through decreased motivation or manifestation of fatigue. The role of patient collaboration in functional assessment has been discussed by Feinstein et al. (1985). The process of psychologic adjustment to physical disability may be hampered by the inconsistent, exacerbating/remitting nature of AIDS. This poor psychologic adjustment has been observed in multiple sclerosis, a relapsing/remitting disease that also affects primarily the young (Hartings et al., 1976). Physical disability and limitation themselves are probably frequent causes for depression in HIV-related illness (Tross & Hirsh, 1988).

Disease Characteristics

The manifestation of HIV infection plays a critical role in the types of HIV-related physical disability, as has already been briefly discussed. Once AIDS has been diagnosed, it is generally progressive, with frequent exacerbations and remissions. Although progression currently occurs over a relatively short period of time, it will increase in the future. The degree of disability at any one time does not necessarily reflect the disability over a period of time. Day-to-day fluctuation of function hampers the ability of rehabilitation professionals to assess the effects of either the disease process or subsequent treatment. The potential fluctuation of individual coping skills may further complicate the assessment. The combination of these factors may manifest as a discrepancy between dysfunction observed by the rehabilitation professional and that related by the patient or family. Intermittent fatigue is a common cause of this day-to-day functional variation and will be an important consideration when conducting longitudinal disability research. The wide variety of multiple impairments in HIV illness makes it difficult to make broad generalizations about HIV disability. When isolated impairments occur, disability management can be approached similarly to that of non-HIV disabled populations. In other words, isolated hemiparesis due to cerebral toxoplasmosis or paraparesis due to HIV myelopathy can be managed similarly to non-HIV stroke or spinal cord injured patient, respectively (see Chapter 9). More likely, however, hemiparesis in AIDS will be accompanied by other nonneurologic impairments such as pulmonary disease, chronic diarrhea, visual loss or complications due to generalized malnutrition. The association of HIV myelopathy with ADC could radically alter the rehabilitation approach and prognosis. One patient with HIV cardiomyopathy may successfully complete a standard cardiac rehabilitation program. Another patient with hemiparesis may complete inpatient rehabilitation, largely within the established model of care for geriatric strokes. The interplay between pulmonary, neurologic and neuropsychologic deficits necessitates an individual approach to patient management.

From a research standpoint, multiple impairment may make population disability studies difficult to interpret unless participants are stratified into similar categories based on complications, presence or absence of severe fatigue or cognitive status. This stratification could pose difficulties in recruiting significant numbers of people within any given category to achieve statistical power.

The neuropsychologic complications and pain management of HIV infection are detailed elsewhere (see Chapters 9 through 11). Cognitive changes seen in HIV infection can

and do have profound effects on high-level intellectual function. The effect on I-ADLs and ADLs in the absence of other disabling impairments needs to be explored. Significant ADL dysfunction due to isolated ADC is rarely seen before the terminal months of life. Neuropsychologic deficits may well affect vocational pursuits, depending on occupation. Nevertheless, the significance of neuropsychologic deficits early in HIV infection has been debated (Saykin et al., 1989). Disability due to pain may be secondary to peripheral neuropathy and pain syndromes later in the course of the disease are usually related to respiratory failure or musculoskeletal complications from prolonged bedrest. A relationship between pain and fatigue has been noted (Laskin, 1988) and deserves further investigation.

FATIGUE AS A SOURCE OF HIV DISABILITY

Fatigue is a clinically common source of physical limitation in patients with HIV infection. It is arguably the most important physical limitation before an AIDS-defining event. Despite this clinical impression, little research has been directed to the study of fatigue in HIV illness. Fatigue was mentioned as a presenting or common constitutional symptom in several studies of generalized lymphadenopathy in homosexual males (Yarchoan et al., 1989; Metroka et al., 1983; Mathur-Wagh et al., 1984; Kalish et al., 1984; Kaslow et al., 1987). No published studies have examined HIV fatigue as a separate entity. Rehabilitation professionals tend to view fatigue as a limitation rather than as a symptom of HIV infection. There are a number of possible etiologies for fatigue among the AIDS and HIV population, including anemia (either primary or secondary to infiltration or pharmacologic treatment), malnutrition, depression and cardiopulmonary insufficiency. Recent research has implicated a human T-lymphocyte virus (HTLV) in the pathogenesis of multiple sclerosis (Kawanishi et al., 1989), a disease where fatigue is also a great source of disability (Freal et al., 1984; Krupp et al., 1988). The pervasiveness of fatigue suggests the possibility of some innate ability of retroviruses to cause fatigue in humans. Efforts to link chronic fatigue syndrome with Epstein-Barr virus infection, however, have been largely unsuccessful (Koo, 1989).

The impact of fatigue on overall function can be significant in persons with relatively few, minor, or no other complications. Moderate-to-severe fatigue may mask other more specific functional deficits. This relationship should be considered in studies of functional assessment in AIDS and HIV illness. From a therapeutic standpoint, the presence of fatigue may prohibit the activity required to regain the strength, endurance or range of motion needed to correct more specific, temporary functional deficits.

Medical treatment of fatigue in multiple sclerosis has been most extensively investigated using amantadine (Murray, 1985). No studies have investigated the use of this drug in HIV disease. Small doses of methylphenidate hydrochloride (Ritalin) have been used with some success to treat fatigue in HIV disease. Dietary supplementation with essential fatty acids has also been reported to improve fatigue in symptomatic HIV individuals (Kahl et al., 1989). Further evaluation of this approach is currently being conducted at The Graduate Hospital in Philadelphia, PA. In the absence of a proven medical approach to the treatment of fatigue, the best approach is probably education in energy conservation and work simplification techniques (O'Connell, 1989).

Further research should be directed toward characterizing the fatigue seen in HIV disease. Fatigue surveys should carefully and completely document disease manifestations, concomitant drug therapy, basic laboratory tests, and effect of fatigue of daily function (see Appendix D). Once the prevalence and impact of fatigue is well documented, funding agencies may be more amenable to providing the needed resources to examine assessment procedures and treatment options.

DISABILITY RELATED TO TREATMENT OF HIV DISEASE

In evaluating HIV-related disability, it is important to remember potential and actual impairments caused by medications. These drugs may lead to new or additional physical disability.

The peripheral neuropathies associated with HIV infection have been well documented (So et al., 1988; Cornblath, 1988; Miller et al., 1988). Despite some suggestion that AZT is beneficial (Dalakas et al., 1988), HIV neuropathy is usually treated only symptomatically for painful paraesthesia. It should be noted that painful peripheral neuropathy is the limiting side effect in DDI (Lambert et al., 1990), and health care professionals may see the increase of the incidence of isolated, disabling peripheral neuropathy. PCP prophylaxis many times consists of administering dapsone, an antibiotic also associated with peripheral neuropathy (Koller, 1977). Chemotherapy as a treatment for KS usually includes vincristine and for *Mycobacterium* (typical and atypical) isoniazid (INH), both of which are well known to produce peripheral neuropathies (Casey, 1973; Victor, 1984). The disability secondary to neuropathy may be lessened or eliminated by discontinuing the inciting agent. Problems are usually limited to the lower extremity and will

affect ambulation and mobility. Painful paresthesia of the hand are seen occasionally, which may influence ADL.

Proximal weakness can be associated with HIV myopathy but has also been seen in AZT use for longer than 9 months (Gertner et al., 1989; Panegyres et al., 1988). This side effect is important to consider when evaluating patient complaints of fatigue and weakness. The presence of shoulder and pelvic girdle weakness should be determined and a history of AZT treatment obtained. Treatment consists of discontinuing the drug.

CONCLUSION

As the impact of HIV grows within the medical community, it will increasingly influence the practice of rehabilitation professionals. Just as diabetes mellitus was once a great killer and subsequently relegated to the status of a chronic disease, resulting in a tremendous range of physical disabilities for those affected, so too may be the future of persons with AIDS.

Research needs to focus on the epidemiology and natural history of physical disability in AIDS and HIV infection. Large longitudinal studies should delineate the types, degree, incidence, prevalence and timing of disability. This information can be used to develop interventional strategies and disease-specific functional assessment tools and to forecast costs related to physical dysfunction. Fatigue is a major source of disability in HIV infection. Today HIV-related disability must be managed clinically, but research is the only mechanism to plan for the future. By organizing and formalizing the "art of observation," essential data can be collected and quality of life enhanced for hundreds of thousands of individuals.

References

Anderson, R.M., and Medley, G. (1988). Epidemiology of HIV infection and AIDS: Incubation and infectious periods, survival, and vertical transmission. *AIDS.* 2:S57.

Arno, P.S., Shenson, D., Siegel, N.F., et al. (1989). Economic and policy implication of early intervention in HIV disease. *Journal of the American Medical Association.* 262:1493.

Aronow, H.A., Brew, B.S., and Price, R.W. (1988). The management of the neurological complication of HIV infection and AIDS. *AIDS.* 2:S151.

Auerback, V., and Jann, B. (1989). Neurorehabilitation and HIV infection: Clinical and ethical dilemmas. *The Journal of Head Trauma Rehabilitation.* 4:23.

Benjamin, A.E. (1989). *Perspectives on a Continuum of*

Care for Persons with HIV Illnesses. Conference Proceedings of New Perspective on HIV-Related Illness: Progress in Health Services Research.. National Center for Health Services Research and Health Care Technology Assessment. (DHHS Publication No. PHS 89-3449). Washington, DC: U.S. Government Printing Office.

Bolognesi, A.P. (1989). Prospects for prevention of and early intervention against HIV. *Journal of America Medical Association.* 261:3007.

Carwein, V.L., and Ray, C.G. (1989). AIDS-Related income losses and implications for policy making. *AIDS Public Policy Journal.* 4:106.

Casey, E.B. (1973). Vincristine Neuropathy. Clinical and electrophysiological observations. *Brain.* 96:69.

Cooley, T.P., Kunches, L.M., Saunders, C.A. et al. (1990). *New England Journal of Medicine.* 322:1340.

Cornblath, D.R. (1988). Treatment of the neuromuscular complication of human immunodeficiency virus infection. *Annals of Neurology.* 23:288.

Cornblath, D.R., and McArthur J.C. (1988). Predominately sensory neuropathy in patients with AIDS and AIDS-related complex. *Neurology.* 38:794.

Cotton, D. (1989). *Synthesis of Conference. Conference Proceedings of New Perspective on HIV-Related Illnesses: Progress in Health Services Research.*. National Center for Health Services Research and Health Care Technology Assessment. (DHHS Publication No. PHS 89-3449). Washington, DC: U.S. Government Printing Office.

Dalakas, M.C., Yarchoan, R., Spitzer, R., et al. (1988). Treatment of human immunodeficiency syndrome-related polyneuropathy with 3'-azido-2', 3' dideoxythymidine. *Annals of Neurology.* 23(supplement):s92.

Dubinsky, R.M., Yarchoan, R., Dalakas, M., and Broder, S. (1989). Reversible axonal neuropathy from the treatment of AIDS and related disorders with 2', 3' dideoxycytidine (ddC). *Muscle and Nerve.* 12:856.

Duckworth, D. (1984). The need for standardized terminology and classification of disablement. In Graham, C.V., and Gresham, G.E. (Eds.): *Functional Assessment in Rehabilitation Medicine.*. Baltimore: Williams & Wilkins.

Dyck, P.J., Thomas, P.K., and Lambert, E.H. (1975). *Peripheral Neuropathy by Seventy-Eight Authorities.* Philadelphia: W.B. Saunders.

Feinstein, A.R, Wells, C.K., Joyce, C.M., and Joseph, B. (1985). The evaluation and sensibility and the role of patient collaboration in clinometric indexes. *Transactions of the Association of American Physicians.* 98:146.

Fischl, M.A., Dickinson, G.M., and LaVoie, L. (1988). Safety and efficacy of sulfamethoxazole and trimethoprim chemoprophylaxis for *Pneumocystis carinii.*

pneumonia in AIDS. *Journal of American Medical Association.* 259:1185.

Fischl, M.A., Richman, D.D., Causey, D.M., et al. (1989). Prolonged zidovudine therapy in patients with AIDS and advanced AIDS-related complex. *Journal of the American Medical Association.* 262:2405.

Francis, R.A. (1989). Moral beliefs of physicians, medical students, clergy and lay public concerning AIDS. *Journal of the National Medical Association.* 81:1141.

Freal J.E., Kraft G.H., and Coryell J.K. (1984). Symptomatic Fatigue in multiple sclerosis. *Archives of Physical Medicine and Rehabilitation.* 65:135.

Gertner E., Thurn J.R., Williams D.N., et al. (1989). Zidovudine-l associated myopathy. *American Journal of Medicine.* 86:814.

Gill, O.N. (1988). Survival analysis of the first thousand cases of AIDS reported in the United Kingdom. Presented at the Fourth International Conference on AIDS. Stockholm Sweden.

Golden, J.A., Chernoff, D., Hollander H., et al. (1989). Prevention of *Pneumocystis carinii.* pneumonia by inhaled pentamidine. *Lancet.* 1:654.

Hartings M.F., Pavlow M.M., and Davis F.A. (1976). Group counseling of MS patients in a program of comprehensive care. *Journal of Chronic Diseases.* 29:65.

Janssen, RS., Saykin, AJ., Connon, L., et al. (1989). Neurological and neuropsychological manifestations of HIV-1 infections: Association with AIDS-related complex but not with asymptomatic HIV-1 infection. *Neurology.* 26:592.

Kahl, P., Golden, S., and Sears, B. (1989). Dietary intervention in ARC patients (abstract Th.B.P.#308). Presented at the Vth International Conference on AIDS, Montreal, Canada.

Kalish, S.B., Ostrow, D.G., Goldsmith, J., et al. (1984). The spectrum of immunologic abnormalities and clinical findings in homosexually active men. *Journal of Infectious Diseases.* 149:148.

Kapantais, G., and Powell-Griner, E. (1989). Characteristics of persons dying from AIDS: Preliminary data from the 1986 National Mortality Followback Survey. *Advance Data from Vitaland Health Statistics.*, Number 173. Hyattville, MD: National Center for Health Statistics.

Kaslow, F.A., Phair, J.P., Friedman, H.B., et al. (1987). Infection with the human immunodeficiency virus: Clinical manifestations and their relationship to immune deficiency. *Annals of Internal Medicine.* 107:474-480.

Kawanishi, T., Akiguchi, I., Fujita, M., et al. (1989). Low-titer antibodies reactive with HTLV-I gag p19 in patients with chronic myeloneuropathy. *Annals of Neurology.* 26:515.

Kaye, B.R. (1989). Rheumatologic manifestations of infection with human immunodeficiency virus (HIV). *Annals of Internal Medicine.* 111:158.

Koller, W.C. (1977). Dapsone-induced peripheral neuropathy. *Archives of Neurology.* 34:644.

Koo, D. (1989). Chronic fatigue syndrome--a critical appraisal of the role of Epstein-Barr virus. *Western Journal of Medicine.* 150:590.

Krupp, L.B., Alvarez, L.A., LaRocca, N.G., and Scheinburg, L.C. (1988). Fatigue in multiple sclerosis. *Archives of Neurology.* 45:435.

Lambert, J.S., Seidlin, M., Reichman, R.C., et al. (1990). 2', 3' -L Dideoxyinosine (ddI) in patients with the acquired immunodeficiency syndrome of AIDS-related complex. *New England Journal of Medicine.* 322:1333.

Laskin, M.E. (1988). Pain management in the patient with AIDS. *Journal of Advanced Medical-Surgical Nursing.* 1:37.

Lawton, M.P. (1971). The functional assessment of elderly people. *Journal of the American Geriatric Society.* 19:456.

Lemp, G.F., Payne, S.F., Neal, D., et al. (1990). Survival trends for patients with AIDS. *Journal of America Medical Association.* 263:402.

Marcusen, D.C., and Sooy, C.D. (1985) Otolaryngologic and head and neck manifestations of acquired immunodeficiency syndrome (AIDS). *Laryngoscope.* 95:401.

Mathur-Wagh, V., Spigland, I., Sacks, H.S., et al. (1984). Longitudinal study of persistent generalized lymphadenopathy in homosexual men: Relation to acquired immunodeficiency syndrome. *Lancet.* 1:1033.

Melvin, J. (1989). Rehabilitation in the Year 2000. *American Journal of Physical Medicine and Rehabilitation.* 67:197.

Metroka, C.E., Cunningham-Rundles, S., Pollack, M., et al. (1983). Generalized lymphadenopathy in homosexual men. *Annals of Internal Medicine.* 99:585.

Meythaler, J.M., and Cross, L.L. (1988). Traumatic spinal cord injury complicated by AIDS related complex. *Archives of Physical Medicine and Rehabilitation.* 69:219.

Miller, R.G., Parry, G.J., Pfaeffl, W., et al. (1988) The spectrum of peripheral neuropathy associated with ARC and AIDS. *Muscle and Nerve.* 11:857.

Murray T.J. (1985). Amantadine therapy for fatigue in multiple sclerosis. *Canadian Journal of Neurological Sciences.* 12:251.

Murray, D., and Mill, R. (1990). State of the art: Pulmonary complications of HIV infections. *American Review of Respiratory Disease.* 141:1356.

O'Connell P.G. (1989). The challenge of AIDS in rehabilitation—new problem in everyday practice, old solutions to a new disease. Presented at the 59th Annual meeting of the American Academy of Physical Medicine and Rehabilitation. Seattle, Washington.

O'Dell, M.W. (1989). Disability in Persons Hospitalized with AIDS. Presented at the 60th Meeting of The American Academy of Physical Medicine and Rehabilitation. San Antonio, Texas.

O'Dowd, M.A. (1988). Psychosocial issues of HIV infection. *AIDS.* 2:S201.

Opitz, J.L. (1990). Continuing physiatric education and our academy: Purpose, past, present, and prospect. *Archives of Physical Medicine and Rehabilitation.* 71:185.

Overton, S.E., Gill, O.N., Marasca, G., and Kennedy, A.R. (1988). Survival Analysis of the First Thousand Cases of AIDS Reported in the United Kingdom (abstract #4593). Presented at the Fourth International Conference on AIDS. Stockholm, Sweden..

Panegyres P.K., Tan N., Kakulas B.A., et al. (1988). Necrotizing myopathy and zidovudine. *Lancet.* 1:1050.

Rankin J.A., Collman R., and Daniels R.P. (1988). Acquired immune deficiency syndrome and the lung. *Chest.* 94:155.

Riggs, R.V., O'Dell, M.W., Turner, I.L., et al. (in press). Reliability of the Karnofsky Performance Status on the HIV Population. Abstract accepted for the Sixth International Conference on AIDS. San Francisco, California.

Saykin, A.J., Janssen, R. (1989). Neuropsychological and Psychosocial Function in Two Cohorts of Gay Men: Relationship to State of HIV-Infection. Presented at the Fifth International Conference on AIDS. Montreal, Canada.

So, Y.T., Holtzman, D.M., Abrams, D.I., and Olney, R.K. (1988). Peripheral neuropathy associated with acquired immunodeficiency syndrome. *Archives of Neurology.* 45:945.

Spector W.D., Katz S., Murphy J.B., and Fulton J.P. (1987). The hierarchical relationship between activities of daily living and instrumental activities of daily living. *Journal of Chronic Diseases.* 40:481.

Spence, D.L., and Brownell, W.W. (1984). Functional assessment of the aged person. In Granger, C.V., and Greshman, G.E. (Eds.): *Functional Assessment in Rehabilitation Medicine (pp. 254-272).* Baltimore: Williams & Wilkins.

Tozzi, V., Dordi, E., Galgani, S., et al. (1989). Fluconazole treatment of cryptococcosis in patient with acquired immunodeficiency syndrome. *American Journal of Medicine.* 87:353.

Tross, S., and Hirsh, D.A. (1988). Psychological distress and neuropsychological complications of HIV infection and AIDS. *American Psychologist.* 43:929.

Victor, M., Adamms, R.D. and Collins, G.H. (1989). The Wernicke-Korsafoff Syndrome and Related Neurologic

Disorders Due to Alcoholism and Malnutrition, 2d ed. Philadelphia: F.A. Davis.

Weinstein, B.D. (1990). Assessing the impact of HIV disease. *American Journal of Occupational Therapy*. 44:220.

Wood, P.H.N. (1988). Classification of impairments and handicaps. document WHO/ICDO/REV-Conf 75*15 Geneva, World Health Organization.

World Health Organization (WHO). (1980). *World Health Organization International Classification of Diseases*. Washington, DC: U.S. Department of Health and Human Services, 1:22.

Yarchoan, R., Mitsuya, H., and Broder, S.(1989). Clinical and basic advances in the antiviral therapy of human immunodeficiency virus. *American Journal of Medicine*. 87:191.

Yarchoan R., and Pluda J.M. (1988). Clinical aspects of infection with AIDS retrovirus: Acute HIV infection, persistent generalized lymphadenopathy and AIDS-related complex. In DeVita, J.T., Jr., Hallaman, S., Rosenberg, S., et al. (1988). *AIDS*, 2d ed. (pp. 107-196). Philadelphia: J.B. Lippincott.

14

Hospice Care

Paul Gustafson, MD, FACP

We should study success by looking at people who survive life-threatening illness. Such "exceptional" patients have certain characteristics in common. We should realize that people want care and healing not necessarily cure.

—Bernie S. Siegel, MD

INTRODUCTION

The care of persons with HIV continues to evolve as the epidemic gathers momentum. With over 130,000 cases of HIV reported to the CDC by March of 1990 (Centers for Disease Control, 1990a), the 270,000 cases predicted by the end of 1991 is fast becoming a reality. Hospitals in many of our largest cities are currently seeing an increasing number of general hospital beds occupied by HIV patients. As caseloads in all risk groups continue to increase, epidemiologists are predicting that the peak of the epidemic will not be reached until the end of 1993 (Centers for Disease Control, 1990b). With this rise in the number of cases and the increased longevity of patients because of effective anti-retroviral therapy (AZT), aerosolized pentamidine, and medical support in general, it is becoming clear that more cost-effective and innovative ways of caring for chronically ill or dying patients with AIDS need to be explored and demonstrated.

These issues are currently being studied by the public and private sector in an attempt to care for those afflicted with this illness and at the same time prevent depletion of limited resources. Efforts to contain costs in this area thus far have focused on various forms of managed health care, which attempt in one way or another to limit access to care. Despite the desire to cut costs, very little has yet been done to address the potential role of traditional hospice care. Because hospice care for patients with HIV infection has not previously been considered a viable alternative, the ability to demonstrate cost savings and efficacy has not been thoroughly appreciated.

DEFINITION OF HOSPICE

Hospice is a concept and not strictly a place. It represents a coordinated program of palliative and supportive care services and provides care for a varied group of patients. These patients include those who are hopelessly ill or dying, many of whom have cancer or HIV disease.

HIV-seropositive patients who are candidates for hospice care include chronically ill demented patients, patients with severe neuropathy or neurologic syndromes such as PML, patients with refractory or untreatable opportunistic infections or malignancies, patients with blindness secondary to progressive refractory cytomegalovirus retinitis, patients too ill to care for themselves, and those without adequate home care. Traditionally, hospice care has been offered to patients with an estimated life span of less than six months. Care is provided either in the home or in an inpatient facility, which may be either free standing or affiliated with an acute care hospital or nursing home. The hospice team is a multidisciplinary team that is physician-directed and implemented primarily by nurses; aides; physical, occupational and speech therapists; counselors; pharmacists; and case managers. The focus of hospice care is the patient and the patient's family and/or significant other. Hospice services include assessment and evaluation; physical, occupational and speech therapy; medical care; teaching and education; social services; pastoral care and counseling; and bereavement counseling. Hospices also provide discharge planning for those who, for one reason or another, recover and are able to return to their home environment.

The history of hospice dates back to ancient times when it was primarily a sanctuary for the sick and needy (Personal communication, 1990). In medieval times, hospices were often run by religious orders. The origin of modern hospice dates back to St. Christopher's Hospital in London in the 1940s and owes much of its heritage to Dr. Cicely Saunders. Modern hospices in the United States began in 1974 when Hospice, Inc. was founded in New Haven, Connecticut, by Florence Wald, RN. Yale University played a prominent role in the founding of this first hospice of the United States.

HOSPICE PHILOSOPHY

Hospice recognizes dying as part of the normal process of living and focuses on maintaining and preserving the quality of life. It prepares patients and their families for death. Hospice attempts to preserve the integrity and autonomy of the patient while attempting to relieve pain and other troubling symptoms such as anorexia, decubitus ulcers, nausea, dysphagia, seizures and fever. Diagnostic tests, x-rays, and blood work are usually kept to a minimum and continuity of care is stressed (Stoddard 1978).

Long ago, hospices were established to provide lodging for travelers. Today, hospice is a concept—a multidisciplinary team providing palliative and support services to both patient and family. The philosophy of hospice is practiced in special hospital units, established hospice nursing homes, and within the patient's home.

Hospice hopes to provide a homelike environment for their patients and includes familiar objects such as pictures and other comforting keepsakes. Emphasis of care is on allowing the patient some control over the situation, reinforcing a sense of worthiness and dignity. Overall, the patient's wishes are the first consideration. Unfortunately, admission into some hospices requires a survival prognosis of less than a month. An alternative approach is the hospices that emphasize living with AIDS, not dying. Ideally, there needs to be a balance, with emphasis on comforting death and rehabilitating life.

PAIN CONTROL

An important goal of hospice care is the control and elimination of pain. Moribund or preterminal patients are often consumed by pain and often seek little more than its elimination. Hospice attempts to provide patients with effective pain relief. As-needed schedules are not used since they, by definition, require patients to experience pain and receive palliation on a schedule. Narcotic analgesics are given on a regular schedule with the goal of rendering patients pain-free at all times. When this goal can be achieved, it uniformly enhances the quality of the patient's remaining life. Because of the necessity to administer medication and the fact that patients will likely be on narcotics until they die, addiction is generally not a concern. This concept is sometimes difficult for both patients and health care workers to understand because our society is so thoroughly educated that drug addiction is, by definition, bad.

Morphine sulfate given by continuous infusion in concentrated doses through IV, subcutaneously, and orally continues to be the most effective means of controlling chronic pain. When morphine is carefully titrated, most patients are able to function without a major change in their mental status and with little alteration in their vital signs. This titration takes very careful attention, and doses need to be escalated slowly. Patients should have the ability to request bolus or extra doses of morphine when breakthrough pain becomes a problem. Use of other psychotropic medications and sedatives can many times complement the use of morphine as an effective analgesic.

TYPES OF MEDICAL CARE

Hospice care is the usual form of medical care offered. This type of care focuses on symptom relief only. A more active form of care generally confused with hospice care is supportive (palliative) care. This care's focus is to sustain, support and extend life; in many instances, it is felt to include provision of intravenous fluids and enteral or parenteral nutrition. It also includes surgery, radiotherapy, chemotherapy and hormonal therapy. Most true hospice patients generally do not choose to pursue this form of care. Blood transfusions and TPN, although traditionally not felt to be consistent with the goals of hospice, are sometimes indicated, if they are perceived to provide comfort. Patients who express the desire to continue to receive supportive care usually have previously not resolved the concept of death and often express a desire to be resuscitated or transferred back to the general hospital should they become ill. Patients requesting hospice care only have generally thought carefully about the issue of resuscitation and have expressed a desire not to be resuscitated if they expire. A smaller group of patients admitted to the modern hospice of the 1990s are indeed capable of rehabilitation and restoration of a sufficient amount of function to allow discharge. These kinds of circumstances arise when patients thought to be near death are transferred out of the general hospital into the hospice, fully expecting to continue to go downhill and expire. Most hospices have documented numerous cases where unexpected recovery has occurred in both moribund HIV patients and cancer patients. Physicians must promptly recognize when this type of recovery occurs and offer both rehabilitative and restorative care. The type of medical care offered to each group of patients must be carefully reviewed with both patients and their families. It must be absolutely clear what the expectations are and, likewise, what the perceived prognosis is. All involved must be in agreement with the plan so that basic misunderstandings do not occur in regard to the provision of terminal care and in the likely event of withholding various interventions that might prolong life.

ROLE OF THE PHYSICIAN

The role of the physician begins with recognizing the need for hospice care and recommending or advising admission to a hospice. The physician is the source of all provided medical care in terms of orders that are written in the patient's charts and general supervision of the hospice team.

Hospice rounds are an integral part of the hospice care and, when compared to general hospital care, are usually less frequent. Generally, hospice rounds two or three times weekly are sufficient to responsibly direct the care of most hospice patients. Hospice rounds are best conducted with the nucleus of the hospice team so that all members of the team can appreciate the changes occurring in the patient's care. The physician must be acutely aware of the natural course of the disease processes of patients admitted to the program. This knowledge allows the physician to make the appropriate decisions about possible interventions. The physician must also be a source of psychologic support and counseling, although these tasks are more actively undertaken by members of the hospice team.

DEATH AND DYING

The concepts of death and dying are not well taught or understood, even in medical and nursing schools. This, along with the natural fear of death, has resulted in medical care that generally seeks to deny the existence of death and dying. These concepts are addressed openly in hospice care from the beginning. They are discussed actively by physicians, nurses and social workers and are viewed as a natural process of life. Counseling in this area is time consuming and highly individualistic and must take into account a patient's religion and social upbringing, as well as fantasies and misconceptions about death. In addition, guilt often needs to be explored. Occasionally, patients misinterpret the goal of preventing and alleviating pain with the use of morphine sulfate and other potent narcotic analgesics. Thus, an occasional family member or caretaker may believe that they have contributed to the death of a loved one by either administering morphine or perhaps requesting that an intervention either be discontinued or not offered (ie., intravenous fluids or nasogastric tube feedings). These treatments, when offered, not offered, or withdrawn, are not felt in and of themselves to be the cause of a patient's death. It must be explained that administering fluids and nutrition through either intravenous or nasogastric tubes is something that artificially and unnecessarily sustains the life of a loved one who otherwise would die from the natural course of the illness. This view of life support systems is an important concept in the current debate over whether medicine and society should allow such behavior to be sanctioned.

COST EFFECTIVENESS

Numerous hospices have already been established for persons living with HIV disease, including the Casey house in Toronto, Canada, the London Lighthouse in England, the Village Nursing Home in New York, Coming Home Hospice in San Francisco, the Shanti Project in San Francisco and CASA—A Special Hospital in Houston.

CASA—A Special Hospital is a free-standing hospice in Houston, Texas. It has an academic affiliation with the University of Texas Medical School in Houston, but is basically a private center to which private physicians admit their patients. It admits a broad spectrum of patients with various medical diagnoses including HIV, cancer, and chronic medical disorders. It also provides interim medical care for numerous other patients who have needs such as blood transfusions, long-term supervised antibiotic therapy and physical therapy.

During 1989, 94 patients were admitted with HIV-related problems. Thirty-five patients (37 percent) died at CASA and 54 (58 percent) were discharged. The longest patient stay was 99 days; the shortest was one day. The average length of stay was 22 days, with 2,039 total patient days. The average cost per day while at CASA was $324.03, as compared with the average cost per day in an acute care hospital in the Houston area for HIV care, which is approximately $1,000.00 per day. This difference results in an average direct savings of $675.97 per day. Calculated total savings on 2,039 patient days was calculated to be $1,378,302.00. Recently, it was calculated that an individual

---

Table 14-1
THE DYING PATIENT'S BILL OF RIGHTS

I have the right to be treated as a living human being until I die.

I have the right to maintain a sense of hopefulness, however changing in focus may be.

I have the right to be cared for by those who can maintain a sense of hopefulness, however changing this might be.

I have the right to express my feelings and emotions about my approaching death in my own way.

I have the right to participate in decisions concerning my care.

I have the right to expect continuing medical and nursing attention even though "cure" goals must be changed to "comfort" goals.

I have the right to die alone.

I have the right to be free from pain.

I have the right to have my questions answered honestly.

I have the right not to be deceived.

I have the right to have help from and for my family in accepting my death.

I have the right to retain my individuality and not be judged for my decisions, which may be contrary to beliefs of others.

I have the right to discuss and enlarge my religious and/or spiritual experiences, whatever these may mean to others.

I have the right to expect that the sanctity of the human body will be respected after death.

I have the right to be cared for by caring, sensitive, knowledgeable people who will attempt to understand my needs and will be able to gain some satisfaction in helping me face my death.

Reprinted with permission of the American Hospital Association, Copyright 1972.

---

patient cost was approximately $100,000.00 less per month during a three-month stay at CASA compared with the general acute care hospital (Personal communication, 1990). This demonstration has led one of the major case management programs in the Houston area to consider more carefully the role of hospice in the care of the chronically ill patient infected with HIV.

Paradoxically, despite these dramatic demonstrated savings, many carriers have no provision for hospice care in their allowed benefits and often refuse to approve payment for hospice care. Rather, they demand that patients be admitted to a general hospital for what is considered to be approved and reimbursed care. The John Alden Life Insurance Company, however, has taken an innovative approach to the care of HIV patients and has established the John Alden Life Case Management Program developed by the AIDS Medical Research Center (Nary, 1989). This program will attempt to incorporate the concept of both inpatient and outpatient hospice as a means of both saving money and delivering appropriate and indicated quality medical care. It is hoped that their experience will further demonstrate the appropriateness of hospice care in this patient population and will lead to an increase in the use of hospice for patients with HIV infection and other catastrophic medical problems. Thoughtful and appropriate use of hospice services for patients with HIV infection should be considered an alterna-

tive in providing care for a significant percentage of patients who are debilitated by this disease. Health care professionals will need to educate themselves about the utility of hospice and incorporate it into their care plan when planning discharge, in general disposition, and during long-term treatment. When this is achieved, patients, families, and the medical care system will benefit.

SUMMARY

This chapter reviewed the hospice concept and cost-effective management of care, with emphasis on living fully with chronic HIV disease. Table 14-1 reviews the Patient's Bill of Rights (Whitman & Lukes, 1975).

References

Centers for Disease Control. (1990a, April). U.S. AIDS cases reported through March 1990. *HIV/AIDS Surveillance*.

Centers for Disease Control. (1990b). Estimates of HIV prevalence and projected AIDS cases: summary of a workshop, October 31- November 1, 1989. *Morbidity and Mortality Weekly Report*. 39(7):110.

Nary, G. (1989). Less costly care for HIV patients. *Best's Review*. 90(6):50.

Robertson, L., Vice President of Affiliated Healthcare, Inc. Personal Communication, 25 January 1990. Personal Communication. March 10, 1990. Stoddard, S. (1978). *The Hospice Movement*. New York: Stein and Day.

Whitman, H., and Lukes, S. (1975). Behavior modification for terminally ill patients. *American Journal of Nursing*. 75:98.

15

Psychosocial Issues of HIV Patients and Health Care Professionals

William Scott, CSW
Mary Hilliard, RN, MS, LPC

Great men are they who see that spiritual is stronger than any material force, that thoughts rule the world.

—Ralph Waldo Emerson

INTRODUCTION

The psychosocial impact of HIV on the lives of people with HIV infection and the professionals that work with this disease process is tremendous (Forstein, 1984). The emotional experiences of the patient facing a life-threatening illness are determined by a number of factors, including the nature of the patient's mental health before the diagnosis of the disease and the quality and extent of life possible (Blaney & Piccol, 1987). Many of the problems that the patients must deal with are, in turn, what the health professionals working with them have to face, only from a different perspective.

HIV PATIENTS

Stigma

Because the disease has been associated with homosexuality and drug abuse, two culturally unacceptable behaviors, society attaches a severe stigma to HIV. The reality that HIV can be transmitted, heightens both rational and irrational fears of contagion. Moreover, the epidemic is surrounded by a sense of blame that society places on homosexuals, drug users, prostitutes and other groups (Forstein, 1984). All of

this affects people living with HIV. They must deal with the negative attitudes of family, friends, health care professionals, employers, landlords and the rest of society. Individuals are often discriminated against, judged and rejected. These reactions may lead to the those living with HIV to internalize the negative attitudes confronting them, further complicating the psychologic problems of dealing with the diagnosis.

Due to these stigmas, it is easy to understand why many persons with HIV do not reveal their diagnosis to their friends, family and loved ones. In attempts to avoid the stigmatism of the disease, many isolate themselves at the exact time that love and support is most needed (Dilley et al., 1985). This fear of disclosure may be very rational because many HIV seropositive individuals have experienced rejection by family and friends upon revealing their diagnosis.

The stigmatism of diagnosis affects people in different ways due to such variables as sex, race, sexual preference, economic status, social status and mental health. Openly homosexual men, for example, may belong to more socially, economically, racially, and politically diverse communities that are more accepting of HIV disease than heterosexual, married males that are secretly addicted to drugs. Women diagnosed with HIV have special problems because the disease is more commonly associated with men. HIV-positive women usually do not have a context in which to discuss their diagnosis, further exacerbating their fears and sense of isolation.

Informational Needs and Education

Individuals living with HIV are deluged with information about the disease process, which they must sort through in order to make informed decisions about their illness. Further compounding the patient's confusion and anxiety are many important questions about prognosis, treatment and the course of the illness that remain unanswered (Dilley et al, 1985). Clients often feel frustrated about the lack of consistent answers and the degree of uncertainty they face. This uncertainty may lead patients to feel anger and resentment toward care givers. Whenever possible, patients need accurate information to feel in control of their future. Many patients also feel angry and afraid because they feel as if they are "being experimented upon."

Educational intervention is essential so that fears and anxieties can be addressed. Patients need to know about modes of transmission; methods of treatment and their side effects; the course of the illness; neuropsychologic complications; infection control; support groups; and medical, psychiatric, legal and social services. The entire medical team can assist in disseminating this information. During periods of high anxiety and fear, the patient often does not remember information presented to them, making repetition necessary. In addition to receiving the information verbally, it is also helpful if the information is presented in written form.

Since 30 to 75 percent of all HIV seropositive persons experience some form of cognitive impairment (Wolcott et al., 1985; Christ et al., 1986), it is essential for them and their families to receive neurologic information about the disease (see Chapter 11). Short-term memory loss, confusion, disorientation, symptoms of depression, thought disorders, delusions and behavioral and personality changes are not uncommon (Dilley et al., 1986). In-service programs about intervention strategies with patients that are experiencing cognitive decline are imperative for the rehabilitation team. Medical and neuropsychologic referrals must be provided in order to discern etiology and possible treatment of the symptoms of each HIV patient. The importance of various interpersonal therapy techniques, such as supportive, insightful, cognitive and behavioral models, cannot be overestimated when discussing dementia. Both patients and the family members must be advised about what to anticipate in both the short and long term. Family members also need to be educated about both practical assistance and developing interventions to help the person who is experiencing these often disturbing neurologic complications. Such interventions include use of large calendars, lists of

daily activities, verbal and written reminders and cues, use of simple language, and labeling of household items.

Patients need to be informed about the diverse adaptive emotional responses that they may experience while trying to cope with HIV disease. Knowing that their reactions are relatively normal and expected helps defer patient fear and anxiety.

Basic Necessities

After testing positive for HIV, many people become immediately concerned with the finances of treatment and survival. Many will need housing, child care, transportation and legal services, in addition to medical and psychologic treatment. Finances must be obtained as quickly as possible due to the ongoing expenses of treatment, as the disease may progress quite rapidly.

Housing is often a primary concern because of the inability to maintain mortgage or rent payments due to the loss of a job, eviction after diagnosis is disclosed, or the need to relocate to a new area in order to receive better medical attention. Without housing, many may need to extend their hospital stay, which adds to increased medical costs. HIV-seropositive women with children have compounded problems finding adequate housing and often have to settle for less than optimal conditions.

Complex legal issues arise around HIV due to the nature of the disease. Wills, child support, powers of attorney, and life support need to be legally documented early in the progression of the disease while patients are still cognitively capable of making such decisions. Legal documentation is especially important for homosexuals who wish their partners to have power of attorney and primary say in major decisions because these relationships are not protected by the law (see Chapter 16).

Patients who do not require full hospital attention should consider alternatives such as home care, outpatient care, or hospice. Though these alternatives are not inexpensive, studies show that they are not as expensive as hospital stays (see Chapter 14).

Psychologic and Emotional Responses

Due to the chronic, progressive nature of HIV, health care professionals must attend to the physiologic, psychologic, and sociocultural needs of patients. It is important to continually assess patients living with HIV in many diverse areas to ascertain where patients may need intervention or awareness. Various approaches can be used. One approach is to implement the following guidelines developed by studying HIV-positive persons in San Francisco and Houston who lived longer than medically predicted, with a diagnosis of advanced disease. Table 15-1 generically applies to most subgroups.

Table 15-1
GUIDELINES FOR APPROACHING PEOPLE LIVING WITH HIV

Working with the doctor	The patient must have a trusting and working relationship with the physician.
Mortality issues	The death and dying processes are different issues. Once dealt with, the patient can go on living (This includes issues of afterlife, wills, etc.).
Hope	Matilda Krin said, "Without hope you have a broken heart."
Spirituality	Not necessarily organized religion. Spirituality is very individualistic, and patients need nonjudgmental acceptance in this area.
Unfinished business	"If you never lied you would never have to remember anything." Most unfinished business (sometimes deception, or cover-ups, etc.) needs completion. (ie, the coming out process for gays and bisexuals at work and/or with family) is often a primary issue.
Relaxation	The practice of applied relaxation can teach patients a coping skill that will enable them to counteract and eventually abort anxiety reactions (Oct. 1987).
Exercise	Exercise has its limitations and patients need to be informed of its benefits and limits. Various forms of exercise are great ways of reducing stress (see Chapter 7).
Dealing with anxiety	Each individual has his/her own way of dealing with anxiety, depression, and stress. As different modalities of treatment are used to address the above, communication with the patient in a manner easily understood is essential.
Healing alternatives	Does the health professional know about alternatives? Are they safe and/or effective? The patient often feels the need to inquire about the professional's opinion on what they are engaging in separate from traditional medicine (ie. yoga, nutrition, meditation, or acupuncture).
Meeting hierarchy of needs	Maintaining control in all areas: a. Social b. Intimacy c. Purpose and Meaning d. Family e. Recreation

Group Therapy

A wide range of group interventions have been found useful for the person facing life-threatening illnesses (Macks, 1987). A short-term, closed-group model can provide consistency, thereby enhancing the development of social support. The structure provides a contained environment that models for the patient the ability to manage overwhelming feelings and provides the context for empowerment and hopefulness. Long-term groups can offer increased opportunities for in-depth therapeutic intervention, but they can be significantly affected by difficulty in maintaining consistent group attendance due to physical illness. The major disadvantage to closed-group models is that significant lag time may occur between the client's initial contact and the beginning of the group. Drop-in groups can be especially useful for persons requiring immediate intervention or for individuals whose emotional and physical state may prevent them from making a commitment to a time-limited or ongoing closed group.

Stages of Illness

The psychosocial needs of people living with HIV vary not only with race, sex and economic status, as mentioned previously, but also with the stage of the illness. In dealing with HIV, three stages of psychologic reaction, each characterized by specific issues and tasks, have been identified (Forstein, 1984; Dilley et al., 1986). The initial stage begins when the individual tests positive for HIV. This stage is often a period of crisis in which the patient may experience feelings of profound anxiety, complete shock and denial, and overwhelming emotion. Emotional responses range from affective numbness to affective discharge. The individual may also feel an impending death, although this is often not an immediate issue. Fears include rejection by family, friends and society. There is often a loss of self-esteem accompanied by feelings of guilt and self-blame due to previous life-style. Patients during this stage commonly feel as if they were to blame for the disease (Dilley et al., 1985). Questions about the future of their sexual experiences, as well as existential searching, are often prevalent. During this initial stage, patients may need crisis intervention. Education and support are essential for patients to resolve returning to their previous level of psychologic and social functioning.

The middle stage is comprised of three parts. The first part, "getting on with life," cannot occur until the patient has overcome the denial of infection. The second part involves dealing with immediate and anticipated losses. During this part of the illness, many homosexuals and substance users, having to inform their family and friends of their life-styles, anticipate the loss of love and support. Patients may feel isolated as a result of the gloves, gowns and masks that health care professionals wear, as well as a lessened sense of intimacy with loved ones. Social withdrawal is common. Ongoing processes, such as taking care of unfinished emotional and practical business, may aid patients in their ability to continue life. During the third part, patients must contend with fluctuating or deteriorating physical states. With the loss of body function, status and control, there is usually a corresponding lack of hope as well as grieving. During this time, health care professionals might easily approach patients about issues such as the extent of treatment, pain control, the use of life support, and, if applicable, treatment for drug use (Dilley et al., 1986).

The final stage is terminal care. Both patients and loved ones may experience immense fear of pain, abandonment and death and dying. There may be a corresponding lack of personal contact due to the family's and friends' fear of death and/or of someone who is dying. Health care professionals, who usually have had more experience with death and dying, can work with loved ones in dealing with these difficult issues. During the natural process of breaking away, health care professionals need to be conscious of neglecting patients that they have become close to and no longer feel they can help. Of primary importance during this last stage of life is for family members, friends and health care workers to honor, if possible, the patient's wishes (see Patient's Bill of Rights, Chapter 14).

Grief

Many of the grieving processes that HIV-seropositive individuals experience are similar to those experienced by cancer and burn patients. The stages of the grief process, as identified by Kubler-Ross (1969), are denial, anger, bargaining, depression and acceptance. As HIV patients experience these stages, they are often on a roller coaster of emotion, harboring both conscious and unconscious fears, anger and sadness. Many of the fears of grieving relate to death and dying; however, many say that they are more afraid of the long, drawn-out process of dying associated with HIV infection than the actual death. Compounding this is the usual young age of this patient population. These patients may not have dealt with death and dying before the time of their infection. Due to this lack of understanding about the dying processes before illness, therapists often stress existentialism and spirituality.

Fear and Anxiety

HIV patients commonly request and require aid in dealing with their feelings and emotions. Patients may feel anger, sadness, frustration, loneliness, hopelessness, despair, loss of control and guilt. Patients may have to abandon their careers and their roles as financial providers, which lead many to feelings of failure. Watching their healthy and physically fit bodies deteriorate is difficult. There is a corresponding loss of self-esteem due to decline in appearance and perceived self-worth. Patients may feel guilty about having acquired the disease. This may possibly be due to unresolved feelings about homosexuality or drug abuse or to the internalization of families', friends', and health care professionals' (either conscious or unconscious) condemnations of homosexuality, substance use or race (Macks, 1988).

These reactions can understandably lead to depression and anxiety in seropositive individuals. Anxiety reactions in which patients feel the intrusion of thoughts about HIV, symptoms, and death associated with panic, sleep disturbances, and somatic complaints are the first signs of depression. If not deferred at this stage, patients will later experience the more severe symptoms of depression, such as sleep disorders, anorexia, apathy, despair and suicidal tendencies. (Macks, 1988).

Most people with HIV have considered suicide. In 1985 in New York City, the relative risk of suicide in men between the ages of 20 and 59 with HIV was 36.3 times that of men of the same age group without HIV disease. Furthermore, the risk was 66.15 times that of the population at large (Marzuk et al., 1988). Health care professionals may have a high index of suspicion for suicide risk in these patients, openly inquire about it and arrange for appropriate intervention. (Rogers, 1988).

Hope and Denial

In living with and managing the course of HIV disease, all involved—patients, family, loved ones and health care workers must maintain hope. Possibilities to consider include getting involved with experimental and complimentary treatments, assisting the patient in establishing future plans, joining support groups and creating a renewed sense of spirituality.

Although denying the reality of HIV by denying it to the self, not disclosing the diagnosis to significant others, not receiving medical treatment, substance use, or continual involvement in risky behaviors is definitely not healthy, some constructive denial is essential for well-being. Constructive denial allows the patient to have breaks from the illness and lessens anxieties and fears. Health care professionals need to keep the denial in check to make sure that it does not become destructive.

Significant Others

While HIV-seropositive patients are experiencing physical and emotional stress due to the illness, their families are often experiencing parallel emotional processes. Not uncommonly, the family is dealing with two new issues at once: the family member's diagnosis of HIV and the knowledge that their loved one is homosexual or a substance user. Families often feel betrayed, embarrassed or angry. Many parents feel guilty, as if they failed as a parent and are somehow to blame for their child's illness. Families may experience denial and may be reluctant to reveal the nature of the family member's illness or are uneasy about receiving family therapy. If family dynamics warrant, or if patients request, the health care professional should recommend intervention to family members. If the patient's significant other or friends are involved in the patient's care, family problems may be compounded. Parents and siblings may not be capable of understanding the nature of their loved one's homosexual relationships and, therefore, diminish their significance.

The patient's lover or spouse is also likely to experience emotional disturbances. In addition to the grief, anger and fear of losing their partner, they must also deal with fears of personal infection; being responsible for their partner's infection; rejection from their family, their partner's family or both; and lack of support from their employees, friends and loved ones who do not acknowledge the significance of the relationship. The patient's friends may overidentify with the patient and develop disease-related anxieties. They may also overcompensate either by becoming intrusive or by distancing to the point of avoidance in attempts to deal with their own fears and anxieties about contagion, HIV disease and death and dying.

HEALTH CARE PROFESSIONALS

Dealing with the Issues

Many health care professionals find that working with HIV patients is both physically and emotionally difficult at times. In order for health care professionals to successfully treat these patients, they must be comfortable with their own feelings about the issues surrounding the disease. These issues include cultural and racial concerns, identity, sexual abuse and incest, spirituality, death, uncertainty in the treatment and course of the illness and limited technology. Health care givers confront difficulties such as information overload, inadequate reimbursements, fear of infection, hopelessness, ethical dilemmas, burnout, dislike of the patient population and homophobia (Cooke & Sande, 1989; Schlotterer, 1989).

Many health care workers identify with their HIV-seropositive patients, who are often young, vibrant people experiencing multiple health changes in the prime of their life. Though some identification is necessary for the therapeutic process, overidentification by the health care worker can cause loss of professional objectivity or periods of irrational fears and vulnerability to the disease (Dunkel & Hatfield, 1986). Health care professionals may distance themselves from patients by concentrating on the differences between them, resulting in unconscious judgment of the patient's life-style, behavior or social class.

Personal fear and shame-based behaviors must be recognized by the health care worker and dealt with appropriately. Common fears of health care professionals include fear of the unknown, fear of contagion, fear of death and dying, fear of homosexuality and/or homosexuals, and fear of substance users (Dunkel & Hatfield, 1986). Education is paramount in combating many of these fears. Shamed based behavior may surface in dealing with a patient who triggers "family secrets" (Sowers, 1988). For example, working with a patient who is (or was) an IV drug user or a prostitute may bring forth painful memories of someone in the health care worker's family who followed the same behavior patterns. To work with patients who have HIV disease, health care professionals need to acknowledge their own misgivings and beliefs in order to give themselves choices.

Acknowledging these feelings is very important for psychosocial intervention. Often verbal acknowledgment with the HIV-positive patient or a co-worker will help health care workers feel more comfortable and capable of the sensitive communication required to help the patient. Professional ethics challenge the health care worker to "let go of the need to feel different from people who have AIDS" (Shernoff, 1989).

As with the patient population, denial on the part of health care professionals is an oxymoron. On one hand, denial aids in providing hope and combating the stress of working with patients living with HIV; on the other hand, denial may lead health care professionals to have unrealistic expectations and to experience guilt and professional failure when these expectations are not met.

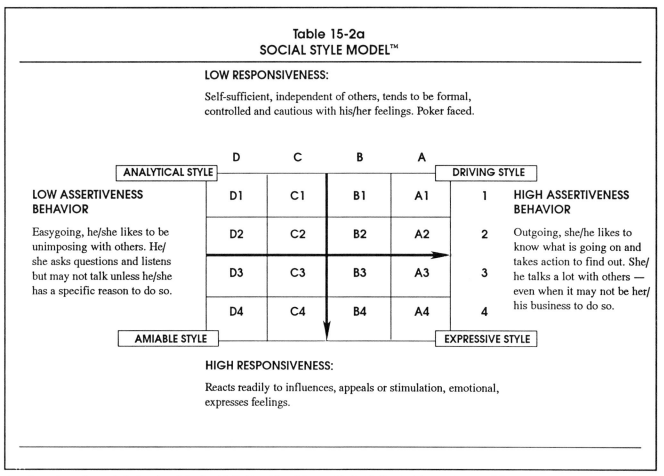

Table 15-2a
SOCIAL STYLE MODEL™

LOW RESPONSIVENESS:

Self-sufficient, independent of others, tends to be formal,
controlled and cautious with his/her feelings. Poker faced.

	D	C	B	A		
ANALYTICAL STYLE						DRIVING STYLE
LOW ASSERTIVENESS BEHAVIOR	D1	C1	B1	A1	1	HIGH ASSERTIVENESS BEHAVIOR
Easygoing, he/she likes to be unimposing with others. He/she asks questions and listens but may not talk unless he/she has a specific reason to do so.	D2	C2	B2	A2	2	Outgoing, she/he likes to know what is going on and takes action to find out. She/he talks a lot with others — even when it may not be her/his business to do so.
	D3	C3	B3	A3	3	
	D4	C4	B4	A4	4	
AMIABLE STYLE						EXPRESSIVE STYLE

HIGH RESPONSIVENESS:

Reacts readily to influences, appeals or stimulation, emotional,
expresses feelings.

An adaptation of materials developed by David W. Merrill and Roger M. Reid. Used with permission of the Tracom Corporation, Denver, Colorado.

Interacting with patients' significant others may also be physically and emotionally exhausting for health care professionals (Dilley & Forstein, 1988). Often, family care givers depend on and work closely with health care professionals to meet the demands of sequence of HIV infection. In its own way, this approach may be the combining of two different styles of dealing with HIV infection: one of a mother, a lover, or a significant other and the person who has HIV. Each will display a different style of communication, education, and social skills, as well as a different style of tolerance for the various stages of loss.

Most people fall into four fairly defined categories of life management behavior. One model to work with is an adaptation of the Social Style Model™ as found in *Personal Style and Effective Performance* (Merrill & Reid, 1981) (Table 15-2a-c). With this information, patients can be divided into categories that might help health care professionals step out of their own peer group and work more effectively when approaching patients and family members

with different behavioral characteristics. By using the following information, a person's style of behavior may be assessed and this information used in working with the patient. The Social Style Model™ is used by rating the individual as A, B, C, or D on the Assertiveness scale, and then rating them as 1, 2, 3, or 4 on the Responsiveness scale. A letter and a number will be arrived at, B 3 for example. The box corresponding to that letter and number lists the characteristics and assesses communication skills. The summation charts help in dealing with the patient on his or her own level.

The Health Care Professionals' Needs

Health care professionals need to admit that they cannot be all things to all people (Shubin, 1989). They must accept professional and personal limits in working with HIV disease. In addition, health care workers should set boundaries and initiate stress reduction for themselves to implement self care.

Table 15-2b
SOCIAL STYLE™ DESCRIPTION

ANALYTICAL STYLE (AN) WHO IS HIV+

Style Determinants:

Person generally has a monotone voice and a slow speech pattern. Their gestures tend to be restrained and they make little use of their hands. In questioning, this person will respond and understand a HOW? question first, then WHAT, WHY, WHO.

They value credibility, information, facts and order. They are concerned about correct methods and following procedures. In decision making, they consider all alternatives, and they are concerned with conserving resources. They have difficulty with timing.

Use WRITTEN COMMUNICATION WITH DOCUMENTATION.

AMIABLE STYLE (AM) WHO IS HIV+

Style Determinants:

Person has a soft manner of speaking and a slow rate of speed when talking. They are excellent listeners, who nod and smile a great deal.

In questioning, this person will respond and understand a WHY? question first, followed by WHO, HOW, WHAT.

They value relationships and feelings and seek a calm environment. They feel they must consider whether people will like their decisions., and will go along with the crowd, concerned about avoiding conflicts.

Use FACE-to-FACE communication, "SHARING IDEAS," and WRITTEN COMMUNICATION highlighting PEOPLE CONCERNS, or VISUAL AIDS.

DRIVER STYLE (DR) WHO IS HIV+

Style Determinants:

Person is concise, direct, and has a fast speech pattern. Their walk is purposeful, and uses gesture of index finger to make point. In questioning, this person will respond and understand a WHAT? question first, then HOW, WHO, WHY.

They value results, setting goals to obtain accomplishments. They are concerned about efficiency and are time minded, and task oriented.

They have tolerance for some chaos in their environment but generally seek to control surroundings.

Use an OUTLINE WITH GOALS, keeping FACE-to-FACE communications brief and timed.

EXPRESSIVE STYLE (EX) WHO IS HIV+

Style Determinants:

Person has a great range of voice inflection and tends to be loud, especially while laughing . They have a rapid walk with expansive use of gestures. They may disrupt things when not getting attention. In questioning, this person will respond and understand a WHO? question first, followed by WHAT, WHY, HOW.

They value their image and looking good. They want to be first or best. They are concerned about how things will look to higher-ups and are usually politically astute. They want recognition for being helpful. They have a great deal of tolerance for chaos, and "better late than never" summarizes their concept of time.

Use FACE-to-FACE communication, with a CHECKLIST. WRITTEN COMMUNICATION with time expectations is helpful, or VISUAL AIDS.

An adaptation of materials developed by David W. Merril and Roger M. Reid. Used with permission of the Tracom Corporation, Denver, Colorado.

Setting Boundaries

Often health care workers have great difficulty in saying "No." If health care workers mistakenly perceive themselves as being the "only hope" for meeting a particular need or providing a particular service, there will be a terrible pressure to always comply with every request, even though feelings of resentment and overwhelmingness may develop. When a health care worker says "No," the patient is often pressured into seeking other resources, which may prove valuable. By stating, "I can't always provide what you want or need," health care professionals free others to find their own solutions and engender more control over their health. Family therapist Carl Whittaker included in a list of hints for therapists this maxim: "Value your impotence as one of your most powerful assets."

Another aspect of setting boundaries is maintaining an identity separate from the helping role. There are other dimension beyond the role of being a health care professional. Many facets, sometimes referred to as "sub-personalities," need to be nurtured and expressed. All of these aspects require attention and means of expression. Because the professional image takes much time and energy

Table 15-2c
SOCIAL STYLE MODEL™
VERBAL AND NON-VERBAL CHARACTERISTICS

ANALYTICAL STYLE (D1,D2,C1,C2)	DRIVER STYLE (B1,B2,A1,A2)	AMIABLE STYLE (D3,D4,C3,C4)	EXPRESSIVE STYLE (B3,B4,A3,A4)
Gestures tend to be controlled.	Will use index fingers to make points.	Gestures generally inward toward body. Open hand gestures.	Great use of hands—expansive out from body.
Monotone—very little variation in pitch. Generally a slow deliberate rate of speed.	Staccato speech pattern. Fast speed and clips sentences.	Voice characterized by softness. Slow rate of speed when talking.	Great range of voice inflection. Loudness. Fast paced.
Tends to ask detailed questions.	May finish others' sentences for them.	Tends to listen rather than talk.	May overtalk points.
Tends to be patient.	Tends to be impatient.	Tends to be patient.	Tends to be impatient.
Walks slowly.	Walk: purposeful and fast paced.	Walk: slow, easy going walk.	Walk: movement tends to be fast, sometimes showy.
Does not show enthusiasm.	Leans forward, ready for action.	Nods a great deal to show feedback.	Overly enthusiastic.
Preoccupied.	Becomes easily bored.	Tends to be attentive.	May disrupt things when not getting attention.
Ponders—must consider everything before making decisions.	Makes quick decisions. Pushes others to make decisions.	May not commit themselves on decisions—decisions may be tentative. May go along with the crowd.	Makes decisions often before thinking things through. Often makes strong stands either for or against.
Concerned with facts and figures. Method conscious.	Focuses on results or outcomes.	Concerned with people's feelings and reactions.	Uses emotional appeals.
Low tolerance for chaos. Seeks order in the environment.	Tolerance for some chaos in environment. Seeks to control environment.	Low tolerance for chaos. Seeks calm and harmony. Can adapt to environment.	Tolerance for great deal of chaos. Can overcome factors in environment.
High time orientation.	High time orientation.	Lower time orientation.	Lower time orientation.

An adaptation of materials developed by David W. Merril and Roger M. Reid. Used with permission of the Tracom Corporation, Denver, Colorado.

and others often see only that role, it is easy for health care workers to become too involved in that aspect at the exclusion of the rest. This separation of personhood from the professional part is crucial for well-being.

It is important for health care workers to realize that they are part of a large network of caring people. Some of their functions can be shared with volunteers, health care agencies and even with the patients.

Stress Reduction

Stress and frustration is inherent in this epidemic, and health care professionals can facilitate methods to appropriately ventilate these emotions. Incorporating mini-breaks and physical activity into every working day may reduce daily stress levels. It is essential that health care professionals leave their work behind them when they complete their day. Health care professionals also benefit by openly recognizing and expressing frustrations, perhaps by yelling or stomping in a private place. In addition, health care workers needs to express sadness, grief, anger and frustration by talking with friends or

participating in a support group for their particular field. Reducing stress can also include various forms of relaxation/imagery to clear the mind or journal keeping. Additionally, involvement in spiritual or religious groups can provide support for health care professionals trying to maintain perspective amidst the tremendous anguish caused by HIV (Dilley & Forstein, 1988).

CONCLUSION

With the ongoing repertoire of drug intervention, health care management for the HIV seropositive person has advanced dramatically, and the quality and longevity of life has become paramount. Today, persons with HIV disease live longer and better with HIV infection, and the health care professional can facilitate this process.

Dr. Torres W. Sullivan, Secretary of the Department of Health and Human Resources, and Dr. Anthony Fauci, Head of the National Institute of Allergy and Infectious Disease, declared that HIV infection should be regarded as a chronic, manageable disease, such as diabetes. In managing the spectrum of HIV disease, patients and health care workers should have hope and a belief that refutes fear, encourages optimism and overcomes negativity. As Matilda Krim stated, "Without hope there is a broken heart." Health care providers should be challenged to become a part of making living with HIV an experience of "living longer and living well" (Pachuta, 1990).

References

Blaney, R.L., and Piccola, G.E. (1987, January). Psychologic issues related to AIDS. *Journal of the Medical Association of Georgia.* 28-32.

Christ, G., Wiener, L., and Moynihan, R. (1986). Psychosocial issues in AIDS. *Psychiatric Annals.* 16:168.

Cooke, M., and Sande, M.A. (1989). The HIV epidemic and training in internal medicine. *New England Journal of Medicine.* 321:1334.

Dilley, J.W., and Forstein, M. (1988). Psychosocial aspects of the human immunodeficiency virus (HIV) epidemic. In Francis, A.J., and Hales, R.E. (Eds.): *American Psychiatric Press Review of Psychiatry,* vol. 7. Washington, DC: American Psychiatric Press.

Dilley, J.W., Ochitill, H.N., Perl, M., et al. (1985). Findings in psychiatric consultations with patients with acquired immune deficiency syndrome. *American Journal of Psychiatry.* 142(1):82.

Dilley, J.W., Shelp, E.E., and Batki, S.L. (1986). Psychiatric and ethical issues in the care of patients with AIDS. *Psychosomatics.* 27(8):562.

Dunkel, J., and Hatfield, S. (1986, March-April). Countertransference issues in working with persons with AIDS. *Social Work,* vol. 31 (114-117).

Forstein, M. (1984). The psychosocial impact of the acquired immunodeficiency syndrome. *Seminars in Oncology.* 11(1):77.

Kubler-Ross, E. (1969). *On Death and Dying.* New York: MacMillan Publishing Co.

Macks, J. (1987). People with AIDS. In Helquist, M. (Ed.): *Working With AIDS: A Resource Guide for Mental Health Professionals (pp. 1-28).* San Francisco: The AIDS Health Project, University of California.

Macks, J. (1988). Psychosocial responses of people with HIV. In Lewis, A. (Ed.): *Nursing Care of the Person with AIDS/ARC.* Rockville, MD: Aspen Publishers.

Marzuk, P.M., Tierney, H., Tardiff, K., et al. (1988). Increased risk of suicide in persons with AIDS. *Journal of the American Medical Association.* 259:1333.

Merrill, D., Reid R. (1981). *Personal Style and Effective Performance: Make Your Style Work for You.* Radnor, PA: Cholton Book Co.

Ost, L.G. (1987). Applied Relaxation: Description of a coping technique and review of controlled studies. *Behavioral Respiratory Therapy.* 25(5):397.

Pachuta, D.M. (1990). AIDS—Living longer and living well: An idea whose time has come. *Maryland Medical Journal.* 39:148.

Rogers, D.E. (1988). Caring for the patient With AIDS. *Journal of the American Medical Association.* 259:1368.

Schlotterer, W. (1989, November 15). Primary care for those with AIDS. *Patient Care.* 15.

Shernoff, M. (1989). Why every social worker should be challenged by AIDS. *Journal of the National Association of Social Workers.* 35:5. Shubin, S. (1989, October). Caring for AIDS patients: The stress will be you. *Nursing,* vol. 19 (pp. 43-46).

Sowers, L. (1988, January 4). Healing shame: How family secrets can mask the problem. *Houston Chronicle.* Lifestyle section, 1-2.

Wolcott, D.L., Fawzy, F.I., and Pasnau, R.O. (1985). Acquired immune deficiency syndrome (AIDS) and consultation-liaison therapy. *General Hospital Psychiatry.* 7:280.

16

AIDS and HIV Infections: Legal Issues Confronting the Health Care Professional

Donald Skipwith, Attorney at Law

I suppose that everyone of us hopes secretly for immortality; to leave, I mean, a name behind him which will live forever in this world. Whatever he may be doing, himself, in the next.

—A. A. Milne

INTRODUCTION

Because of our reluctance to address the consequences of AIDS in our society, lawmakers have been slow to respond to this growing medical and social crisis. Our state legislatures and Congress, preoccupied with their perception of the opinions of a majority of their constituents, have been slow to perceive and react to personal tragedies brought on by this disease and to its grave implications for all of us. In conformity with the 1980s, a decade marked by society's denial of the implications of AIDS and HIV infection, laws have been enacted only with great reluctance and usually at half measure.

It is little comfort that similar medical and social crises have confronted us in the past; just in this century, influenza and tuberculosis epidemics have swept the United States and threatened to decimate our population. However, because AIDS and HIV infection were totally unforeseen 10 years ago, no profession or discipline had any prior knowledge or experience relevant to the unique issues raised by this mysterious virus and the population it has stricken. Likewise, we have little to learn from legal response to past epidemics in view of our changing health care system and, on a positive note, our growing national commitment to the disabled and handicapped.

From the onset of this virus, you, the health care professional, are compelled to do your job, notwithstanding many unanswered questions about the legal ramifications of AIDS and HIV infection as it relates to you, to the patient, and to our medical care system as a whole. Some of the legal issues of HIV are testing and consent, duty to warn those at risk, the obligation to treat, implications of the American Disabilities Act, and legal documents that can help you cope with your responsibilities in this area of medical treatment.

TESTING AND CONSENT ISSUES

It is of primary importance to remember that in many states, failure to disclose to your patient that he or she is being tested for HIV infection may expose you to legal recourse and penalty.

As medicine continues to address more effectively HIV infection, more and more people who identify themselves as "high risk" are coming forward for HIV testing before the onset of any AIDS-related symptoms. The methodology of HIV testing, for the asymptomatic individual particularly, presents special considerations; medical and social implications cannot be overemphasized. Potentially life-saving medical intervention may, in fact, be denied by the medical financing systems because of positive test results.

Anonymous vs Confidential Testing

Most states allow HIV testing at anonymous test sites with no requirement for identification other than by pseudonym or assigned number. Some private physicians have developed their own systems to provide for anonymous testing. Anonymous test results are never traceable to the individual. The test is properly preceded by counseling and followed up with counseling once the test results are known, regardless of whether the test is positive or negative.

As distinguished from anonymous testing, confidential HIV testing is handled like most other medical information. That is, test results are recorded in the patient's file and made available to health care providers and to anyone else to whom the patient authorizes disclosure, such as an insurance company. When applying for insurance or making claims under an existing insurance policy, the applicant or policyholder usually is compelled to authorize the release of medical information in order to obtain coverage or receive benefits. Thus, confidentiality is waived, and an individual with positive test results will likely be judged uninsurable and so identified on the national insurance computer network used for storing information about persons who have been rejected for insurance.

More and more, insurance policies are reflecting total exclusion or minuscule dollar caps placed on benefits related to HIV treatment. Therefore, the initial choice of anonymous or confidential testing, most particularly for the HIV-positive, asymptomatic individual, is far-reaching and has lifelong consequences.

Non-Consent Testing

Some instances of medical trauma do not allow time for the luxury of consent and test results before critical medical intervention occurs. In such instances, you should use all available safeguards in treatment of the individual as if HIV infection was already diagnosed (Centers for Disease Control Guidelines).

DUTY TO WARN THOSE AT RISK

To promote an environment that encourages testing, most states have not imposed "contact tracing" of sexual partners (for example, those mandated for sexually transmitted diseases such as syphilis). However, in states where contact tracing is the law, the duty to warn rests with the state and not with the medical practitioner.

The question of a duty to warn remains in the vast majority of states that have not adopted contact tracing as a component to HIV testing. Some jurisdictions, for instance, provide that the spouse of a person testing positive for HIV

should be informed of the otherwise confidential test results if the physician who ordered the test makes the notification. Likewise, the same statute may allow for the release of a test result to medical practitioners who have a legitimate need to know of a test result for their protection and to provide for the patient's health and welfare. (For illustration purposes only, the Texas Statute addressing confidentiality is included, see Appendix D).

Aside from these types of constantly changing requirements, which vary from state to state, the duty to warn can become an issue for the medical professional. There may seem to be an unclear determination both ethically and legally. The confidentiality mandated to the patient must be weighted against those instances in which there is factual knowledge or reasonable belief that the patient continues unsafe practices.

Your own conscience can weigh the confidentiality you owe to your patient against the slim possibility that your patient may continue unsafe practices in spite of positive test results. This dilemma of "duty to warn" can be placed squarely with the patient, provided he or she has the benefit of appropriate counseling before and after HIV testing. If you decide that extended counseling is needed, then you should refer your patient to a counselor who is familiar with HIV-related issues. Taking these steps should protect you from possible legal liability imposed by a failure to warn and will satisfy your obligation of confidentiality to your patient. Such a "duty to warn," which appears to be in conflict with most laws and professional ethics was recognized by the landmark California case of *Tarasoff v. Regents* (1976). In this case, the court found that the psychotherapist had a duty to warn an identifiable third party who the patient was likely to harm. Such a scenario is analogous to a health practitioner's duty to warn. On occasion, you may encounter patients who you believe may not be exercising responsible behavior toward third parties. The relationship between medical practitioner and patient should be extremely confidential, as generally mandated both by law and professional codes of ethics. Only in the most extreme case should a well-founded factual knowledge of inappropriate behavior require a breach of this confidentiality. In most instances, there are existing statutes about reporting individuals with communicable diseases who pose a public health risk. Caution in breaching confidentiality should certainly be exercised. However, in addition to conflicts with laws and codes of ethics, your relationship with the patient will no doubt be sabotaged by such a breach. The "duty to warn" should be placed squarely with the patient, and appropriate counseling will familiarize the patient with the precautions that should be exercised in contact with others. Further, in some states "partner notification programs" provide the opportunity for the patient to permit the state to notify sexual partners about the HIV-positive individual. Most often discussion of these programs is a component of post-test counseling.

Only in the most extreme situations should procedures, which are law in all jurisdictions, be undertaken that allow for judicial action to control an individual who has a communicable disease such as HIV and is reasonably suspected to be a threat to public health.

For illustrative purposes, following are case examples that would be consistent with the Section 81.103 of the Texas Health and Safety Code:

Patient John is HIV-positive, asymptomatic, and under Dr. Smith's care. Dr. Smith, a general practitioner, notices that some routine dermatologic care should be addressed and refers John to Dr. Jones, a dermatologist. Dr. Smith legitimately believes that John's HIV status is relevant to both Dr. Jones' protection and patient John's treatment. In such a case, confidentiality would not be breached by advising Dr. Jones of John's HIV status.

Over time, as Dr. Smith regularly monitors John's condition, John develops a familiar relationship with the office staff. In discussion with Dr. Smith, John states that he has developed a new relationship but that he can't bring himself to discuss his health condition with his new partner. He states that he practices safer sex but doesn't use a condom. In further discussion, it becomes apparent that John really does not fully understand the practice of "safer sex." Dr. Smith reiterates the importance of the use of condoms and of responsible sexual behavior. He provides John with information resources about safer sex through counseling and safer sex workshops. In a later visit, Dr. Smith learns that John still has not discussed his health status with his partner. John admits that his intercourse continues unprotected. John becomes recalcitrant to any further guidance regarding protected sex; he states that he has never felt better in his life, he looks great, and he is going to have "a good time" as long as he can. In such a case, John has clearly become unmanageable and poses a threat to public health. After information is presented to the proper governmental agency, the health care provider obtains an application to have John managed so as to address public health concerns through the judicial process.

OBLIGATION TO TREAT

AIDS has brought out the best and worst in our society. The medical profession is no exception. Some medical professionals and institutions, legally and ethically bound to provide medical care, refuse treatment to people who have HIV. Others have met the challenge in spite of a clear stigma that can attach to those who treat HIV infection.

Refusal to treat HIV-seropositive persons for reasons of prejudice or bias against AIDS can be unlawful. Professional medical codes from state to state generally mandate treatment without regard to race, creed, national origin, sex, age, handicap, social status, financial status or religious affiliation (see Chapter 17). In some states, the code of medical ethics operates with the force of law. Further, few medical institutions exist today without some form of federal funding (including Medicare or Medicaid) which imposes the obligation to treat through the Federal Rehabilitation, Comprehensive Services, and Development Disabilities Act of 1978. This Act prohibits discrimination against handicapped persons under any program receiving federal funding. Clearly, an individual diagnosed with AIDS fits the definitional criteria of an "individual with handicap." Less clear is the situation involving a patient with symptomatic HIV disease or one who tests positive for HIV. Such a patient may not be classified as handicapped or found to have a substantial impairment, even though mere infection may be perceived by some as creating a handicap.

IMPLICATIONS OF THE AMERICANS WITH DISABILITIES ACT

Legal protection for HIV-seropositive persons as handicapped persons has been enacted at state levels. Most state laws mirror federal laws and, depending on the jurisdiction, may even be more protective of the handicapped.

The Americans with Disabilities Act enacted by Congress has attempted to resolve legal loose ends left dangling in protecting the rights of the disabled and handicapped, including persons living with HIV disease. The rights of handicapped and disabled individuals will be uniformly protected by this federal legislation at levels basically coequal with constitutional protection that forbids discrimination based on race, creed, national origin, sex, age and religion. Protection of these rights will no longer be contingent upon a nexus to federal funding. In the interim, however, codes of ethics and existing laws should discourage any medical professional from withholding treatment from a patient because of suspected HIV infection.

LEGAL DOCUMENTS TO AID THE MEDICAL PRACTITIONER

The medical community has at its disposal various programs and schools that offer training in the specialized area of treating the patient living with HIV. Likewise, such specialized guidance is available to the legal community.

Most often, the medical professional is first in the line of intervention and will be asked by the patient to advise him or her on legal matters.

Just as no lawyer must practice medicine, no medical professional need practice law, but a little knowledge can provide your patient with some of the best and most effective therapy in terms of smoothing the progress of medical treatment and contributing to peace of mind. Urge your patient to seek the advice of an attorney. Most legal issues, excepting insurance and employment, are not time-consuming and can be resolved by the execution of a few simple documents. Once completed, these documents relieve you and your patient from the imperative of making grave decisions under stress and without time for consideration. The Durable General Power of Attorney, the Health Care Power of Attorney, and the Directive of Physicians ("Living Will") may very well save both you and your patient much anguish and uncertainty in the future.

In the Durable Power of Attorney document, the patient identifies the person who, during the patient's lifetime, can act in virtually any capacity to conduct the patient's affairs. As a "durable" document, it remains effective if the patient is later judged to be incompetent. It eliminates the necessity of costly and burdensome court-imposed guardianship proceedings otherwise necessary to conduct the affairs of an incompetent person.

The Durable Power of Attorney for Health Care is a legal document which gives the person named therein the authority to make any and all health care decisions for the designating party once such party is no longer capable of making decisions for him or her self. The term "health care" means any treatment, service or procedure used to maintain, diagnose or treat the physical or mental condition of the designating party. The document gives the agent the power to make a broad range of health care decisions such as consent, refusal to consent, or withdrawal of consent to medical treatment, and withdrawal or withholding life sustaining treatment. The law provides that a treating physician must comply with the designated agent's instructions or allow the designating party to be transferred to another physician.

Most states have adopted legislation allowing for a Directive to Physicians (living will). Simply put, the law stipulates that if the patient is terminally ill or comatose, conditions to be determined by the agreement of two physicians, artificial life sustaining devices will not be used to sustain life. Without this living will, such a decision usually falls in the following priorities: 1) legal guardian, if one is appointed; 2) spouse; 3) majority of adult children; 4) parents; and 5) next living relative. In the absence of a living will, it is not uncommon for health care professionals and institutions to take the conservative and safe approach and order the use of artificial life support systems. In some instances, removal of the system requires the cost and ordeal of litigation. Through the living will, the patient relieves you, his or her loved ones, and family by making this most difficult of decisions in advance.

Copies of these executed documents should be made part of your patient's record to avoid the confoundment that can arise during the exigent times when medical considerations alone should be your only concern.

CONCLUSION

We are still far from approaching the HIV virus as just another medical affliction, albeit a grave one. While taking the necessary precautions to protect yourself from exposure of the virus and from potential legal liabilities, you must at the same time take care that you do not succumb to the discrimination often directed against HIV-seropositive persons. Extreme caution must be used in recording impressions about the patient's life-style because patient records follow the patient forever. Unless it is an absolute medical necessity that such impressions be documented, you best serve your patient by resisting written comments that may be, on close examination, nondiagnostic and unrelated to treatment.

Finally, every state and virtually every city has agencies and organizations to address the social issues raised by HIV infection. Through them, you can locate attorneys in your community who are experienced in addressing the legal issues raised by your patient's affliction. Legal professionals can advise you about state laws that address the concerns raised by HIV infection and can provide expert consultation on other issues that could affect you or your patient, such as employment, entitlement programs, insurance and estate planning.

References

AIDS Update. New York: Lambda Legal Defense and Education Fund.

AIDS Policy and Law. Washington, DC: Bkuraff Publications.

AIDS and Public Policy Journal. Frederick, MD: University Publishing Group.

American Academy of Hospital Attorneys. *AIDS Task Group, AIDS and the LAW: Responding to the Special Concerns of Hospital.* Chicago: American Hospital Association.

Douglas, C., Kalman, T., Kalman, C., et al. (1985) Homophobia among physicians and nurses: An empirical study. *Hospital and Community Psychiatry* (December 1985) (Study of attitudes of health care personnel dealing with AIDS patients) 36:1309.

Exchange, The. San Francisco: National Lawyers Guild AIDS Network.

Gunderson, M., Mayo, D., and Rhame, F. (1989). *AIDS: Testing and Privacy.* Salt Lake City: University of Utah Press.

Kennedy, I., and Grub, A. *Medical Language Techniques & Materials.* London: Butterworth and Company.

Lesbian/Gay Law Notes. New York: Bar Association for Human Rights of Greater New York.

Mental and Physical Disability Law Reporter. Washington, DC: American Bar Association.

Newsletter of the AIDS Legal Council of Chicago. Chicago: AIDS Legal Council of Chicago.

Parry. (1989, March-April). Life services planning for persons with AIDS-related mental illnesses, *Mental and Physical Disability Law Reporter.* 13:82.

Rubenfeldt, A. *AIDS Legal Guide.* Lambda Legal Defense and Education Fund Inc. New York, NY (1987).

Tarasoff vs Regents of the University of California, 17 California. Third 425, 551 p. 2d 334(1976).

17

Ethics: Decision Making and AIDS

Ann Giffin Monson, MS, PT

The unexamined life is not worth living.

—Socrates

INTRODUCTION

Health care professionals face daily moral dilemmas. Moral dilemmas for health care providers are those clinical situations that are complicated by interpersonal relationships and differing individual or community values. Perhaps none is more difficult than those punctuated by the emotions surrounding individuals who are infected with HIV. Most of us remember a time in our lives when we thought "doing the right thing" was fairly clear cut. We knew how to distinguish between right and wrong. Frequently in health care, however, the "right" decision is no longer so obvious. The most apparent clinical decision may be clouded by patient preference, facility policy, or financial responsibility. By learning to distinguish between moral and nonmoral judgments, between technical and ethical judgments, and between competing ethical principles, clinical decision making can be enhanced. This process does not necessarily make the decision easier. The process, however, may illuminate the center of the dilemma and focus the energies of the health care professional on an acceptable solution.

The study of ethics can be primarily theoretical, such as examining the meaning of value concepts. Ethics, on the other hand, can be as practical as helping decide what to do.

PERSONAL VALUES AND DECISIONS

Moral vs Nonmoral Judgments

Each of us has a history. We have developed throughout our personal lives a set of attitudes that guide us in all of the choices we make. Some of those attitudes have been carefully considered, whereas we hardly recognize others as our own. Those attitudes are perhaps more easily understood when categorized as either moral or nonmoral judgments.

In examining personal values, consider your response to the following situation. You are a graduate student living in a house with three roommates. Each of you has limited resources and are barely meeting financial obligations. One roommate suddenly informs you that he/she is leaving school mid-semester because of a family illness. The roommate who is leaving, however, has found someone else to move into the house. The new roommate is a hemophiliac who is HIV positive. What will be your response? Would your reaction differ if the new roommate was a rehabilitated IV drug-user who is HIV positive? What if the new roommate was a sexually active bisexual, HIV status unknown?

We each make decisions about what is valuable to us. We set individual goals for our lives, and we make plans as to how to accomplish those goals. We usually support those decisions with reasons or information to confirm our choices. These decisions are evaluative judgments that are considered to be nonmoral. They are individual choices. We might choose to live in a house with other graduate students because we prefer the space and companionship that might not be found in a dorm or apartment. This decision is not one we would consider "right" or "wrong," but simply the best thing to do considering our choices and preferences. In that case, any new roommate might be acceptable.

We do, however, make moral evaluative judgments about ourselves and other people when we make character judgments. These are judgments we make about actions, motives, and the capacity to do good. They give us insights as to our own motives and the kind of person we ought to be. This kind of judgment would perhaps enter into your response to your new roommate. You might find the person with hemophilia acceptable as a roommate because of her/his courage to attend graduate school despite health problems. You might agree to have the rehabilitated IV-drug user as your roommate because you admire her/his strength in overcoming addiction. On the other hand, you might reject the bisexual because you consider promiscuity immoral. You would be guided by what you thought was admirable to do.

Another type of moral judgment is one of obligation or duty and involves issues of what we should do or what action is required by us. We most often find ourselves caught in a dilemma when we have conflicting obligations or duties. In the example of the graduate student accepting a new roommate, there is an obligation to the other students to uphold the financial arrangement previously agreed upon. Perhaps you are receiving financial support from your parents who would object to either of the HIV positive roommates, as well as to the bisexual roommate. Do you also have an obligation to your parents? How do you resolve this conflict in obligations? What is the right thing to do?

You are beginning to see how difficult it is to balance judgments of nonmoral evaluation, moral character, and moral obligation, even when you have accurately categorized them. This is where ethical theories can be of assistance.

Ethical Theories

Ethical theories can be said to have two primary functions: 1) they can help us to explain why we chose something as right or wrong, and 2) they can guide us in discovering the right (or best) thing to do when the decision is not obvious. Ethical theories can be broadly grouped into two categories: duty-based or deontologic and goal-based or teleologic.

An example of an absolute duty-based position would be that it is always wrong to tell a lie. We have a duty not to lie because the person to whom we might consider lying has a right to the truth. Additionally, our respect for the other person requires us to tell the truth and accept a just response. For example, as the graduate student described previously, you rely on your parents for their financial support. You

determine that you must be completely honest with your parents about your new roommate and accept the consequences of their response. You trust them to be fair.

This deontologic theory of absolute duties was described by Immanual Kant (1959). He maintained that it is absolutely right and always wrong to treat persons as a means rather than an end. We should not impose anything on a person against their will. We should help them further their own goals. We should never treat them as an object and always respect them as a person. Therefore, according to Kant, you would simply be using your parents as a means of financial support if you did not inform them of the status of your new roommate.

Another approach to duties is not to consider them as absolute but rather within their context. This approach is a way to address duties when they conflict with one another. Suppose we have a list of our duties. This list may be based on prior promises, indebtedness, gratitude, justice, beneficence, self-improvement or avoiding harming others (Ross, 1930). As we consider a particular action, we need to examine all the features of the action and list the duties that apply to that particular activity. We would then weigh the duties against one another and determine which duty carried the greater obligation in this situation. Personal preference or convenience should not enter here. As the graduate student faced with an obligation to roommates, to parents, and perhaps to the new roommate, you would have to decide which duty carried the greatest weight.

Goal-based or teleologic theories of moral action are based on judgments about action that would produce the most good and avoid the most harm. It focuses on side-effects and consequences of our actions, as well as actual outcomes. These theories attempt to merge the right thing to do with the best thing to do. This contrasts with deontologic theories that may place the right action and the best action in conflict. Goal-based theories vary in how they define good or bad. They also differ as to who is included in a particular moral reference group. Some versions try to determine standards of action, whereas others consider each situation separately. For example, if you were a hedonist, good is determined as happiness or pleasure, bad as pain or unhappiness. You may be the only person in your moral reference group and each experience is viewed separately. Relying on our graduate student roommate experience again, as a hedonist, you would have to consider the balance of happiness over unhappiness with each possible resolution. You may be concerned with your happiness only or you may want to consider your parents and roommates as well. As you can see, there is an obvious problem measuring "happiness" and "unhappiness."

What if you consider other values important, independent of the happiness they might bring? This position of considering more than one intrinsic good is known as pluralism. It may include a long list of items valuable in and of themselves, such as knowledge, freedom, justice and beauty (Frankena, 1973). You would resolve a dilemma differently depending on which value you could justify as having priority in a particular situation. If justice held the greatest importance for you in the graduate student roommate dilemma, your resolution would probably be different than if you held happiness as the only intrinsic good. It will be helpful for you in clinical problem solving to make a list of the "goods" that are important to you.

Once you have identified what you consider as "good" or "goods" and the moral reference group for application, you still need to determine whether a policy can be developed from your deliberations. These steps are followed by a Rule Utilitarian.

1. Are there any "rules" that would assist you in similar situations? Make a list of these rules.
2. Predict the consequences of following these rules in a specific situation.
3. Evaluate the consequences.
4. Choose the action that gives you the greatest good over bad.

Perhaps you believe that every situation is too different to formulate rules. In that case you would be considered an Act Utilitarian and would take the following steps:

1. Look at as many aspects of the situation as you possibly could.
2. List all the alternatives.
3. Predict the consequences of each alternative.
4. Evaluate the consequences.
5. Compare your alternatives and choose the one that shows the greatest balance of good over bad.

At this point, you should review your own style of moral decision making to see which theory it most closely resembles. Do you focus on duties or outcomes? Which duties or goals are more important? Most of us do not fall into one category all the time. We may also vary over time based on our own experiences and priorities. Identifying our own values and understanding how we make our personal decisions are important before we consider professional and patient values and decisions. Take some time to do this before you read further. The case study below may help you. The Smiths are an attractive young couple in their twenties who began coming to the church you attend several months ago when they moved to your city. They have three active youngsters, ages 18 months, 3 years and 5 years. Sally Smith, the wife, has taken an active role in coordinating nursery volunteers. Both she and Sam, the husband, have offered to teach in Church School next year, she on the primary grade level and he on the junior high level.

Sam has been sick a good bit since they moved to town,

having been hospitalized twice with pneumonia. Recently, the rumor has begun circulating that Sam has AIDS. A church member with acquaintances in the town the Smiths moved from reports that it was "common knowledge" there that Sam had been diagnosed with AIDS and that Sally was HIV positive. The children were not infected as far as anyone was aware.

How should you, as a member of the church, react to these rumors?

PROFESSIONAL VALUES AND DECISIONS

What is a profession? Rather than focusing on the variety of answers, let's accept as a working definition a rather traditional definition of a profession.

1. A profession can be said to have a unique body of knowledge. There is a theoretical construct for technical performance. In other words, there is a why as well as a what.
2. A profession meets some need in society.
3. A profession exerts control over its members. It monitors professional performance in some manner.

A corollary to the above definition would seem to require the professional to exhibit ethical as well as technical competence. Technical competence alone is insufficient for the health care professional when there are no guidelines for determining, for example, when to discontinue treatment, how to handle delicate confidential information, what to do about an unethical colleague, or where and when to challenge a team decision. For this reason, there are societal expectations that a professional will meet the minimal legal requirements for technical competency and at the same time strive to uphold ethical ideals to which the profession is committed.

What characteristics would you expect of a professional? Perhaps some of the morally admirable characteristics you thought of earlier would apply. Is there a different standard of morality for health care professionals? Some argue that being a health care professional makes no ethical difference (Goldman, 1980). Perhaps the patient as client has the ultimate control of health care decisions and the care giver only carries out those wishes.

On the other hand, there may be unique ethical characteristics for the health professions because of public promise, mutual valuation of health, duty of promoting health, and because the lack of good health inhibits autonomy. Pelligrino and Thomasma (1988) call this characteristic beneficence in trust, to find the middle ground between paternalism and autonomy (Pellegrino and Thomasma, 1988).

Another paradigm characteristic of the health care professional that has been offered is integrity. Even when more carefully defined, however, this concept offers little as a means of conflict resolution unless duties or goals are also defined and placed in priority.

What, then, is the moral background of our commitment as health professionals to care for patients? One principle that seems foremost is the moral principle of beneficence, which can be interpreted as our duty to promote the interests and well-being of others in the medical setting, and especially to promote the well-being of those who are ill or are entrusting us with their care. Among the meanings of beneficence are the terms mercy, kindness and charity.

As health care professionals we assume that our primary goal is to assist the patient wherever possible in achieving a favorable state of health. Whenever a favorable state of health is not possible, we assume a role of assisting in care that promotes the highest quality of life possible. In other words, our activities should benefit the patient.

Does our commitment to beneficence also entail personal risk in the treatment of the patient? There has been a rich history of care givers providing care when there was certain exposure to infectious diseases. Should we hold this self-sacrifice as an expectation? Perhaps the martyr is not an appropriate model for the care giver, especially given the other personal responsibilities most people have. There is, however, a certain amount of risk assumed in the care of any patient. Procedures to protect the care giver have been developed based on the best information that can be gathered about the spread of HIV. Failure to follow established precautions can certainly be faulted as careless. Refusal to treat patients simply because they are HIV positive seems contradictory to the expectations about the health care professional.

A second moral principle that goes hand in hand with beneficence in the health care setting is patient autonomy. One reason we promote the patient's interests is so that the patient may act freely in determining his or her life plans and then seek to fulfill these plans. Acknowledging this principle of autonomy reflects a sense of dignity for ourselves as well as others. We recognize the value we place on individual liberty, privacy, freedom of choice and moral responsibility.

Consider the following situation. A young man has been coming into your outpatient facility for rehabilitation of a nonsurgical knee injury. You have spent a good deal of time together and this patient trusts you. One day the patient says, "You would keep anything I told you secret, wouldn't you?" He then tells you he is gay and begins to reveal his fears about AIDS. He has refused to have a test for HIV, stating that he simply does not want to know, even though he is sexually active. What should you do?

As we have already noted, frequently we find ourselves in a conflict unique to the health professional. We are called on to mediate between conflicting duties and goals. We respect the young man's autonomy and his desire to make his own decisions. The care giver has given a promise not to violate the patient's trust. We know, however, that it would be in the patient's best interest, as well as those with whom he has had sexual contact, to submit to the test for HIV. We might even be tempted to adopt an attitude of paternalism in order to "help" the patient by contacting his physician, but this would mean violating the patient's autonomy and trust. How do we weigh these ethical principles in order to resolve the dilemma?

One means of understanding our allegiance to the principles of beneficence and autonomy is to refer to the codes of professional conduct developed by individual professional organizations. Historically, these codes were more rules of etiquette than conduct. Their more contemporary roles are as an educational tool that lists desirable behaviors for the professional. They may also be useful in analyzing the profession for its priorities. Politically speaking, codes are a stamp of professionalism, an external symbol. Cynics might call this purpose an ideologic smoke screen, masking economic self-interest and social power.

One idealistic purpose of professional codes is to provide a framework for making ethical decisions and setting forth professional expectations. Certainly broad professional expectations can be described; however, no code can be written to detail how a specific dilemma should be resolved. In a comparative study, five codes were analyzed, including medicine, nursing, pharmacy, physical therapy and social work. A review of portions of the codes related to patient interaction recognizes five distinct categories (Yeaworth, 1985).

Statements on human dignity were the very first statements in three different codes (medicine, nursing and physical therapy), suggesting its prime importance in the giving of care. Privacy and confidentiality were mentioned next in medicine, nursing, pharmacy and social work. Safety for the patient was third in order of priority for nursing and pharmacy. Fourth included the sharing of information and honesty in medicine, pharmacy and physical therapy. The fifth common theme was individuality in medicine, nursing and social work. One of the most interesting statements reflecting the value of autonomy for the patient is found in the nursing code: "The nurse shall have respect for uniqueness of client, unrestricted by consideration of social or economic status, personal attributes, or nature of health problems."

Codes of ethics for health care professionals may reaffirm the commitment to autonomy and beneficence in patient care. They do not, however, actually help to mediate the tension between paternalism and autonomy so aptly drawn in the preceding study. To do this, we must also include the patient's values as part of the process in clinical decision making.

PATIENT VALUES AND DECISIONS

The past 25 years have been an age of the individual. Facilitated by the Civil Rights Movement, the Women's Movement, and most recently, the Human Rights Movement, a whole new language has developed. This is a language of rights. Newspaper headlines abound with claims of rights. Just what does it mean to issue a claim to a particular right?

First of all, rights are the domain of entitlements or those things that we can rationally assert to be our due. Second, if someone validates a particular right, this claim logically entails someone else having an obligation to fulfill that claim.

There are a number of problems in asserting rights. First, there are conflicts of rights. When two individuals both have a legitimate claim, how do you assess one right over another? An example would be a parent declining medical care for an ill child based on religious grounds. The courts have been asked to determine whose right takes precedence, the parent's right to religious freedom or the child's right to medical care.

Second, there is frequently a question as to who has the status to claim a right. Does a fetus have the same status as a pregnant woman? Does the HIV-infected individual have the same right to elective coronary by-pass surgery as the individual who is HIV negative?

Third, if a right is acknowledged, who is to perform the correlative duty? If health care is a right, then who has the duty to provide it and at what level? Who will provide funding for research on HIV and hospice care?

Finally, are there limits in satisfying rights? How do we allocate scarce resources, whether they be goods or services? The implications of and conflicts about health care are obvious. One response by the health care industry to the cry from patients for recognition of their rights has been to develop a list of patient rights.

Bioethical Principles

Patient rights are based on accepted principles of medical ethics. These principles have been developed and refined by philosophers responding to the needs of health care. For centuries, the health care giver played a unique fiduciary role in providing service. With the advent of technology and increased consumer information, the patient in many cases demanded an equal role in health care decisions. This shift was awkward for both the care giver and the patient. The role of the philosopher/medical ethicist often is to clarify the ground rules of this new relationship.

The principle of autonomy, or the right to self-rule, has been a key theme in shifts in health care policy. This principle asserts that no one can know better than the competent individual what is best for that individual. Since the health care provider is frequently in possession of information that would assist the individual in making a decision about the course of that individual's care, informed consent becomes the key concept in the execution of patient autonomy.

What are the functions of informed consent? It is intended to promote patient autonomy by providing accurate and understandable information about medical tests, diagnosis, prognosis and treatment options. After receiving this information, the patient should be better prepared to make decisions about their care. This process also protects the patient from fraud and duress. It also encourages self-scrutiny by medical personnel regarding the values they express in the information they choose to share with patients. The complications to autonomy, however, come into play when the patient refuses treatment that under most circumstances would seem to be the preferred course. The ultimate complication is the patient considering autonomous suicide. This option is one that is at least considered by many victims of AIDS. Why is this viewed as a failure?

Autonomous suicide borders on the controversial issue of euthanasia. After more than three decades of discussion in the medical community, there is still no consensus. Practitioners seem to find that their individual positions on euthanasia are more closely tied to their personal and professional values than on any other issue. A detailed discussion of euthanasia can be found in *Bio-ethics* (Edwards & Graber, 1988).

Beneficence has already been identified as a primary ethical principle supporting the role of the health care professional. Beneficent actions are identified as those intended to help. Helping is traditionally defined in the health professions as improving health status and, where possible, curing illness. When a patient refuses what appears to be the logical course of treatment, the care giver frequently feels frustrated and even rejected. The reaction may be one of paternalism, which is the desire to act for the patient in what the care giver believes is the patient's best interest.

There seems to be no justification for strong paternalism, that is, deciding what is best for the patient irrespective of the competent patient's wishes. An example would be for a physician to decide to treat a patient with AIDS aggressively, despite the patient's explicit instructions to the contrary. Perhaps there can be an element of justification for weak paternalism when the patient, for some reason, is not fully competent. This occurs frequently when the care giver determines that the patient, when fully informed, would choose the course of treatment the care giver has selected. The key here is to seek as much information as possible about the patient's wishes, rather than for the care giver to rely on personal preference.

It seems important when tackling the ethical issues related to the treatment of individuals who have AIDS or disorders related to HIV to discuss the ethical principle of justice. Justice can be described as giving someone what they are due. In health care we recognize a need for some means of determining fairness when there is a conflict between individuals, institutions or an individual and an institution. Decisions based on this sense of fairness may be determined on a number of things, including: 1) an equal share, 2) individual or institutional need, 3) individual or institutional effort, 4) societal contribution, 5) merit, 6) opportunity and 7) availability of resources. Each of these items comes into play when we consider how to allocate and pay for health care services. For example, you may provide an excellent justification and a plan for implementation of a research design to develop a promising new drug for combating HIV. The project, however, is very expensive. The funds required for the research could also be used to provide a pediatric treatment team and medical supplies for a Third World country for an extended period of time. These are the kinds of competing goods faced in health care delivery. The decisions cannot be made without carefully examining the values, duties and goals wherever possible. Even then, the decisions are very difficult.

Another important bioethical principle to examine is confidentiality. A long-held tradition in health care is the expectation that the care giver will keep secret any information shared during the course of treatment. Generally, this promise is not hard to keep. In the case of a disease as potentially lethal as AIDS, however, this may be more difficult. We have already seen in one case mentioned previously that the obligation to keep information confidential may be at odds with the value placed on public health and safety. Should we reveal information to sexual partners about someone's HIV status when the individual refuses to do so? What should our public policy be in order to balance confidentiality, privacy and justice?

CONCLUSION

How do we approach a resolution of the ethical dilemmas created by HIV? How do we review the conflict in order to make sense of what we ought to do? The health care professional, by the very nature of the commitment to help, must come to a decision. The theoretical, therefore, must become practical.

The following steps present a systematic framework for viewing all the available information. It will not make the decision for you, however. It will only help you to determine whether all the alternatives have been considered before committing to a plan of action.
1. Identify that you have an ethical problem. It may not be clear where the conflicts lie; however, recognize that the situation is not simply one that requires a technical decision.
2. Gather all the relevant information. We frequently want to react as if we have a medical emergency and react quickly before we have all the facts.
3. Determine all the individuals with a legitimate interest in this dilemma.
4. Identify the values and obligations of each individual involved in this situation.
5. Estimate the consequences of the actions proposed by each individual.
6. Determine where the conflicts lie. Are they between values, duties, or consequences?
7. Decide what to do after reviewing the alternatives and their consequences.
8. Carry out the plan. At its completion, review the whole process in order to learn both personally and professionally from the experience.

The following case study (Levine, 1989) should be reviewed with these steps in mind. Dr. Lois Dorsey, a psychiatry resident, was paged by an intern from the Medical Intensive Care Unit (MICU) for an emergency psychiatric consultation. Gary Davidson, a 28 year-old gay man, had been hospitalized 11 days earlier for an initial episode of PCP. One week earlier he had been told that the presumptive diagnosis for his illness was AIDS.

On the day Dr. Dorsey was called, the medical team discussed with Mr. Davidson the need for a Swann-Ganz catheter, which would be inserted in his pulmonary artery. Mr. Davidson refused permission for placement of the catheter and requested that medical treatment be stopped. "Take the tubes away and let me die with dignity," he declared.

The medical team discussed the clinical status and prognosis in detail with Mr. Davidson, his lover, his parents and his sister. Mr. Davidson had a 50 percent chance of surviving the current illness. However, people with AIDS rarely survive more than five years, and Mr. Davidson could expect several bouts of severe illness during his remaining life span. The medical team also pointed out that rapid advances were being made in understanding the pathophysiology of AIDS and offered the prospect for a future treatment as a result of current research efforts.

With the support of his lover and family, Mr. Davidson continued to insist on cessation of treatment, citing as his reasons "quality of life" and the "right to die with dignity." In the presence of witnesses he signed a living will and statement of competency. The legal formalities were carried out; however, for "legal reasons" and "completeness," the medical team was waiting for a psychiatric assessment before complying with the patient's request.

Dr. Dorsey reviewed Mr. Davidson's records and interviewed him. Mr. Davidson reaffirmed his belief that quality of life was more important than quantity of life and that he wished to die with dignity. He admitted that he was feeling pain, fear, loss of control, extreme discomfort on the respirator and sleeplessness. He added that he was distressed by his inability to eat due to the respirator. When Dr. Dorsey asked how he might feel should he recover from the pneumonia, the patient noted that he knew he had AIDS and that he would die within one or two years. Therefore, he said, he did not deserve to take up a bed in the hospital and continue to receive medical treatment that could better benefit another patient.

The patient had no psychiatric history and had never attempted suicide. He had no prior personal experience with death or dying among family or friends. He could not speak because of the respirator tubes, but he communicated by writing notes and nodding his head. He was alert, oriented, wrote clearly and logically, and initiated his own statements and topics for the interview. He was not tearful and appeared anxious. In his own eyes, he did not want to commit suicide but wanted to be allowed to die.

Dr. Dorsey concluded that the patient showed no evidence of confusion, psychosis or delusional thinking but that he did show symptoms consistent with depression, probably secondary to his underlying medical condition.

Mr. Davidson, then, was legally competent, understood the consequences of his decision to refuse treatment, and had the support of those closest to him. Yet, because of the patient's age and depression, the availability of treatment for the current illness, and the possibility that some treatment for AIDS may become available within the next few years, Dr. Dorsey hesitated. Should Mr. Davidson's treatment be stopped as he wished?

References

Beauchamp, T., and Childress, J. (1983). *Principles of Biomedical Ethics*, 2nd ed. New York: Oxford University Press.

Edwards, R., and Graber, G. (1988). *Bio-ethics*. Orlando, FL: Harcourt Brace Jovanovich.

Frankena, W. (1973). *Ethics*, 2nd ed. Englewood Cliffs, NJ: Prentice-Hall.

Goldman, A. (1980). *The Moral Foundations of Professional Ethics*. Totowa, NJ: Rowman and Littlefield.

Graber, G., Beasley, A., and Eaddy, J. (1985), *Ethical Analysis of Clinical Medicine*. Baltimore: Urban and Schwarzenberg.

Herbison, G. (1988). Ethics and rehabilitation, *Archives of Physical Medicine* 69:311.

Kant, I. (1959). *Foundations of the Metaphysics of Morals*. Translated by Lewis White Beck, Indianapolis: Bobbs-Merrill.

Levine, C. (1989). *Cases in Bioethics*. New York: Saint Martin's Press.

Pellegrino, E., and Thomasma, D. (1988). *For the Patient's Good*. New York: Oxford University Press.

Purtilo, R., and Cassel, C. (1981). *Ethical Dimensions in the Health Professions*. Philadelphia: W.B. Saunders.

Ross, W.D. (1930). *The Right and the Good*. Oxford: The Clarendon Press.

Yeaworth, R. (1985, Summer). The ANA code: A comparative perspective. *Image, The Journal of Nursing Scholarship*. 94.

18

The Patient in the Home Setting

Deirdre McDowell, PT

What would life be if we had no courage to attempt anything?
—Vincent Van Gogh

SAFETY ASSESSMENT OF THE HOME

Addressing Architectural Barriers and Interior Hazards

This chapter provides direction for the rehabilitative health care team and assists the patient and care giver upon discharge. It concentrates on items that will enhance functional ability and is arranged to promote a sequential assessment of needs before discharge.

Inspection of the home setting for obstructive hazards and architectural barriers is essential to the safety and functional well-being of the patient. It should be completed, if possible, before the patient is discharged. Inspection should consider the following components: 1) the physical capabilities of the patient, 2) the physical layout (floorplan) of the home, and 3) the functional objectives to be performed on a daily basis. Because each component is quite complex, an integrative tool may facilitate creative problem solving in the home setting. One tool would be a tour the of the home setting as viewed through the eyes of the patient. The following questions illustrate some of the issues raised during such a tour.

- The initial obstacle to the patient returning home may be the driveway. If the patient has a walker, cane or any other assistive device, will he or she be able to get it out of the car? Could the patient trip on broken pavement, steps or gravel? Is the distance too far to negotiate in one trip? If so, is there a place for the patient to sit and rest?

- Are there steps? If so, how many? Are they deep enough to accommodate a walker? Is the patient able to lift legs over the height of the step riser?
- Is the patient capable of unlocking the front door?
- Are there hand rails on both sides? (A hemiplegic patient will need a rail on the strong side if he or she cannot use a cane).
- Does the door open in so that the patient can walk straight in? If the door opens out, the patient will have to back up before proceeding straight in.
- Is there room in the hallway for the patient and all the needed or attached equipment (ie. I-Med pole, walker, cane, wheelchair)?
- Can the patient maneuver around the kitchen and prepare meals? Does the patient have difficulty carrying items from the refrigerator to the table?
- Can the patient tell how hot the water is, or should the thermostat be turned down to avoid scalding?

After the tour, items that were seemingly nonhazardous, in actuality, can be quite complex to negotiate. The tour, like any other objective evaluation, is a fact-finding mission. The facts (in this case hazards and barriers) are assessed and solutions become more readily available.

Realistically, one cannot change the architectural layout of the edifice. However, some orderly rearranging of objects may provide a vastly improved area for functional activities.

SUGGESTIONS FOR IMPROVEMENT OF FUNCTION AND SAFETY AT HOME

- Remove throw rugs as they may prove to be a needless obstacle to someone with a foot drop or shuffling gait.
- Move any item located at waist height or above, that may be unsteady if "grabbed" when walking. People tend to hold on to things for a sense of security without thinking about whether they will provide support during a loss of balance.
- Pick up any extension cords, telephone cords or appliance cords that are in a high traffic area.
- Push any chairs used for sitting against the wall or be sure they have good floor friction. Try to use chairs of a moderate height with arm rests and good support in order to facilitate ease of transfers.
- Turn on lamps by wall switches or a noise-activated box. These switching devices can help avoid fumbling in the dark.
- Arrange furniture in such a way as to allow access to supported rest stops. The rest intervals should be at distances within the work capacity and fatigue level of the patient. For example, place a chair along the wall at the midpoint of the hallway. The chair should be easy to pass but handy if needed.
- Use a bath bench. A chair is also adequate, but a bench allows safe transfers and decreased slippage. The patient should sit on the end of the bench and swing legs over the edge onto the tub and then scoot to the center.
- Use a hand-held shower head with the mount within reach while bathing.
- Use a raised toilet seat to decrease muscular energy needed to stand.
- To avoid scalding, lower the thermostat on the water heater if sensation is not intact.
- Put frequently used kitchen utensils conveniently within arm's reach. Provide an uncrowded work surface with a sturdy chair.
- Use plastic/paper cups and plates if fine motor coordination or upper extremity strength is a problem, as they are much lighter and cannot break.
- Review standing and stooping with upper extremity support when using an assistive gait device. Put a small basket or bag on the walker to enable transportation of items.
- Have phone and most frequently used numbers in large print on easily reached bed side table.
- Plan two exits from the bedroom in case of emergency and notify fire/police department that someone with strength, mobility, or endurance problems resides in the home. A sticker should be applied to the outside of the patient's bedroom window to help with rapid identification and location of the patient.
- Review the necessary precautions of oxygen use with the patient and family. Post oxygen hazard signs in visible locations.
- Remind patient of slip/slide possibilities of assistive devices on wet surfaces.
- Keep a piece of Dicem™ handy in the kitchen. It is good for opening items or placing under plates.
- Use glove mitts rather than pot holders to avoid burns.
- Place a grab bar in the bathroom by the toilet, tub or sink.
- Install hand rails at both sides of any steps.
- Have a step stool handy in some central location. Review the up-from-floor-to-chair technique with patient using stool.
- Install a sufficiently illuminated front door with a "peep" hole to provide additional security for patients with loss of independence.
- Install ramps to replace steps.

POSITIONING AND SKIN CARE

Frequent repositioning of the patient at two-hour intervals: 1) prevents pressure sores and contractures, 2) minimizes the deconditioning effects of prolonged bed rest, 3) provides rest and relief of pain, and 4) decreases abnormal stiffness or synergistic patterns.

The individual with a decubitus ulcer requires considerably more skilled care than one with healthy intact skin. Problems of the skin, joint stiffness, and consequent loss of active movement limit the progression of rehabilitation programs. These problems of joints and skin may occur when prolonged pressure placed on an area blocks the microcapillary circulation. Subsequently, shearing forces can also break down tissue by creating friction between the bone and outlying skin. Nutritional deficits also influence maintenance of skin integrity because they affect synthesis of adenosine triphosphate (ATP), bone matrix, and the integument (see Chapter 6).

The care giver must understand that the process of breakdown and formation of decubitus ulcers starts in underlying tissue and works its way outward. The beginning signs are soreness or redness over bony prominences, which does not disappear within 30 minutes to one hour once the pressure has been removed. If the care giver observes prolonged redness, every attempt should be made to avoid undue pressure or irritation of the areas. If the skin is intact, it should be kept clean and dry but well moisturized, or a piece of Duoderm may be applied. Inform the physician if it becomes an open sore.

Contractures are also common among nonmobile individuals, the most common being ankle plantarflexion, knee flexion, hip flexion, and cervical flexion. Unless they occur in decerebrate or decorticate posturing, the contractures result from viscous changes in the colloidal nature of cytoplasm, causing an often permanent reduction in the resting length of soft tissue. Appropriate intervention helps to prevent the irreversibility of this reaction. Other deformities may also occur, including scoliosis or any other type of bony malalignment secondary to prolonged alteration of ligamentous length or muscle contractile ability.

The patient's overall condition must be considered when implementing a positioning program. The following questions should be posed when determining the appropriate activities:

- Is the person conscious?
- Does the person have pain or lack sensation? In what areas and to what degree?
- Does the person lack proprioception?
- Does the person have muscle function? Is there any position which decreases it?
- Is there edema?
- Does the patient have any cuts, burns or abrasions?
- Does the skin have redness?
- Is the skin oily or dry?
- Does the patient have bowel or bladder incontinence?
- Is the patient well nourished?
- Does the patient have contractures or deformities?
- What is the body type?
- What is the psychologic state?
- Is the patient mentally alert?

A good positioning program addresses all aspects and characteristics of the patient's condition and provides for ease of daily activities of the patient. Consider the following considerations as you formulate a plan, and review the illustrated positions for help. A sample program is located at the end.

Whenever positioning a patient use a chair that provides good back and seat support and, if possible, has arm rests. When the patient is assisted into the chair, the patient's hips, knees and ankles should be in 90 degrees of flexion, with the heel firmly planted on a flat surface. Position and support the upper extremities and trunk in such a way as to maintain good vertebral alignment against gravity and good functional positioning of the arms and head.

If the patient is hemiplegic, be sure to use a small folded towel on the pillow behind the affected scapula to protract it, pillows or a lap trap under the elbow to maintain glenohumeral approximation, and a pillow on the affected side to prevent trunk shortening and leaning toward that side. Don't be afraid to use more pillows if necessary to align the patient correctly.

Also remember to position in such a way as to encourage cervical rotation and awareness toward the affected side.

If the hand appears edematous, use an Isotoner glove turned inside out for external compression. The lower extremity on the same side may also need some sort of compressional support while it is in a dependant position. A Jobst or antiembolitic stocking should be applied before getting the patient out of bed to avoid fluid pooling in the foot and ankle. A bed positioning program should be initiated when the patient is unable to reposition independently secondary to weakness, fatigue, decreased consciousness, abnormal tone, contractures or poor skin integrity. Begin by assessing the extent and location for pressure relief. For individuals with low body weight, poor skin integrity, and contractures, additional equipment may be warranted, (such as a flexicare KinAire bed or Roho mattress). A two-inch block foam egg crate mattress or sheep skin could be used for the less involved patient. When positioning the patient in the supine position, maintain good spinal alignment as in sitting. One medium-sized pillow under the head is sufficient; avoid putting pillows under both knees if possible. Foot alignment must also be addressed. If a foot board is not feasible use high-top tennis shoes or prefabricated ankle foot orthoses (AFO) with shoes. If the patient is a hemiplegic, try to position the uninvolved side in a pattern out of synergy, and encourage the family to address the patient from the involved side. The patient may be one-half or three-fourths turned when placed in side lying. Rotate the patient from supine by flexing the opposite knee and bring the opposite shoulder toward you. While stabilizing at the hip, tuck the long edge of a pillow under their side, from shoulder to hip, and then turn the other side under. Let the patient gently fall back onto the pillow; roll and position the upper extremities, with the underside shoulder protracted and flexed and the topside shoulder and arm resting on a folded pillow or sheet. Flex the upper leg and place pillows between the knees and lower leg and ankle.

To place the patient in the prone position, roll the patient from side lying. Rotate the head toward the involved side and lace small towel rolls under both lateral clavicles and humeral heads. Place a small pillow roll at ankles to allow dorsiflexion. Figure 18-1a-j presents examples of proper positioning.

EDUCATING THE CARE GIVER

The role of primary care giver is an important and time consuming. It requires stamina, strength, patience and a talent for organizing daily activities. A sense of humor is also an often needed asset for those times when things just don't seem to run smoothly. The following common sense principles can be applied to anyone attending someone with

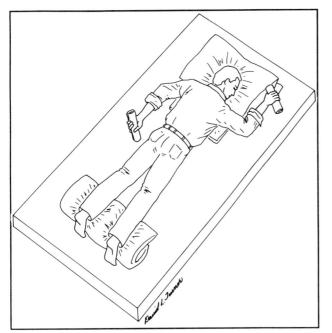

Figure 18-1a. Proper position in prone.

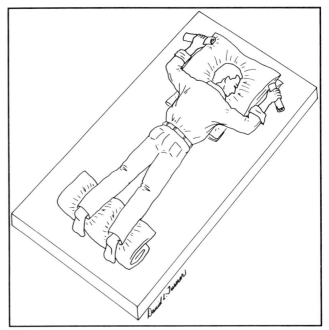

Figure 18-1b. Prone positioning with arms overhead.

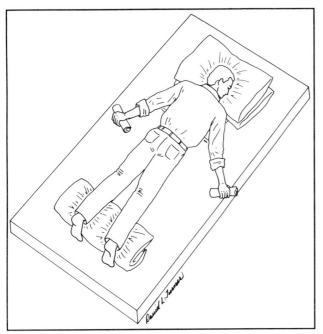

Figure 18-1c. Optimum support in prone with arms extended.

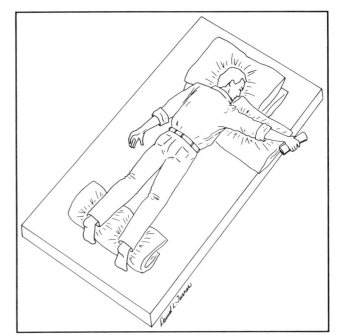

Figure 18-1d. Affected side elevated and positioned to maintain skin integrity.

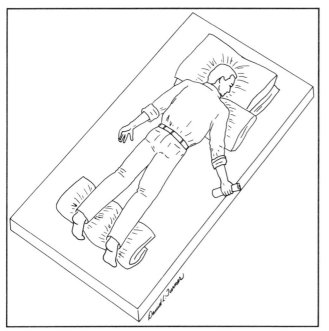

Figure 18-1e. Glenohumoral support of the involved extremity.

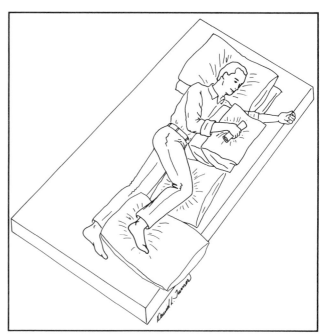

Figure 18-1f. Sidelying with optimum positioning of right extremities.

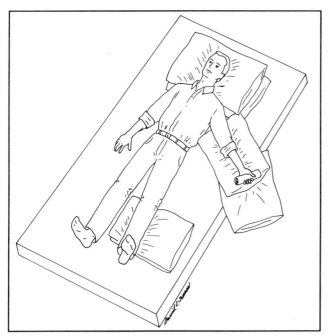

Figure 18-1g. Supine position for left extremity involvement.

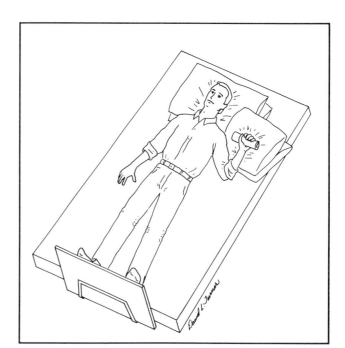

Figure 18-1h. Maintenance of neutral ankle position and left upper extremity support in extreme rotation.

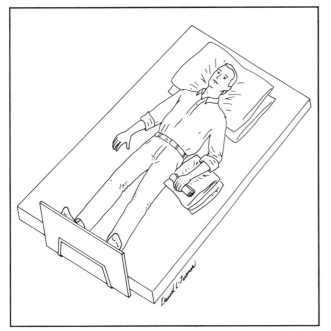

Figure 18-1i. Footboard placement to prevent plantarflexion contractures. Left upper extremity support with internal rotation.

special needs.

- Do not shout at someone who is ill unless he or she has a hearing problem. Rather, speak clearly and concisely. Neurologically involved individuals usually respond better to calm, quiet voices.
- Always speak and listen to the person in need with respect. Be patient. Hearing is easy; listening is an art.
- When assisting with dressing, feeding, bathing, or positioning, think: "Would this position/movement be comfortable to me?"
- When dealing with the manifestations of stroke or other CNS involvement, make sure to call attention continually to the affected side. This may require addressing the patient from the affected side to stimulate the senses, with the patient ultimately acknowledging and/or facilitating movement responses.
- Help the individual remain cognizant and informed of activities and events. A plan of daily activities, as well as general information, such as what day it is, what time it is, or what is happening in the local news, is helpful.
- Do not leave someone unattended without a safety restraint unless you are sure there is absolutely no possibility of any mishap. Patients (particularly those with AIDS dementia) can fall out of chairs or bed when asleep, pull out/off needed supportive equipment, wander aimlessly if confused, or attempt unsafe acts if impulsive or not safety conscious. *Be alert!*

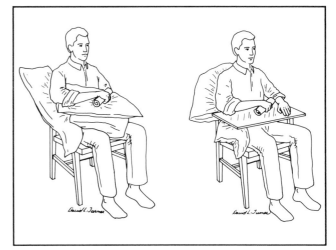

Figure 18-1j. Supported sitting positions with pillows and lapboard.

- Establish a consistent daily routine, but be flexible enough to accommodate the individual:
    1. Establish a good sleep/wake cycle.
    2. Encourage the patient to dress, get up and go outside if possible. This will help raise the patient's spirits, increase alertness.
    3. Establish a mealtime routine to aid with bowel and bladder regularity and increase comfort. Scheduled naps help replenish energy reserves.
- Consult members of the health care team and don't be afraid to ask questions. You may be the most reliable source for amending the individual's daily routine and the most able to implement changes.

It is important to remember that care giving may require the patience of a saint, and there will invariably be times when nothing goes right. Recognize your own human limitations, talk about critical issues, seek the support of others, and take a break.

LOWER EXTREMITY EXTERNAL SUPPORT SYSTEMS

There are four basic categories of external bracing devices for the lower extremity, each named for the body part it supports or controls: 1) foot orthosis (FO); 2) ankle, foot orthosis (AFO); 3) knee, ankle, foot orthosis (KAFO); and 4) hip, knee, ankle, foot orthosis (HKAFO).

The most commonly used device is the AFO. Several variations are available and each is used to address a specific problem. The prefabricated AFO is used for a person who needs help in keeping the ankle in a neutral position when

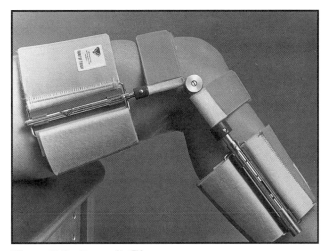

Figure 18-2a. Dynasplint™.

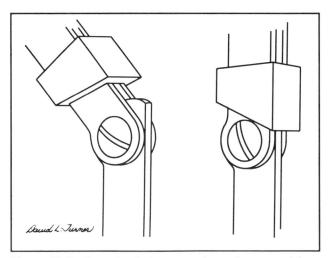

Figure 18-2b. Drop-ring lock commonly used to control knee flexion.

walking so the forefoot does not drag the floor. The AFO is worn for a limited time under these circumstances, and the patient exhibits no other neurologic deficits such as an increase in tone, a strong Babinski's reflex, or clonus. These persons may exhibit a steppage gait, which is a combination of external rotation, abduction, and hip hiking, in order to bring the affected foot through the swing phase of gait.

The plain custom AFO is usually recommended for individuals who could manage with a prefabricated brace, but who require a built-in moveable ankle or will be wearing the brace for long periods of time. There is less chance of skin breakdown with custom orthotics, and a moveable ankle with a plantar flexion stop will allow for dorsiflexion on steps and during swing through of the opposite foot. This device costs considerably more than the prefabricated variety.

The neuromuscular or inhibitive AFO is designed for persons with increased tone and/or other accompanying neurologic signs such as those previously mentioned. It helps to keep the ankle neutral rather than in rigid plantar flexion and decreases the occurrence of clonus and toe curling in weight bearing. This type of AFO uses a protruding metatarsal notch built into the bottom, which allows it to make uniform contact over the foot while holding in alignment.

The total contact AFO completely surrounds the foot and ankle like a glove and may also have a metatarsal notch. This device works well for individuals who have very little to support good bony alignment during weight bearing, possibly due to weakness or severe hypotonia. Because the fit is snug, however, the patient or care giver may experience difficulty in donning and doffing the brace independently, as both sides must be pulled apart in order to get the foot in.

The floor reaction AFO is a relatively new approach to the old problem of crouched gait secondary to weakness of the gastrocnemius and soleus, quads, and/or hip extensors. This weakness maybe accompanied by an increase in tone and other CNS signs such as Babinski or clonus. The AFO works primarily by applying the lever arm in a posterior motion through the anterior tibia during the stance weight bearing phases, thus blocking dorsiflexion of the ankle and partial flexion of the knee. Donning and doffing is easily managed and a metatarsal notch may electively be included. This AFO may not be appropriate for heavy persons due to the weight tolerance of the metatarsals.

The KAFO consists of two metal uprights that extend from an AFO to mid thigh. Leather calf and thigh bands provide anteroposterior support, with the knee lock providing the needed extension at the knee joint. These braces are used predominantly to assist weight bearing activities and are differentiated by the type of lock.

The other KAFOs typically consist of two metal uprights as previously described and can be locked by drop locks or bail locks. Drop locks move up or down over a ball bearing to encase both ends of the upright and require locking and unlocking on both sides of the knee it. Bail locks work through for knee extension and will automatically unlock when external pressure is applied to the brace behind the knee (ie. backing up to a chair to sit). The Dynasplint™ is a brace used for the stretching of moderate to severe contractures (see Chapter 5, patient with KS) but is not usable for weight bearing and support. It is light weight and relatively simple to use and applies a gradual but constant stretch on contracted tissues. They are readily available and can be adapted for each extremity (Figure 18-2a-e).

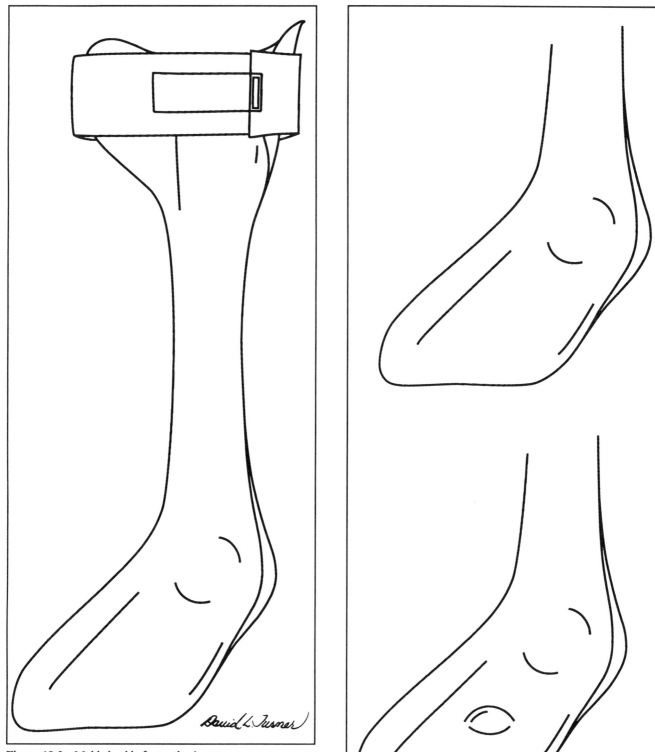

Figure 18-2c. Molded ankle foot orthosis.

Figure 18-2d. Inhibitive ankle foot orthosis.

PRACTICAL EXERCISE FOR IMPROVED PERFORMANCE

Exercise requires an output of energy through the musculoskeletal system. It may be walking, running or simply sitting up in a chair. It may be done for a specific purpose, such as improving strength or muscle mass, or for a routine daily action, such as pulling the mail from the post box. Regardless of the reason it is performed, every activity that requires energy expenditure affects the individual to varying degrees.

Practically speaking, most patients do not need to be able to do ten quad sets or ten straight leg raises successfully in order to brush the teeth or use the toilet. While conventional resistance training has its place, it is not easily integrated by the patient into the functional ability sorely needed. Transforming those exercises into daily activities is a more realistic way to approach strengthening, endurance training and balance difficulties and allows the patient to experience success while helping them develop more independent living.

When developing a home program, the primary goal is to give the patient activities that 1) can be done in his or her own surroundings, 2) will eventually decrease dependency on others, and 3) improve the ability to participate in enjoyable activities.

FIVE BASIC GUIDELINES FOR ESTABLISHING A HOME PROGRAM

1. Start with a good specific baseline assessment. It gives a standard to show improvement and helps determine where to begin.

2. Set measurable goals that are challenging and inclusive of the patient's goals.

3. Use groups of exercises that work on specific functions and end the exercise with a specific task or movement. The exercises performed should prepare the patient to accomplish a preselected activity. Example: anterior weight shift and gradual lower extremity loading exercises for sit to stand transition.

4. Give the patient a written, illustrated home program. Have the care giver and patient reverse roles.

5. Set up a time to reassess the program and the patient's progress if possible. If you are unable to see the patient again, ask the patient or family to call and report progress or difficulties in one week or less.

With these five guidelines in mind, several tasks can be performed for each problem. Be creative and adjust every exercise activity for each individual. For the patient with

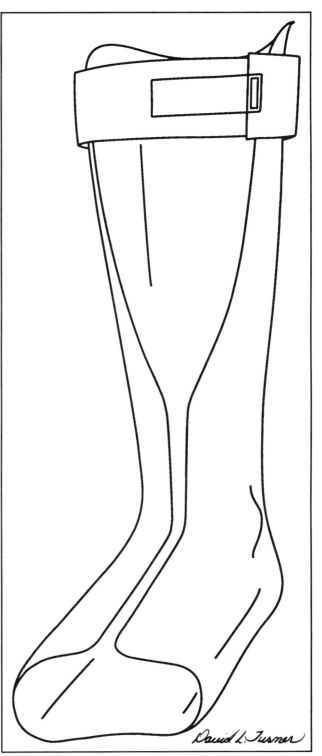

Figure 18-2e. Custom ankle foot orthosis to provide increased medial lateral support.

poor proprioceptive feedback or some types of peripheral neuropathies, a magnification of joint receptor and cutaneous receptor feedback may help. Try some simple joint approximation techniques using tights, bike shorts, elastic ankle braces with soft cotton socks and firmly laced up tennis shoes, or cuff weights around the wrist or ankle. Stomping feet and clapping hands also seems to assist in awareness of body positioning.

Balance in Sitting (Figure 18-3)
Items Needed: Bench or chair, firmly planted so that it will not slide
Activity: Diagonal reaching down to floor as if to obtain an item
Desired Action: Lateral weight shift with trunk rotation and elongation, increased weight bearing in both lower extremities with stimulated plantar flexion

Balance in Sitting (Figure 18-4)
Items Needed: Bench or chair firmly planted so that it will not slide
Activity: Lateral reaching as if to obtain item
Desired Action: Lateral weight shift with trunk elongation and increase in lower extremity weight bearing on the same side; righting reactions of opposite leg and arm

Balance in Standing (Figure 18-5)
Items Needed: Kitchen counter
Activity: Single leg standing
Desired Action: Increased co-activation around hip, knee, and ankle; righting reactions to help accommodate for postural change

Balance in Standing (Figure 18-6)
Items Needed: Kitchen counter
Activity: Heel-toe standing with partial squat
Desired Action: Increased co-contraction around hips, knees, and ankles; accommodation to gradual postural change; righting reactions with both lower extremities; controlled eccentric and concentric lower extremity contractions

Balance in Walking (Figure 18-7)
Items Needed: Kitchen counter
Activity: Braiding
Desired Action: Coordination of movement of both lower extremities; righting reactions of both lower extremities; integrated single leg standing balance; sequencing of activity

Balance in Walking (Figure 18-8)
Items Needed: Kitchen counter
Activity: Heel-toe walking

Desired Action: Coordination of movement of both lower extremities; righting reactions both lower extremities; integrated single leg standing balance; sequencing of activity

Anterior Weight Shift with Graded Lower Extremity Weight Bearing (Figure 18-9)
Items Needed: Step by hand rail or foot stool by counter
Activity: Step standing with weak leg up
Desired Action: Anterior weight shift over leg with most of weight bearing on uninvolved extremity; righting reactions; integrated single leg standing balance

Anterior Weight Shift with Graded Lower Extremity Weight Bearing (Figure 18-10)
Items Needed: Chair firmly planted so it will not slide
Activity: Sit-to-stand transition with both arms held out in front
Desired Action: Anterior weight shift over both lower extremities; shoulder protraction of involved extremity; assisted shift of center of gravity (COG) down and forward for better sequencing of movement

Anterior Weight Shift with Graded Lower Extremity Weight Bearing (Figure 18-11)
Items Needed: Two chairs, planted firmly so they will not slide
Activity: Forward shift onto extended arms with partial knee extension
Desired Action: Weight bearing on both upper extremities; forward weight shift over both lower extremities; enforced even weight distribution over both lower extremities; down and forward shift of COG stressed

Enforced Weight Bearing Through the Affected Side (Figure 18-12)
Items Needed: Wall free of obstacles
Activity: Leaning on forearm while standing next to wall
Desired Action: Weight shift over lower extremity; weight bearing through upper extremity; trunk elongation; standing balance

Enhanced Weight Bearing Through the Involved Side (Figure 18-13)
Items Needed: Five small items (ie. cans of soup), countertop, and shelf
Activity: Diagonal reaching for items and placing them on the opposite surface with visual follow of hand
Desired Action: Lateral weight shift over and below

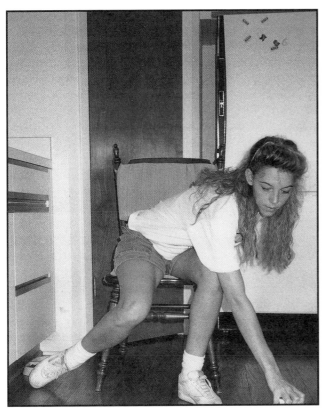

Figure 18-3. Balance in sitting for lateral weight shift with trunk rotation and elongation.

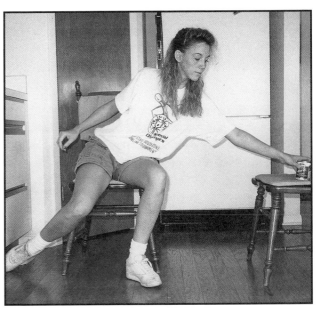

Figure 18-4. Balance in sitting for lateral with trunk elongation and increase lower extremity weightbearing.

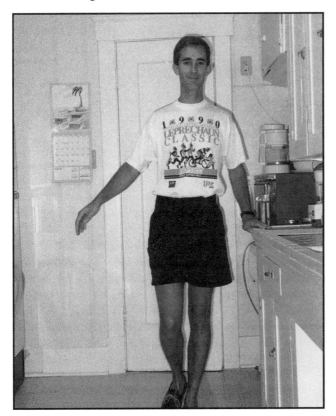

Figure 18-5. Balance in standing to increase co-activation around hip, knee and ankle.

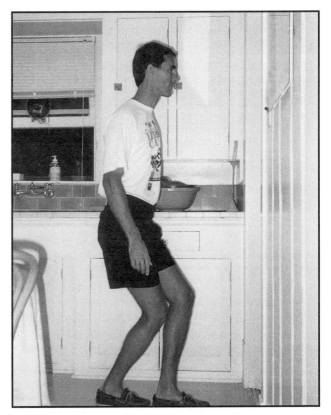

Figure 18-6. Balance in standing to increase co-contraction around hip, knee and ankle.

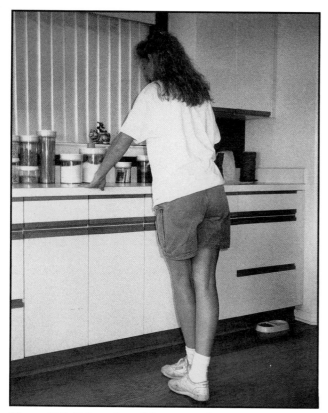

Figure 18-7. Balance in walking to coordinate movement of both lower extremities.

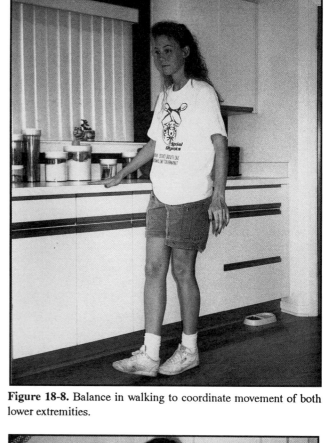

Figure 18-8. Balance in walking to coordinate movement of both lower extremities.

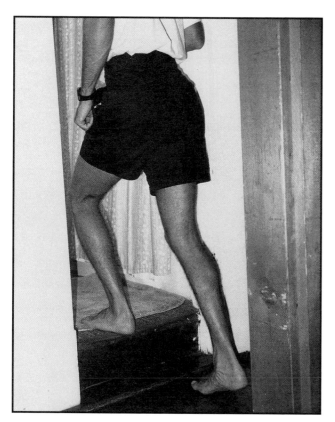

Figure 18-9. Anterior weight shift with graded lower extremity weight bearing on one lower extremity.

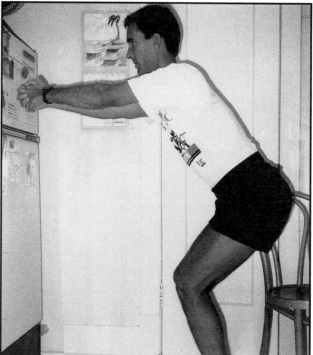

Figure 18-10. Anterior weight shift with graded lower extremity weight bearing on both lower extremities.

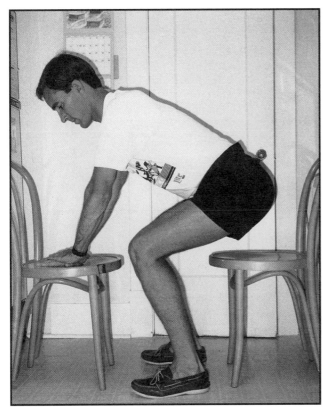

Figure 18-11. Anterior weight shift with graded lower extremity weight bearing on both lower extremities.

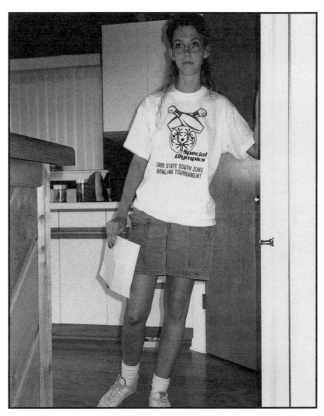

Figure 18-12. Enforced weight bearing through the affected side.

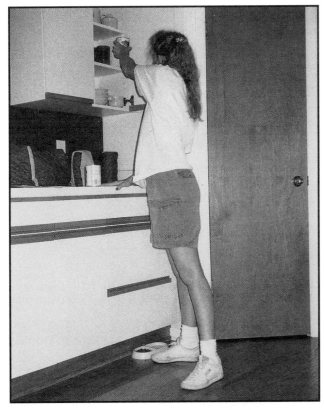

Figure 18-13. Enhanced weight bearing through the involved side.

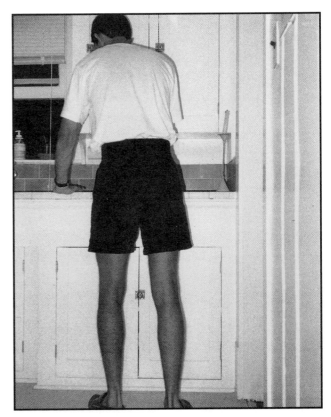

Figure 18-14. Enhancing weight bearing through the affected side.

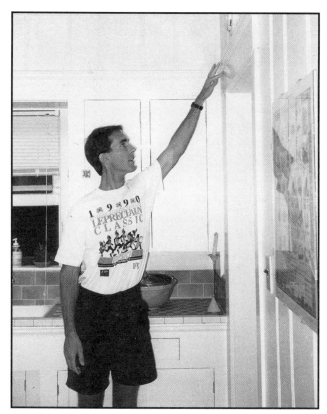

Figure 18-15. Spinal extension with shoulder flexion and scapular protraction.

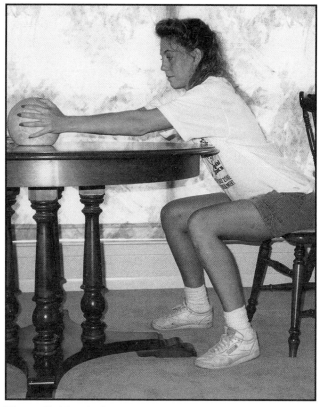

Figure 18-16. Spinal extension with shoulder flexion and scapular protraction.

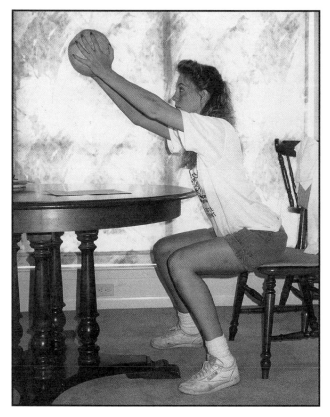

Figure 18-17. Spinal extension with shoulder flexion and scapular protraction.

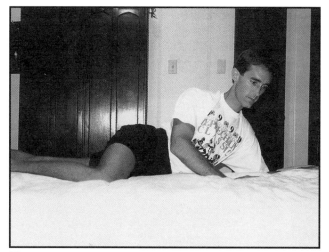

Figure 18-18. Weight bearing through both upper extremities while prone.

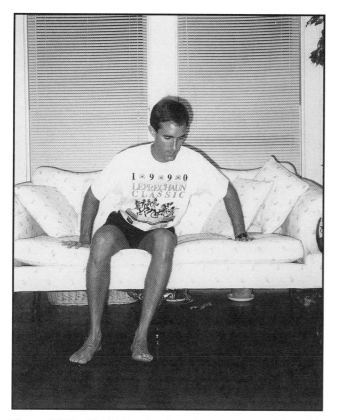

Figure 18-19. Weight bearing through upper extremities with lateral weight shift.

extremities; trunk rotation and elongation; cervical rotation, flexion and extension; standing balance; upper body strengthening

Enhancing Weight Bearing
Through the Affected Side (Figure 18-14)
Items Needed: Kitchen table
Activity: Side stepping around table toward affected side
Desired Action: Side-to-side weight shift; weight bearing both upper extremities and both lower extremities; integrated single leg standing balance

Spinal Extension With Shoulder Flexion
and Scapular Protraction (Figure 18-15)
Items Needed: Wall free of obstacles
Activity: Walking fingers up wall
Desired Action: Shoulder flexion with elbow extension and wrist extension; weight bearing both lower extremities; spinal extension

Spinal Extension With Shoulder Flexion
and Scapular Protraction (Figure 18-16)
Items Needed: chair, kitchen table, and small ball

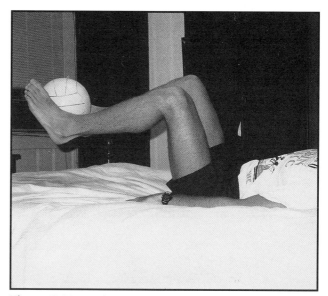

Figure 18-20. Trunk activation with controlled movement of both lower extremities.

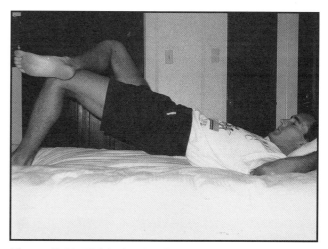

Figure 18-21. Weight bearing through Lower extremities while supine.

Activity: Sliding ball forward on table with both upper extremities
Desired Action: Forward weight shift over both lower extremities; scapular protraction and shoulder flexion; enhanced palmar arch with partial resistance through hands; spinal extension

Spinal Extension With Shoulder Flexion
and Scapular Protraction (Figure 18-17)
Items Needed: Chair and small ball
Activity: Raising ball over head

Desired Action: Forward weight shift over both lower extremities; scapular protraction with shoulder flexion; enhanced palmar arch with partial resistance through hands; spinal extension

Weight Bearing Through Both
Upper Extremities While Prone (Figure 18-18)
Items Needed: Bed
Activity: Rolling prone on elbows to side-propped position
Desired Action: Use of amphibian reactions; weight bearing through both upper extremities; trunk rotation; cervical stabilization; lateral weight shift; preparation for rolling

Weight Bearing Through Upper Extremities
With Lateral Weight Shift (Figure 18-19)
Items Needed: Bed
Activity: Side scooting
Desired Action: Weight bearing through both upper extremities; lateral shift and partial weight bearing both lower extremities; trunk elongation; sequencing of activity

Trunk Activation With Controlled Movement
of Both Lower Extremities (Figure 18-20)
Items Needed: Bed and small ball, or bean bag
Activity: Picking up ball with feet and moving it to edge of bed

Desired Action: Activation of transverse abdominis; graded movement of both lower extremities; co-contraction around hips, knees, and ankles; increased resistance at feet

Weight Bearing Through
Lower Extremities While Supine (Figure 18-21)
Items Needed: Bed
Activity: Unilateral bridging
Desired Action: Activation of trunk and hip extensors; weight bearing through lower extremities with lateral weight shift; preparation for rolling from supine

FUNCTION AFTER DISCHARGE

Several aspects of dealing with the long-term ramifications of AIDS need to be addressed long before the patient is discharged from the hospital. Patients need to be prepared for potential challenges at home and in their outside environment. Care givers also need to be educated about what their role is and how to fulfill it successfully and efficiently. This chapter should serve as a template for home setting evaluations, home exercise and positioning programs, lower extremity orthotic devices assessment, and as a resource base for health care giver's creativity at the time of patient discharge.

19

Living Well, Living Long: Patient Perspectives

Mary Lou Galantino, MS, PT

Although the plague clouds our thoughts and our eyes, we must always remember that AIDS is what has happened to us, not who we are. What we do as a society will be measured not by the depth of our grief but by the depth of our commitment to those who suffer.

—Robert M. Mehl, 1988

INTRODUCTION

My colleagues and I have presented a number of treatment regimens, therapeutic approaches, scientific studies, and psychosocial issues. This chapter presents the essence of my work: the person living with HIV disease.

We live in a society conditioned to deny death. We seldom use illness as an opportunity to investigate our relationship with life or to explore our fear of death. Seldom do we use the news of another's death as a recognition of the impermanence of all things and the inevitability of change. Yet the acknowledgment of impermanence holds within it the key to life itself.

In my experience, it seems that suffering does not have to accompany the concept of death. There is not a morbid preoccupation with death but rather a staying in the loving present with a life that focuses on each precious moment. Through my work as a physical therapist, persons living with HIV continuously explore their hearts and minds in preparation for whatever might come next, be it illness or death, grief or joy.

We speak of dying in wholeness, yet we see there are aspects of ourselves that have never fully seen the light of day. My patients have allowed me to explore many states of mind throughout this process each day. It is they who speak in this chapter.

To be whole, to live life fully and to die fully, we must deny nothing. I can no longer deny you a glimpse of the minds and hearts of my patients.

BRAD

Brad was referred to me for orthopedic management. He had postcervical laminectomy with right upper extremity limitation in range pain. At the time of surgery, Brad was informed that he tested seropositive for HIV. He was in total shock and experienced great rejection.

As a school teacher, he is experiencing fatigue mid-day; however, he wishes to be more effective. His search for complementary therapies is ongoing. He participates in our HIV fitness program and contributes thought-provoking ideas to the group. He is very introspective.

Brad is a writer and the following is a beautiful expression of his innermost thoughts. He has profound insights; many of his emotions were revealed while unmasking himself through writing.

At this time AIDS is associated with a group of people popularly despised for their sexual activity and with a group seen in dark alleys or smelly rooms shooting up illegal drugs. In the popular opinion of this country, homosexuals get AIDS. Drug users who share needles get AIDS. I know that we have come around for the brave young man, Ryan White, who fought AIDS and received a deserved blessing from entertainers and heads of State. We have felt compassion for a number of AIDS victims, but the disease continues with a unique fanfare and flourish that no other ailment carries.

The shame attached to AIDS translates readily into the difficulties that dramatically affect the area of health care. Along with the many selfless and generous people working with people with AIDS (PWA), there are those with attitudes that work against the best interests of the patient. I would like to point out two unfortunate encounters I have had with members of the medical profession, encounters that have accomplished at least two things. They have made me potentially distrustful of doctors, at least until I have a chance to test out their humanity, and they have brought out the fighter in me, making me an active participant in the healing process.

Toward the end of February, 1989, I had surgery on my upper spine for a pinched nerve. My surgeon informed me in his office a week after my surgery that I was HIV positive and that he wanted to terminate our relationship as soon as possible because he wanted nothing to do with AIDS patients or people on their way to contracting AIDS.

A second surgeon, who performed a biopsy on me, explained the possible results of the kinds of cancer that I might have. He thought I had the kind that he could operate on, thereby buying me time, to the tune of perhaps a year, after which I could expect to die. He was professional in his delivery of the verdict and I was professional in my acceptance of it, that is, I did not know of any agency I could report him to, so I kept my silence. It is imperative for people involved in the care of PWA to know this brand of insensitivity exists. It can be helpful to attempt some compensatory news on an upbeat note. The notion of hope has been around long enough to suggest it might have some validity to it.

It is unfortunate that a few members can give

a black eye to the larger community of medical practitioners, but the black eye is deserved until the community can police its ranks and suggest better tactics for the few who insist on the malpractice of denying hope to their patients.

There is good coming out of the many shared experiences of PWA. I am sure of it. There are many groups throughout the country that are talking about something new, new at least to many of us. We are beginning to understand that the way we think and act makes an important difference in the way we feel. We are listening to tapes and renting videos designed for promoting health, investigating alternative methods of healing, and reading and discussing the books of Bernie Siegel, Blair Justice, Laurence Badgley, and Norman Cousins. We are finding out that there are things we can do to foster well-being, empower our thoughts, and enhance the quality of our actions. We are learning, above all, that we are not powerless. It is the first time we have felt capable of making a difference in the health of our lives. We have begun to understand something of the correspondence among our physical, mental, emotional, and spiritual needs.

The recognition of the inseparability of mind and body is beginning the rounds. It is an understanding that is getting there but it is not here soon enough. The news media need to be hammering home the most obvious ways to help people promote their own health. The medical community needs to help push the news.

How many PWA know about the importance of diet and exercise for enhancing the immune system? Information on diet is available and neatly packaged in health food stores and through health care professionals. It can make a difference between sickness and health. Exercise programs are an ongoing concern in many cities. Support groups include knowledgeable people and frequently invite speakers from various areas of health care, both traditional and holistic.

MICHAEL

Michael's spirit lives on. He was totally blind in one eye, had contractures of his right hip and knee secondary to radiation necrosis for treatment of extensive KS, distal neuropathy pain as a result of side effects of chemotherapy and a T-cell count of six.

Michael often exclaimed, "Let's exercise. I am determined to straighten this leg and walk better, walk without a cane!" Placing a Dynasplint on his right leg, using microcurrent therapy to manage his neuropathic pain, and starting an interval training program incorporating visual stimulation, kept us busy.

His talent in music filled our clinic with saxophone melodies on occasion, when he was not performing locally. His sense of musical creativity compensated for his deteriorating vision. He listened with greater depth throughout all aspects of his life.

Despite the effects of many opportunistic infections, he still expressed the very joy of his existence, his thoughts, and his appreciation. Slated to be co-facilitator of a community HIV fitness program, he passed away before it was implemented. I was angry at the disease for taking away such a vital entity in my professional world. He continues to provide reason for forging on in my work with this group.

Since I have had full blown AIDS, I have had pneumonia twice, a collapsed lung twice, KS, CMV retinitis, and I am presently experiencing peripheral neuropathy in my finger tips. One thing that I have not had a lot of has been weight loss. I just have basically become a field day for any and all opportunistic infections.

The different drugs that I have used have been fairly effective at times inhibiting the growth of the virus. I started AZT, and I was only able to take it for six months because it decreased many of my white blood cells. I have had quite a problem with KS from the waist down. It has engulfed my legs quite a bit. I did get radiation therapy on one of my legs, and it caused radiation necrosis, which, in turn, makes it difficult to walk.

As of October, 1989, I started seeing a physical therapist. I also started to develop peripheral neuropathy in my finger tips in the same fall. We tried microcurrent stimulation, which helped with the pain.

Since I became ill, some drugs have worked rather well while some have had little or no effect. The main drug now available is AZT, and I have not been able to take it for the past year because it lowered my white blood cell count. The chemotherapy that I have been taking has been vinblastine and vincristine. I have relatively good success with that because it slowed the growth of the KS without making me sick to my stomach, but that drug had to be abandoned when the peripheral

neuropathy and lack of circulation developed in my fingers. Another drug that I have taken is called aerosolized pentamidine; I have had the best luck with this one. I have taken it twice a week for a year and a half and have only had two cases of pneumonia, only one of which was severe. I have also had cobalt radiation treatment and have been on DHPG as well. Out of all these drugs, the combination of DHPG and AZT diminished my white blood cell count to below 1,000. In combatting thrush, I have had extremely good success with nizoral. There have been several other drugs that I have taken which do not affect the virus but just treated the symptoms. AZT and DdI are the only drugs available to treat my virus.

Having AIDS has had its good side also. Before I became sick, I was a workaholic and an alcoholic, working 70 hours a week. The only place I could escape from work was the bars. After my diagnosis of AIDS, I have realized my priorities; I have given up alcohol, smoking, and work. Instead of looking at it as leaving the work force, I look at it as a career change since I am now a musician. I am playing my saxophone now, doing what I always really wanted to do.

AIDS has also given me a new perspective on living in the now moment; I do not worry about the future. I have developed more appreciation for my friends, strangers, and the sun, and, surprisingly enough, I am now a happier person for the most part then before I became sick. I am more in touch with my feelings and into what matters, and I am closer with my family and friends. It is no bed of roses; it is a lot of hard work and a lot of pain. There is a lot of suffering, sorrow, and a lot of disappointments, but you must keep the faith so that you will continue to live until they find a cure. This is the hope we all hold on to. A positive attitude also sustains your mental state. I just thank God every day that I wake up and that I can see the sun shining. I say, ''I am not going to have a bad day,'' and then, I don't.

BYRON

Byron is extremely informed and well aware of the ravages of HIV infection on his central nervous system. He is a professor at the university and continues to teach, despite his altered coordination and balance. He is a gorgeous man; I have to wonder about his self-image. He teaches me and constantly sends articles on advancements in research and medical technology for me to review for consideration in his team management of care.

We have implemented a multitherapeutic approach: PNF patterns to stabilize the trunk, therapeutic exercises on a ball for dynamic activities, and balance exercises. A flair of creativity through various movement therapy approaches includes the Feldenkrias and Laban techniques. The combination of plasmapheresis and rehabilitation has improved his overall function, and he has further organized seminars and educational series in his home town, stressing the importance of physical activity. Coordinating his therapy with the department at the university has facilitated good carry-over for Byron to enhance his functional abilities. He continues to teach so many people through his determination.

At Thanksgiving, 1989, I went to San Francisco. My brother had a cottage he leased to a psychologist involved with Project Inform, a clearinghouse of AIDS information based in San Francisco. My brother thought he might be aware of some new treatment for the problem I was having with my legs and trunk.

He said he was aware of a procedure called plasmapheresis that had been developed at Children's Hospital in San Francisco to treat peripheral neuropathy, which he said looked like my problem. Yes, I had remembered them saying peripheral neuropathy was part of my problem. But it was the weekend, and I was scheduled to return home Monday morning.

I delayed my flight one day and met Monday with one of the researchers at Children's who had done work with the plasmapheresis. He had none of my records, but, based on what he saw, he thought the treatment would help. He gave me the journal article on the procedure and the protocol Children's followed. To his knowledge the treatment had not been tried outside of the city.

Armed with this envelope of hope, I returned home. My doctor in Alabama was receptive to the treatment, which would cost approximately $25,000, and wrote a letter to my insurance company seeking authorization for the procedure, but the big test would be when I would see my other doctor, the AIDS specialist, and my neurologist. I was disappointed when both told me during my appointments that, first, they had not read the material I had sent them, and, second, that

plasmapheresis would not help my condition.

In January, a letter from my insurance company arrived that told me that they considered the treatment, which was approved by the FDA, to be experimental and that they would not pay for it. So the vote was in and it was 2-0 against what I considered to be my only hope for improvement. I could not get a new insurance company, but I could get a new doctor. That is where I started.

I found a young neurologist at the university where I taught whose enthusiasm for research and experimentation more than compensated for his lack of HIV expertise. He told me my condition did not look like typical peripheral neuropathy, but he agreed to conduct an NCV [nerve conduction velocity] test to determine if indeed I had such a condition. To his surprise, the test documented the neuropathy, and he agreed to pursue the plasmapheresis.

Now the insurance company: A careful reading of my policy pointed out that if I were to have the medical workup performed at my university's hospital, no precertification was required. In other words, I could have it done and they would reimburse the bill.

By the time February came and my plasmapheresis had started, I felt like I knew as much about the procedure as any doctor. I could probably have operated the machine myself and would have, if necessary. It was not fun, but it seemed to do some good. I was determined that it would help. I had not gone to hell and back for it not to work. Improvement was not dramatic, but I was now walking without a cane and feeling more confident. My neurologist noticed it. My physical therapist noticed it. My friends noticed it.

I know I am doing all that I can to fight something that we all know so very little about. But I am confident because I have found people, "partners in the healing process" as Bernie Siegel would call them, who are not afraid of exploring alternatives that might help me. They are receptive to anything, even if it was not their idea. And they talk to one another, each taking a unique yet vital role in my care. But I am the show director.

I now consider my illness to be a gift. Without it, I would not have been able to see so easily what is important in my life, and what is not. Who is important, and who is not. It has given me the ability to live each day completely, as if it is my

last, but not worrying that it may be. I am not
afraid of dying. More importantly, I am no longer
afraid of living.

CHRISTINE

Christine recently ceased her hectic, adventurous life-
style because of a one-month hospitalization for what she
thought was acute abdominal pain. Unfortunately, she was
wrong. She had esophageal candidiasis and AIDS. How can
this vibrant, married female contract this virus?

Most of my patients have been gay males. It really
touched me when this atypical patient came to my clinic
with HIV diagnosis. She could barely rise from sit to stand
and her muscles ached terribly. Despite severe proximal
muscle weakness from myopathies, her determination impressed me. She quickly gained strength and endurance
through interval training. Many people unaware of her
diagnosis were impressed with her performance in the gym.
After writing a federal grant, I had received funds to start a
community fitness program for the HIV population in
Houston. She was the perfect candidate and is now the
co-facilitator and best cheerleader.

It is so wonderful to be alive!

*One morning, probably in 1987 or 1988, I
heard on the way to work that if you have had a
blood transfusion, that you should have an HIV test
done. I had heard of AIDS, but I did not really pay
too much attention; I never had female diseases, let
alone something that was going to kill me. Neither
was my husband. We had been together nine years,
had not been to bed with anyone else, and did not
use drugs. In 1981, I gave birth to a son who was
born dead, and I had to have some blood
transfusions. This is the only thing that had ever
been wrong with me. What do you do when
someone says you are HIV positive? I did not do
anything. I was very quiet for a few minutes, then I
turned around and asked my doctor, "Where do we
go from here?"*

*Your life changes instantly, nothing is the
same. You are numb all over. It was like instantly,
every emotion was shut off. I can remember laying
there thinking about how sick I was and trying to
comprehend everything that was being done to me,
let alone the HIV diagnosis. I was not expecting to
die. All I wanted was instantaneous knowledge
about this disease. I was not concerned about the*

*dying part; I was concerned about the part that
came between the day I was diagnosed to the day I
died.*

*My daughter asked me if my life was worth it.
I said, "yes," and she said, "Well Mom, you have
to die of something." It just kind of bing, bang,
drums went off, bells rang, whistles, light bulbs:
that is it! I have to die of something, if it was not
AIDS it could be something else. It could be one of
these new viruses, cancers, or a heart attack. It
could be anything.*

*I have got to get better. I gave up on
succumbing to the pain and not being able to do
anything. I have had very few bouts of depression.*

*There is one thing I have told both my
daughters, my mother, and my husband. There are
not going to be any extraordinary measures made
if I get sick enough that I have to go to the hospital.
I could be maintained by one little IV to prevent me
from being dehydrated and possibly medication to
keep me out of pain and then just let me die.
Everybody knows, including my doctors, that when
and if the time comes, just let me sleep because I
am not going to be sick like that.*

*Maybe you have to die of a disease because
everybody has to die of something. But you do not
have to suffer. You do not have to have all these
illnesses that are associated with AIDS. All you
have to do is be careful. Be environmental. I wish
I could put this feeling into words. It is so
wonderful to be alive and so sad.*

STUART

Stuart has painful peripheral neuropathies. Function is
always the first goal of our treatment regimens. First and
foremost, I had to assist him in managing the pain. Stuart
gives an excellent, succinct account of our pain management
techniques.

*There is no doubt in my mind that emotional
co-factors contribute to the onset of illness.
Stereotypical symptoms began: persistent fevers,
severe night sweats, and shivers that became
quakes to the point that I feared I might bounce
myself out of bed. Add to this the unimaginable
intense fear regarding telling my family, friends,
and most of all my employer, stir well, and you*

have a recipe for a living nightmare.

My healing first began when I mustered up the courage to tell my family, friends, and employer what was happening to me. My painful secret was so terrible, so horrible that it was literally consuming me emotionally while the opportunistic infections were consuming me physically. Quite literally, as soon as I let go of my secret, come what may, I felt a tremendous sense of relief.

I began to hear talk of the benefits of physical therapy. Many of my fellow HIV-positive friends were mentioning the name of Mary Lou Galantino and praising the benefits perceived from her attention. I was skeptical.

I was noticing an unusual sensation in my feet. In the course of two or three weeks I fell hard to the ground three times and frightened myself considerably. My feet just gave out from under me. I finally went on my own to Mary Lou. I was happy that she wanted to liaise and coordinate with my doctor. That gave me a sense that what I was doing was medically acceptable and therapeutic.

We began microcurrent therapy, and over the next week or two I began to feel much more comfortable. For the next month or two I continued to see Mary Lou twice a week, receiving microcurrent therapy and relaxing manual therapy. I was eventually given a portable microcurrent unit for use at home.

I am quite sure that microcurrent therapy was working. I left Houston to come to Northern Minnesota. I basically stopped using my home unit

for about three weeks. My feet were not bothering me too much. I felt guilty about not using my unit. Then, I felt significant pain again and was very grateful that I had the unit and hooked it up as soon as possible. The next day I felt significant amelioration.

I have always been a firm believer in the overall benefits of physical exercise. My doctor said he was convinced that I would have surely died in my first round of PCP and TB had I not been in such excellent shape. I am sure he was right.

I have a tremendous sense of urgency to accomplish my innermost goals and make life as worthwhile as possible. I am living on borrowed time now.

CONCLUSION

These are just a few of the many wonderful encounters with patients living with HIV disease. I have been with those whose illness brought them fully into life and strengthened their confidence in something sensed to be ongoing and untouched by the demise of their bodies. I have seen those, whose lives had been fearful, come to the moment of death with a new openness that allowed them a sense of completion they had seldom known before. It is through their candid sharing that emotions unfold, breakthroughs are realized, and patients become teachers to those around them.

Appendix A

Walter Reed (WR) Staging System

	HIV antibody or antigen	Chronic lymphadenopathy	T-helper cells/mm3	Delayed hypersensitivity	Oral thrush	Opportunistic infection
WR0	-	-	>400	NORMAL	-	-
WR1	+	-	>400	NORMAL	-	-
WR2	+	+	>400	NORMAL	-	-
WR3	+	+/-	<400	NORMAL	-	-
WR4	+	+/-	<400	PARTIAL	-	-
WR5	+	+/-	<400	COMPLETE CUTANEOUS ANERGY AND/OR THRUSH		-
WR6	+	+/-	<400	PARTIAL TO COMPLETE	+/-	-

Source: Redfield, R.R., et al. (1986). *New England Journal of Medicine,* 314:131.

Appendix B

Universal Infection Control Guidelines

The increasing prevalence of HIV increases the risk that health care workers will be exposed to blood from patients infected with HIV, especially when blood and body-fluid precautions are not followed for all patients. Thus, this document emphasizes the need for health care workers to consider all patients as potentially infected with HIV and/or other blood-borne pathogens and to adhere rigorously to infection control precautions for minimizing the risk of exposure to blood and body fluids.

The recommendations contained in this document consolidate and update CDC recommendations published earlier for preventing HIV transmitted in health care settings; precautions for clinical and laboratory staffs and precautions for health-care workers and allied professionals; recommendations for preventing HIV transmission in the work place and during invasive procedures; recommendations for preventing possible transmission of HIV from tears; and recommendations for providing dialysis treatment for HIV-infected patients. The recommendations contained in this document have been developed for use in health-care settings and emphasize the need to treat blood and other body fluids from all patients as potentially infective. These same prudent precautions also should be taken in other settings in which persons may be exposed to blood or other body fluids.

UNIVERSAL PRECAUTIONS

Since medical history and examination cannot reliably identify all patients with HIV or other blood-borne pathogens, blood and body-fluid precautions should be consistently used for all patients. This approach, previously recommended by CDC, and referred to as "universal blood and body-fluid precautions" or "universal precautions" should be used in the care of all patients, especially including those in emergency-care settings in which the risk of blood exposure is increased and the infection status of the patient is usually unknown.

1. All health care workers should routinely use appropriate barrier precautions to prevent skin and mucous-membrane exposure when contact with blood or other body fluids of any patient is anticipated. Gloves should be worn for touching blood and body fluids, mucous membranes, or non intact skin of all patients, for handling items or surfaces soiled with blood or body fluids, and for performing venipuncture and other vascular access procedures. Gloves should be changed after contact with each patient. Mask and protective eyewear or face shield should be worn during procedures that are likely to generate droplets of blood or other body fluids to prevent exposure of mucous membranes of the mouth, nose and eyes. Gowns or aprons should be worn during procedures that are likely to generate splashes of blood or other body fluids.

2. Hands and other skin surfaces should be washed immediately and thoroughly if contaminated with blood or other body fluids. Hands should be washed immediately after gloves are removed.

3. All health care workers should take precautions to prevent injuries caused by needles, scalpels and other sharp instruments or devices during procedures when cleaning used instruments; during disposal of used needles; and when handling sharp instruments after procedures. To prevent needlestick injuries, needles should not be recapped, purposely bent or broken by hand, removed from disposable syringes or otherwise manipulated by hand. After they are used, disposable syringes and needles, scalpel blades and other sharp items should be placed in puncture-resistant containers for disposal; the puncture-resistant containers should be

located as close as is practical to the use area. Large-bore reusable needles should be placed in a puncture-resistant container for transport to the reprocessing area.

4. Although saliva has not been implicated in HIV transmission, to minimize the need for emergency mouth-to-mouth resuscitation, mouthpieces, resuscitation bags or other ventilation devices should be available for use in areas in which the need for resuscitation is predictable.

5. Health care workers who have exudative lesions or weeping dermatitis should refrain from all direct patient care and from handling patient-care equipment until the condition resolves.

6. Pregnant health care workers are not known to be at greater risk for contracting HIV infection than health care workers who are not pregnant; however, if a health care worker develops HIV infection during pregnancy, the infant is at risk for infection resulting from perinatal transmission. Because of the risk, pregnant health care workers should be especially familiar with precautions to minimize the risk of HIV transmission.

Implementation of universal blood and body-fluid precautions for all patients eliminates the need for use of the isolation category of "Blood and Body-Fluid Precautions" previously recommended by the CDC for patients known or suspected to be infected with blood-borne pathogens. Isolation precautions (eg. enteric, "AFB") should be used as necessary if associated conditions, such as infectious diarrhea or tuberculosis, are diagnosed or suspected.

ENVIRONMENTAL CONSIDERATION FOR HIV TRANSMISSION

No environmentally mediated mode of HIV transmission has been documented. Nevertheless, the precautions described here should be taken routinely in the care of all patients.

STERILIZATION AND DISINFECTION

Standard sterilization and disinfection procedures for patient-care equipment currently recommended for use in a variety of health care settings including hospitals, medical and dental clinics and officers, hemodialysis centers, emergency-care facilities, and long-term nursing-care facilities are adequate to sterilize or disinfect instruments, devices, or other items contaminated with blood or other body fluids from persons infected with blood or other body fluids.

Instruments or devices that enter sterile tissue or the vascular system of any patient or through which blood flows should be sterilized before reuse. Devices or items (that contact intact mucous membranes should be sterilized or receive high-level disinfection, a procedure that kills vegetative organisms and viruses but not necessarily large numbers of bacterial spores. Chemical germicides that are registered with the U.S. Environmental Protection Agency (EPA) as "sterilants" may be used either for sterilization or for high-level disinfection, depending on contact time.

SURVIVAL OF HIV IN THE ENVIRONMENT

The most extensive study on the survival of HIV after drying involved greatly concentrated HIV samples, ie. 10 million tissue-culture infectious doses per milliliter. This concentration is at least 100,000 times greater than that typically found in the blood or serum of patients with HIV infection. HIV was detectable by tissue-culture techniques one to three days after drying, but the rate of inactivation was rapid. Studies performed at the CDC have also shown that drying HIV causes a rapid (within several hours) one to two log (90 - 99 percent) reduction in HIV concentration. In tissue-cultured fluid, cell-free HIV could be detected up to 15 days at room temperature, up to 11 days at 37 degrees celsius (98.6 degrees Fahrenheit) and up to 1 day if the HIV was cell associated.

When considered in the context of environmental conditions in health care facilities, these results do not require any changes in current recommended sterilization, disinfection or housekeeping strategies. When medical devices are contaminated with blood or other body fluids, existing recommendations include the cleaning of these instruments, followed by disinfection or sterilization, depending on the type of medical device. These protocols assume "worst-case" conditions of extreme virologic and microbiologic contamination, and whether viruses have been inactivated after drying plays no role in formulating these strategies. Consequently, no changes in published procedures for cleaning, disinfecting or sterilizing need to be made.

HOUSEKEEPING

Environmental surfaces, such as walls and floors are not associated with transmission of infections to patients or health care workers. Therefore, extraordinary attempts to disinfect or sterilize these environmental surfaces are not necessary. However, cleaning and removal of soil should be done routinely.

Cleaning schedules and methods vary according to the area of the hospital or institution, type of surface to be cleaned, and the amount and type of soil present. Horizontal surfaces (eg. bedside tables and hard-surfaced flooring) in patient-care areas are usually cleaned on a regular basis, when soiling or spills occur and when a patient is discharged. Cleaning of walls, blinds and curtains is recommended only if they are visibly soiled. Disinfectant fogging is an unsatisfactory method of decontaminating air and surfaces and is not recommended.

Disinfectant-detergent formulations registered by the EPA can be used for cleaning environmental surfaces, but the actual physical removal of microorganisms by scrubbing is probably at least as important as any antimicrobial effect of the cleaning agent used. Therefore, cost, safety and acceptability by housekeepers can be the main criteria for selecting any such registered agent. The manufacturer's instructions for appropriate use should be followed.

CLEANING AND DECONTAMINATING SPILLS OF BLOOD OR OTHER BODY FLUIDS

Chemical germicides that are approved for use as "hospital disinfectants" and are tuberculocidal when used as recommended dilutions can be used to decontaminate spills of blood and other body fluids. Strategies for decontaminating spills of blood and other body fluids in a patient-care setting are different from those for spills of cultures or other materials in clinical, public health or research laboratories. In patient-care areas, visible material should first be removed, and the area should then be decontaminated. With large spills of cultured of concentrated infectious agents in the laboratory, the contaminated area should be flooded with a liquid germicide before cleaning, then decontaminated with fresh germicidal chemical. In both settings, gloves should be worn during the cleaning and decontaminating procedures.

LAUNDRY

Although soiled linen has been identified as a source of large numbers of certain pathogenic microorganisms, the risk of actual disease transmission is negligible. Rather than rigid procedures and specifications, hygienic and common-sense storage and processing of clean and soiled linen are recommended. Soiled linen should be handled as

little as possible and with minimum agitation to prevent gross microbial contamination of the air and of persons handling the linen. All soiled linen should be bagged at the location where it was used; it should not be sorted or rinsed in patient-care areas. Linen soiled with blood or body fluids should be placed and transported in bags that prevent leakage if hot water is used with detergent in water at least 71 degrees Celsius (160 degrees Fahrenheit) for 25 minutes. If low-temperature (<70 degrees Celsius [158 degrees Fahrenheit]) laundry cycles are used, chemicals suitable for low-temperature washing at proper use concentration should be used.

INFECTIVE WASTE

There is no epidemiologic evidence to suggest that most hospital waste is any more infective than residential waste. Moreover, there is no epidemiologic evidence that hospital waste has caused disease in the community as a result of improper disposal. Therefore, identifying wastes for which special precautions are indicated is largely a matter of judgment about the relative risk of disease transmission. The most practical approach to the management of infective waste is to identify those wastes with the potential for causing infection during handling and disposal and for which some special precautions appears prudent. Hospital wastes for which special precautions appear prudent include microbiology laboratory waste, pathology waste and blood specimens or blood products. Although any item that has had contact with blood, exudates, or secretions may be potentially infective, it is not usually considered practical or necessary to treat all such waste as infective. Infective waste, in general, should either be incinerated or should be autoclaved before disposal in a sanitary landfill. Bulk blood, suctioned fluids, excretions and secretions may be carefully poured down a drain connected to a sanitary sewer. Sanitary sewers may also be used to dispose of other infectious wastes capable of being ground and flushed into the sewer.

BODY FLUIDS TO WHICH UNIVERSAL PRECAUTIONS APPLY

Universal precautions apply to blood and to other body fluids containing visible blood. Occupational transmission of HIV and hepatitis B virus (HBV) to health care workers by blood is documented. Blood is the single most important source of HIV, HBV and other blood-borne pathogens in the occupational setting. Infection control efforts for HIV, HVB and other blood-borne pathogens must focus on preventing exposures to blood as well as on delivery of HBV immunization.

Universal precautions also apply to semen and vaginal secretions. Although both of these fluids have been implicated in the sexual transmission of HIV and HBV, they have not been implicated in occupational transmission from patient to health care worker. This observation is not unexpected, since exposure to semen in the usual health care setting is limited to laboratory analysis, and the routine practice of wearing gloves for performing vaginal examinations protects health care workers from exposure to potentially infectious vaginal secretions.

Universal precautions also apply to tissue and to the following fluids: cerebrospinal fluid (CSF), synovial fluid, pleural fluid, peritoneal fluid, pericardial fluid and amniotic fluid. The risk of transmission of HIV and HBV from these fluids is unknown; epidemiologic studies in the health care and community setting are currently inadequate to assess the potential risk to health-care workers from occupational exposures to them. However, HIV has been isolated from CSF, synovial fluid, amniotic fluid and peritoneal fluid. One case of occupational HIV transmission was reported after a percutaneous exposure to bloody pleural fluid obtained by needle aspiration. Whereas aseptic procedures used to obtain these fluids for diagnostic or therapeutic purposes protect health care workers from skin exposures, they cannot prevent penetrating injuries due to accidents from contaminated needles or other sharp instruments.

BODY FLUIDS TO WHICH UNIVERSAL PRECAUTIONS DO NOT APPLY

Universal precautions do not apply to feces, nasal secretions, sputum, sweat, tears, urine and vomitus unless these substances contain visible blood. The risk of transmission of HIV and HBV from these fluids and materials is extremely low or nonexistent. HIV has been isolated and hepatitis B surface antigen (HBsAg) has been demonstrated in some of these fluids; however, epidemiologic studies in the health-care and community setting have not implicated these fluids or materials in the transmission of HIV and HBV infections. Some of the above fluids and excretions represent a potential source for nosocomial and community-acquired infections with other pathogens, and recommendations for preventing transmission of nonblood-borne pathogens have been published.

PRECAUTIONS FOR OTHER BODY FLUIDS IN SPECIAL SETTINGS

Human breast milk has been implicated in perinatal transmission of HIV, and HBsAg has been found in the milk of mothers infected with HBV. However, occupational exposure to human breast milk has not been implicated in the transmission of HIV or HBV infection to health care workers. Moreover, the health care worker will not have the same type of intensive exposure to breast milk as the nursing neonate. Whereas universal precautions do not apply to human breast milk, gloves may be worn by health care workers in situations where exposures to breast milk might be frequent, for example, in breast milk banking.

Saliva of some persons infected with HBV has been shown to contain HBV DNA at concentrations 1/1,000 to 1/10,000 of that found in the infected person's serum. HBsAg-positive saliva has been shown to be infectious when injected into experimental animals and in human bite exposures. However, HBsAg-positive saliva has not been shown to be infectious when applied to oral mucous membranes in experimental primate studies or through contamination of musical instruments or cardiopulmonary resuscitation dummies used by HBV carriers. Epidemiologic studies of nonsexual household contacts of HIV-infected patients, including several small series in which HIV transmission failed to occur after bites or after percutaneous inoculation or contamination of cuts and open wounds with saliva from HIV-infected patients, suggest that the potential for salivary transmission of HIV is remote. One case report from Germany has suggested the possibility of transmission of HIV in a household setting from an infected child to a sibling through a human bite. The bite did not break the skin or result in bleeding. Since the date of seroconversion of HIV was not known for either child in this case, evidence for the role of saliva in the transmission of virus is unclear.

Universal precautions do not apply to saliva. General infection control practices already in existence, including the use of gloves for digital examination of mucous membranes and endotracheal suctioning and handwashing after exposure to saliva, should further minimize the minute risk, if any, for salivary transmission of HIV and HBV. Gloves need not be worn when feeding patients and when wiping saliva from skin.

Special precautions, however, are recommended for dentistry. Occupationally acquired infection with HBV in dental workers has been documented, and two possible cases of occupationally acquired HIV infection involving dentists have been reported. During dental procedures, contamination of saliva with blood is predictable, trauma to health care workers hands is common, and blood spattering may occur.

Infection control precautions for dentistry minimize the potential for nonintact skin and mucous membrane contact of dental health care workers to blood-contaminated saliva of patients. In addition, the use of gloves for oral examina- tion and treatment in the dental setting may also protect the patient's oral mucous membranes from exposures to blood, which may occur from breaks in the skin of dental workers' hands.

Sample Protocol for Whirlpool Treatments

PART ONE: Actual Patient/Wound Care
1. Bring supplies to area including dressings, disposal bag (may be identified by a specific color), tape, scissors and sterile gloves.
2. Explain procedure to the patient and make the patient as comfortable as possible. Discuss with the patient the need to maintain infection control guidelines to establish a comfortable setting.
3. Wash hands and put on gloves.
4. Remove dressing from patient's wound and dispose of soiled dressing in disposal bag.
5. Place wound in whirlpool for treatment.
6. Dispose of gloves and wash hands after whirlpool session.
7. Assist patient out of whirlpool.
8. Put on clean sterile gloves.
9. Dry area around wound and debride if necessary.
10. Dress wound as indicated and apply tape to hold dressing in place.
11. Place all disposable items, including gloves, into a plastic bag and seal.
12. Make patient comfortable before leaving unit.

PART TWO: Disinfecting of Hydrotherapy Equipment
1. Completely drain the Hubbard Tank or whirlpool.
2. Leave the equipment in the tank (ie. stretcher lift for Hubbard Tanks, whirlpool seats) that has contacted the patient or water.
3. Spray tank and all equipment with hospital-approved disinfectant, allow all areas to stand 5 minutes for disinfectant to take effect, and wipe down with a towel.
4. Rinse with clear, hot water (at least 115 degrees Fahrenheit). Remove all equipment.
5. Loosen any debris from the agitator and turbine by spraying and abrading surface with a towel.
6. Immerse the jet of the agitator in a bucket of disinfectant solution and run the agitator for five minutes. Rinse by running agitator for one minute in a bucket of clear water, (115 degrees Fahrenheit).
7. Clean all accessible parts of drains with a towel removing any debris that has accumulated. Close drain and fill with a disinfectant. Allow to stand five to ten minutes, and then rinse with clear hot water (greater than 115 degrees Fahrenheit).
8. Rinse all sides of tank and equipment with full strength calcium hypochlorite (bleach) and rinse well with hot water.

Note: A culture should be taken monthly on all Hubbard Tank and whirlpool equipment and a record kept of the results.

Appendix C

Activities of Daily Living Checklist for People With HIV Infection

Key: I= independent;   min A= minimal assistance;   mod A= moderate assistance;   max A= maximal assistance

Physical task	I	min A	mod A	max A	Describe Performance
Feeding					
Grooming/ Hygiene					
Bathing					
Dressing					
Mobility/ Transfers					
Communication					
Continence					

Psychosocial Considerations: (eg. chosen dependence on care giver, anger, withdrawal from task performance, patient does not value activity).

Environmental Considerations: (eg. bathes bedside, wheelchair bound, uses lap tray to eat in bed).

Biomedical Considerations: (eg. ROM, strength, endurance).

Adaptive equipment needed: _____

_____

_____

Functional Independence Measure

FUNCTIONAL INDEPENDENCE MEASURE

FIM

L E V E L S	7 Complete Independence (Timely, Safely) 6 Modified Independence (Device)	NO HELPER

	Modified Dependence
	    5 Supervision
	    4 Minimal Assist (Subject = 75%+)
	    3 Moderate Assist (Subject = 50%+)
	Complete Dependence
	    2 Maximal Assist (Subject = 25%+)
	    1 Total Assist (Subject = 0%+)
		HELPER

	ADMIT	DISCHG	FOL-UP
Self Care			
A. Eating	☐	☐	☐
B. Grooming	☐	☐	☐
C. Bathing	☐	☐	☐
D. Dressing-Upper Body	☐	☐	☐
E. Dressing-Lower Body	☐	☐	☐
F. Toileting	☐	☐	☐
Sphincter Control			
G. Bladder Management	☐	☐	☐
H. Bowel Management	☐	☐	☐
Mobility			
Transfer:			
I. Bed, Chair, Wheelchair	☐	☐	☐
J. Toilet	☐	☐	☐
K. Tub, Shower	☐	☐	☐
Locomotion			
L. Walk/wheel Chair	w/c ☐	w/c ☐	w/c ☐
M. Stairs	☐	☐	☐
Communication			
N. Comprehension	a/v ☐	a/v ☐	a/v ☐
O. Expression	v/n ☐	v/n ☐	v/n ☐
Social Cognition			
P. Social Interaction	☐	☐	☐
Q. Problem Solving	☐	☐	☐
R. Memory	☐	☐	☐
Total FIM	☐	☐	☐

NOTE: Leave no blanks; enter 1 if patient not testable due to risk.

HIV Evaluation Form

C - 3   **HIV EVALUATION FORM**

Patient Name: _____ Date: _____ Time: _____

Physician Diagnosis: _____ PT Diagnosis: _____

Previous Admission: _____ Age: _____ Sex: _____

Referred For: _____

Precautions: _____ Referring Physician: _____

History: _____

Meds: (Circle Choice(s))   AZT   DDI   DDC   ANTINEOPLASTIC

Comments: _____

Opportunistic Infections: (Key: C = current   P = Past)

PCP _____ Cryptococcus Menigitis _____ Lymphoma _____ Kaposi Sarcoma _____ CMV _____ Other _____

- -

SUBJECTIVE:

Patient's Support System(s): (Circle Choice(s))   Family   Friends   Organizations   Others:_____

Patient's Chief Complaint(s): (Circle Choice(s))   Fear & Anxiety   Discomfort   Inability to Function   Others:_____

Do you have any pain?   Yes   No   If yes, where is the pain located? _____

What is the nature of your pain? _____

How would you rate the pain? |—|—|—|—|—|—|—|—|—|—|
                             0   5   10

What type of Diet was ordered? _____ Did you have a nutritionist consult with you? Yes   No

- -

OBJECTIVE: | JOINT   RANGE OF MOTION / STRENGTH / PAIN |

SHOULDER:	RIGHT	LEFT
Flexion	/	/
Extension	/	/
Abduction	/	/
Adduction	/	/
Ext. Rotation	/	/
Int. Rotation	/	/

ELBOW:		
Flexion	/	/
Extension	/	/
Supination	/	/
Pronation	/	/

WRIST:		
Flexion	/	/
Extension	/	/
Ulnar Devi.	/	/
Radial Devi.	/	/

HIP:	RIGHT	LEFT
Flexion	/	/
Extension	/	/
Abduction	/	/
Adduction	/	/
Ext. Rotation	/	/
Int. Rotation	/	/

KNEE:		
Flexion	/	/
Extension	/	/

ANKLE:		
Plantar Flex	/	/
Dorsi Flex	/	/
Inversion	/	/
Eversion	/	/

HEAD & NECK:	RIGHT	LEFT
Flexion	/	/
Extension	/	/
Rotation	/	/
Lat. Flexion	/	/

TRUNK		
Flexion		
EXtension	/	/
Rotation	/	/
Lat. Flexion	/	/

PELVIC:		
Flexion	/	/
Extension	/	/
Rotation	/	/
Lat. Flexion	/	/

KEY: Range of Motion

MIN. = < 25% limitation
MOD. = > 25% < 50%
MAX. = > 50% limitation

KEY: Muscle Strength

O =	No contraction	= 0
T =	Trace	= 1
P =	Poor	= 2
F =	Fair	= 3
G =	Good	= 4
N =	Normal	= 5

Circle to indicate pain

continued . . .

C - 3   **HIV EVALUATION FORM**

SPINAL/ POSTURE EVALUATION

Pain Key:

Numbness ||| Moderate

Severe ///   Shooting

Palpation Key:

Tender X   Hypomobile |

Pain Referred ////   Hypermobile

Central Pain (X)   Spasm

POSTURE: _____

_____

Gait Deviation: _____

_____

Comments: _____

_____

FUNCTIONAL STATUS

	MAX	MOD	MIN	SBA	Ind
Rolling	___	___	___	___	___
Supine to Sit	___	___	___	___	___
Sit to Stand	___	___	___	___	___
Transfer	___	___	___	___	___
Ambulation	___	___	___	___	___
(Flat Surface)					
(Stair)	___	___	___	___	___

Assistive Devices: _____

ACTIVITIES OF DAILY LIVING

	MAX	MOD	MIN	SBA	IND
Hygiene	___	___	___	___	___
Dressing	___	___	___	___	___
Food Acquistion	___	___	___	___	___
Food Preparation	___	___	___	___	___
Household Maintance	___	___	___	___	___
Ability to use					
Transportation Service	___	___	___	___	___
Ambulation	___	___	___	___	___

PATIENT'S ACTIVITY LEVELS

ENERGY	ACTIVITY	Previous	Current
< 1.5 METS	Sitting		
1.5 - 2 METS	Standing	___	___
2 - 3 METS	Walking 2 mph	___	___
3 - 4 METS	Walking 3 mph	___	___
4 - 5 METS	Walking 3.5 mph	___	___
5 - 6 METS	Walking 4 mph	___	___
6 - 7 METS	Walking 5 mph	___	___
7 - 8 METS	Jogging 5 mph	___	___
8 - 9 METS	Running 5.5 mph	___	___
10 + METS	Running 6+ mph	___	___

BODY COMPOSITION

% Lean Body Mass: _____ % Body Fat_____

CARDIORESPIRATORY

Pt. Age:_____ Resting HR:_____ Target HR_____

Blood Pressure:_____ / _____

Est. Max. HR = (220 - Pt. Age)

HR Reserve = Est. Max HR - Resting HR

Target HR = (HR Reserve x .6) + Resting HR

NEUROLOGICAL:

REFLEXES:

L / R

Biceps	___/___
Triceps	___/___
Brachiorradialls	___/___

KEY:

0 = Absent
1+ = Diminished
2+ = Normal
3+ = Increased
4+ = Clonus

Knee	___/___
Ankle	___/___
Babinski	___/___

SENSATION:

Light Touch	intact	diminished	absent
Pain & Temp	intact	diminished	absent
Proproception	intact	diminished	absent
Position Sense	intact	diminished	absent

Area Tested: _____

Skin Integration: _____

VISION: Intact   diminished   absent

BOWEL &   Continent   incontinent
BLADDER

BALANCE:

Sitting	Poor	Fair	Good
Standing	Poor	Fair	Good
Romberg	(+)	(-)	NT

COGNITION: ORIENTED TO:

Time _____ continued . . .
Place _____
Person _____

C - 3

HIV EVALUATION FORM

Initial Treatment Given: _____

_____

Plan of Care Discussed with Patient and Family: _____

_____

Assessment _____

_____

PATIENT GOALS

Physical Therapy Goals	Problem List	Patient Goals	STG ___Days / Weeks	LTG ___Weeks / Month
1. Increase Strength	___	___	___	___
2. Increase Range of Motion	___	___	___	___
3. Increase Coordination	___	___	___	___
4. Increase Endurance	___	___	___	___
5. Decrease Pain	___	___	___	___
6. Decrease Muscle Spasm	___	___	___	___
7. Decrease Spasticity	___	___	___	___
8. Decrease Swelling	___	___	___	___
9. Decrease Chest Congestion	___	___	___	___
10. Improve Posture	___	___	___	___
11. Heal Soft Tissue Lesions	___	___	___	___
12. Ind. Ambulation	___	___	___	___
13. Decrease Gait Deviation	___	___	___	___
14. Ind. in Functional Activity	___	___	___	___
15. Ind. in Elevated Activity	___	___	___	___
16. Ind. in Transfer Activity	___	___	___	___
17. Teach Pt. & Family Home Program	___	___	___	___
18. Prevent Contracture	___	___	___	___
19. Prevent Deformities	___	___	___	___
20. Maintain Strength	___	___	___	___
21. Decrease Abnormal Sensory Feedback	___	___	___	___

Rehabilitation Potential: Poor   Fair   Good   Excellent

Reassessment Frequency: _____

Plan: _____

_____

_____

_____ PT   License # _____   Date: _____

_____ MD   Date: _____

Role Checklist

ROLE CHECKLIST

NAME _____ AGE _____ DATE _____

SEX: ☐ MALE   ☐ FEMALE   ARE YOU RETIRED: ☐ YES   ☐ NO

MARITAL STATUS: ☐ SINGLE   ☐ MARRIED   ☐ SEPARATED   ☐ DIVORCED   ☐ WIDOWED

The purpose of this checklist is to identify the major roles in your life. The checklist, which is divided into two parts, presents 10 roles and defines each one.

PART I

Beside each role, indicate, by checking the appropriate column, if you performed the role in the past, if you presently perform the role, and if you plan to perform the role in the future. You may check more than one column for each role. For example, if you volunteered in the past, do not volunteer at present, but plan to in the future, you would check the past and future columns.

ROLE	PAST	PRESENT	FUTURE
STUDENT: Attending school on a part-time or full-time basis.			
WORKER: Part-time or full-time paid employment.			
VOLUNTEER: Donating services, *at least once a week,* to a hospital, school, community, political campaign, and so forth.			
CARE GIVER: Responsibility, *at least once a week,* for the care of someone such as a child, spouse, relative or friend.			
HOME MAINTAINER: Responsibility, *at least once a week,* for the upkeep of the home such as housecleaning or yardwork.			
FRIEND: Spending time or doing something, *at least once a week,* with a friend.			
FAMILY MEMBER: Spending time or doing something, *at least once a week,* with a family member such as a child, spouse, parent or other relative.			
RELIGIOUS PARTICIPANT: Involvement, *at least once a week,* in groups or activities affiliated with one's religion (excluding worship).			
HOBBYIST/AMATEUR: Involvement, *at least once a week,* in a hobby or amateur activity such as sewing, playing a musical instrument, woodworking, sports, the theater or participation in a club or team.			
PARTICIPANT IN ORGANIZATIONS: Involvement, *at least once a week,* in organizations such as the American Legion, National Organization for Women, Parents Without Partners, Weight Watchers, and so forth.			
OTHER: _____ A role not listed that you have performed, are presently performing, and/or plan to perform. Write the role on the line above and check the appropriate column(s).			

PART II

The same roles are listed below. Next to *each* role, check the column which best indicates how valuable or important the role is to you. Answer for *each* role, even if you have never performed or do not plan to perform the role.

ROLE	NOT AT ALL VALUABLE	SOME-WHAT VALUABLE	VERY VALUABLE
STUDENT: Attending school on a part-time or full-time basis.			
WORKER: Part-time or full-time paid employment.			
VOLUNTEER: Donating services, *at least once a week,* to a hospital, school, community, political campaign and so forth.			
CARE GIVER: Responsibility, *at least once a week,* for the care of someone such as a child, spouse, relative or friend.			
HOME MAINTAINER: Responsibility, *at least once a week,* for the upkeep of the home such as housecleaning or yardwork.			
FRIEND: Spending time or doing something, *at least once a week,* with a friend.			
FAMILY MEMBER: Spending time or doing something, *at least once a week,* with a family member such as a child, spouse, parent or other relative.			
RELIGIOUS PARTICIPANT: Involvement, *at least once a week,* in groups or activities affiliated with one's religion (excluding worship).			
HOBBYIST/AMATEUR: Involvement, *at least once a week,* in a hobby or amateur activity such as sewing, playing a musical instrument, woodworking, sports, the theater, or participation in a club or team.			
PARTICIPANT IN ORGANIZATIONS: Involvement, *at least once a week,* in organizations such as the American Legion, National Organization for Women, Parents Without Partners, Weight Watchers and so forth.			
OTHER: _____ A role not listed which you have performed, are presently performing, and/or plan to perform. Write the role on the line above and check the appropriate column(s).			

Occupational Therapy Service, Department of Rehabilitation Medicine, Clinical Center, National institutes of Health

☆U.S. GOVERNMENT PRINTING OFFICE: 1985-526-620:30339

Activity Record

Activity Record

Name _____ Age ___ Day/Date ___ I.D. # ___

Day 1 — Morning

Page 1 of 6

Key#	Half-Hour Beginning At	Category	Activity	Question 1 — During This Time I Felt Pain (1=Not At All, 2=Very Little, 3=Some, 4=A Lot)	Question 2 — At The Beginning Of This Half-Hour I Felt Fatigue (1=Not At All, 2=Very Little, 3=Some, 4=A Lot)	Question 3 — I Think That I Do This (1=Very Poorly, 2=Poorly, 3=Average, 4=Well)	Question 4 — I Find This Activity To Be (1=Very Difficult, 2=Difficult, 3=Slightly Difficult, 4=Not Difficult)	Question 5 — For Me This Activity Is (1=Not Meaningful, 2=Slightly Meaningful, 3=Meaningful, 4=Very Meaningful)	Question 6 — This Activity Causes Fatigue (1=Not At All, 2=Very Little, 3=Some, 4=A Lot)	Question 7 — I Enjoy This Activity (1=Not At All, 2=Very Little, 3=Some, 4=A Lot)	Question 8 — I Stopped To Rest During The Activity (1=Yes, 2=No)
	4:30 AM			1 2 3 4	1 2 3 4	1 2 3 4	1 2 3 4	1 2 3 4	1 2 3 4	1 2 3 4	1 2
	5:00 AM			1 2 3 4	1 2 3 4	1 2 3 4	1 2 3 4	1 2 3 4	1 2 3 4	1 2 3 4	1 2
	5:30 AM			1 2 3 4	1 2 3 4	1 2 3 4	1 2 3 4	1 2 3 4	1 2 3 4	1 2 3 4	1 2
	6:00 AM			1 2 3 4	1 2 3 4	1 2 3 4	1 2 3 4	1 2 3 4	1 2 3 4	1 2 3 4	1 2
	6:30 AM			1 2 3 4	1 2 3 4	1 2 3 4	1 2 3 4	1 2 3 4	1 2 3 4	1 2 3 4	1 2
	7:00 AM			1 2 3 4	1 2 3 4	1 2 3 4	1 2 3 4	1 2 3 4	1 2 3 4	1 2 3 4	1 2
	7:30 AM			1 2 3 4	1 2 3 4	1 2 3 4	1 2 3 4	1 2 3 4	1 2 3 4	1 2 3 4	1 2
	8:00 AM			1 2 3 4	1 2 3 4	1 2 3 4	1 2 3 4	1 2 3 4	1 2 3 4	1 2 3 4	1 2
	8:30 AM			1 2 3 4	1 2 3 4	1 2 3 4	1 2 3 4	1 2 3 4	1 2 3 4	1 2 3 4	1 2
	9:00 AM			1 2 3 4	1 2 3 4	1 2 3 4	1 2 3 4	1 2 3 4	1 2 3 4	1 2 3 4	1 2
	9:30 AM			1 2 3 4	1 2 3 4	1 2 3 4	1 2 3 4	1 2 3 4	1 2 3 4	1 2 3 4	1 2
	10:00 AM			1 2 3 4	1 2 3 4	1 2 3 4	1 2 3 4	1 2 3 4	1 2 3 4	1 2 3 4	1 2
	10:30 AM			1 2 3 4	1 2 3 4	1 2 3 4	1 2 3 4	1 2 3 4	1 2 3 4	1 2 3 4	1 2
	11:00 AM			1 2 3 4	1 2 3 4	1 2 3 4	1 2 3 4	1 2 3 4	1 2 3 4	1 2 3 4	1 2
	11:30 AM			1 2 3 4	1 2 3 4	1 2 3 4	1 2 3 4	1 2 3 4	1 2 3 4	1 2 3 4	1 2
	12:00 PM			1 2 3 4	1 2 3 4	1 2 3 4	1 2 3 4	1 2 3 4	1 2 3 4	1 2 3 4	1 2

Activity Record
NIH-2637 (7-87)

Department of Rehabilitation Medicine
National Institutes of Health

Activity Record

Name _____ Age _____ Day/Date _____ I.D.# _____

Day 1 — Afternoon

Key#	Half-Hour Beginning At	Category	Activity	Question 1 During This Time I Felt Pain 1 = Not At All 2 = Very Little 3 = Some 4 = A Lot	Question 2 At The Beginning Of This Half-Hour I Felt Fatigue 1 = Not At All 2 = Very Little 3 = Some 4 = A Lot	Question 3 I Think That I Do This 1 = Very Poorly 2 = Poorly 3 = Average 4 = Well	Question 4 I Find This Activity To Be 1 = Very Difficult 2 = Difficult 3 = Slightly Difficult 4 = Not Difficult	Question 5 For Me This Activity Is 1 = Not Meaningful 2 = Slightly Meaningful 3 = Meaningful 4 = Very Meaningful	Question 6 This Activity Causes Fatigue 1 = Not At All 2 = Very Little 3 = Some 4 = A Lot	Question 7 I Enjoy This Activity 1 = Not At All 2 = Very Little 3 = Some 4 = A Lot	Question 8 I Stopped To Rest During The Activity 1 = Yes 2 = No
	12:30 PM			1 2 3 4	1 2 3 4	1 2 3 4	1 2 3 4	1 2 3 4	1 2 3 4	1 2 3 4	1 2
	1:00 PM			1 2 3 4	1 2 3 4	1 2 3 4	1 2 3 4	1 2 3 4	1 2 3 4	1 2 3 4	1 2
	1:30 PM			1 2 3 4	1 2 3 4	1 2 3 4	1 2 3 4	1 2 3 4	1 2 3 4	1 2 3 4	1 2
	2:00 PM			1 2 3 4	1 2 3 4	1 2 3 4	1 2 3 4	1 2 3 4	1 2 3 4	1 2 3 4	1 2
	2:30 PM			1 2 3 4	1 2 3 4	1 2 3 4	1 2 3 4	1 2 3 4	1 2 3 4	1 2 3 4	1 2
	3:00 PM			1 2 3 4	1 2 3 4	1 2 3 4	1 2 3 4	1 2 3 4	1 2 3 4	1 2 3 4	1 2
	3:30 PM			1 2 3 4	1 2 3 4	1 2 3 4	1 2 3 4	1 2 3 4	1 2 3 4	1 2 3 4	1 2
	4:00 PM			1 2 3 4	1 2 3 4	1 2 3 4	1 2 3 4	1 2 3 4	1 2 3 4	1 2 3 4	1 2
	4:30 PM			1 2 3 4	1 2 3 4	1 2 3 4	1 2 3 4	1 2 3 4	1 2 3 4	1 2 3 4	1 2
	5:00 PM			1 2 3 4	1 2 3 4	1 2 3 4	1 2 3 4	1 2 3 4	1 2 3 4	1 2 3 4	1 2
	5:30 PM			1 2 3 4	1 2 3 4	1 2 3 4	1 2 3 4	1 2 3 4	1 2 3 4	1 2 3 4	1 2
	6:00 PM			1 2 3 4	1 2 3 4	1 2 3 4	1 2 3 4	1 2 3 4	1 2 3 4	1 2 3 4	1 2
	6:30 PM			1 2 3 4	1 2 3 4	1 2 3 4	1 2 3 4	1 2 3 4	1 2 3 4	1 2 3 4	1 2
	7:00 PM			1 2 3 4	1 2 3 4	1 2 3 4	1 2 3 4	1 2 3 4	1 2 3 4	1 2 3 4	1 2
	7:30 PM			1 2 3 4	1 2 3 4	1 2 3 4	1 2 3 4	1 2 3 4	1 2 3 4	1 2 3 4	1 2
	8:00 PM			1 2 3 4	1 2 3 4	1 2 3 4	1 2 3 4	1 2 3 4	1 2 3 4	1 2 3 4	1 2

Department of Rehabilitation Medicine
National Institutes of Health

Activity Record
NIH-2637 (7-87)

Developed by Gloria Furst, MPH, OTR/L and Lynn Gerber, MD, Occupational Therapy Service, National Institutes of Health. Used with permission. SLACK Incorporated, 6900 Grove Road, Thorofare, NJ 08086-9447.

Activity Record

Name _____ Age _____ Day/Date _____ I.D.# _____

Day 1 Evening

Key#	Activity / Category	Half-Hour Beginning At	Question 1 During This Time I Felt Pain 1 = Not At All 2 = Very Little 3 = Some 4 = A Lot	Question 2 At The Beginning Of This Half-Hour I Felt Fatigue 1 = Not At All 2 = Very Little 3 = Some 4 = A Lot	Question 3 I Think That I Do This 1 = Very Poorly 2 = Poorly 3 = Average 4 = Well	Question 4 I Find This Activity To Be 1 = Very Difficult 2 = Difficult 3 = Slightly Difficult 4 = Not Difficult	Question 5 For Me This Activity Is 1 = Not Meaningful 2 = Slightly Meaningful 3 = Meaningful 4 = Very Meaningful	Question 6 This Activity Causes Fatigue 1 = Not At All 2 = Very Little 3 = Some 4 = A Lot	Question 7 I Enjoy This Activity 1 = Not At All 2 = Very Little 3 = Some 4 = A Lot	Question 8 I Stopped To Rest During The Activity 1 = Yes 2 = No
		8:30 PM	1 2 3 4	1 2 3 4	1 2 3 4	1 2 3 4	1 2 3 4	1 2 3 4	1 2 3 4	1 2
		9:00 PM	1 2 3 4	1 2 3 4	1 2 3 4	1 2 3 4	1 2 3 4	1 2 3 4	1 2 3 4	1 2
		9:30 PM	1 2 3 4	1 2 3 4	1 2 3 4	1 2 3 4	1 2 3 4	1 2 3 4	1 2 3 4	1 2
		10:00 PM	1 2 3 4	1 2 3 4	1 2 3 4	1 2 3 4	1 2 3 4	1 2 3 4	1 2 3 4	1 2
		10:30 PM	1 2 3 4	1 2 3 4	1 2 3 4	1 2 3 4	1 2 3 4	1 2 3 4	1 2 3 4	1 2
		11:00 PM	1 2 3 4	1 2 3 4	1 2 3 4	1 2 3 4	1 2 3 4	1 2 3 4	1 2 3 4	1 2
		11:30 PM	1 2 3 4	1 2 3 4	1 2 3 4	1 2 3 4	1 2 3 4	1 2 3 4	1 2 3 4	1 2
		12:00 AM	1 2 3 4	1 2 3 4	1 2 3 4	1 2 3 4	1 2 3 4	1 2 3 4	1 2 3 4	1 2
		12:30 AM	1 2 3 4	1 2 3 4	1 2 3 4	1 2 3 4	1 2 3 4	1 2 3 4	1 2 3 4	1 2
		1:00 AM	1 2 3 4	1 2 3 4	1 2 3 4	1 2 3 4	1 2 3 4	1 2 3 4	1 2 3 4	1 2
		1:30 AM	1 2 3 4	1 2 3 4	1 2 3 4	1 2 3 4	1 2 3 4	1 2 3 4	1 2 3 4	1 2
		2:00 AM	1 2 3 4	1 2 3 4	1 2 3 4	1 2 3 4	1 2 3 4	1 2 3 4	1 2 3 4	1 2
		2:30 AM	1 2 3 4	1 2 3 4	1 2 3 4	1 2 3 4	1 2 3 4	1 2 3 4	1 2 3 4	1 2
		3:00 AM	1 2 3 4	1 2 3 4	1 2 3 4	1 2 3 4	1 2 3 4	1 2 3 4	1 2 3 4	1 2
		3:30 AM	1 2 3 4	1 2 3 4	1 2 3 4	1 2 3 4	1 2 3 4	1 2 3 4	1 2 3 4	1 2
		4:00 AM	1 2 3 4	1 2 3 4	1 2 3 4	1 2 3 4	1 2 3 4	1 2 3 4	1 2 3 4	1 2

Department of Rehabilitation Medicine
National Institutes of Health

Activity Record
NIH-2637 (7-87)

Page 3 of 6

Developed by Gloria Furst, MPH, OTR/L and Lynn Gerber, MD, Occupational Therapy Service, National Institutes of Health. Used with permission. SLACK Incorporated, 6900 Grove Road, Thorofare, NJ 08086-9447.

Activity Record

Name _____   Age _____   Day/Date _____   I.D.# _____

Day 2 — Morning

Half-Hour Beginning At	Activity (Key# Category)	Question 1: During This Time I Felt Pain (1=Not At All, 2=Very Little, 3=Some, 4=A Lot)	Question 2: At The Beginning Of This Half-Hour I Felt Fatigue (1=Not At All, 2=Very Little, 3=Some, 4=A Lot)	Question 3: I Think That I Do This (1=Very Poorly, 2=Poorly, 3=Average, 4=Well)	Question 4: I Find This Activity To Be (1=Very Difficult, 2=Difficult, 3=Slightly Difficult, 4=Not Difficult)	Question 5: For Me This Activity Is (1=Not Meaningful, 2=Slightly Meaningful, 3=Meaningful, 4=Very Meaningful)	Question 6: This Activity Causes Fatigue (1=Not At All, 2=Very Little, 3=Some, 4=A Lot)	Question 7: I Enjoy This Activity (1=Not At All, 2=Very Little, 3=Some, 4=A Lot)	Question 8: I Stopped To Rest During The Activity (1=Yes, 2=No)
4:30 AM		1 2 3 4	1 2 3 4	1 2 3 4	1 2 3 4	1 2 3 4	1 2 3 4	1 2 3 4	1 2
5:00 AM		1 2 3 4	1 2 3 4	1 2 3 4	1 2 3 4	1 2 3 4	1 2 3 4	1 2 3 4	1 2
5:30 AM		1 2 3 4	1 2 3 4	1 2 3 4	1 2 3 4	1 2 3 4	1 2 3 4	1 2 3 4	1 2
6:00 AM		1 2 3 4	1 2 3 4	1 2 3 4	1 2 3 4	1 2 3 4	1 2 3 4	1 2 3 4	1 2
6:30 AM		1 2 3 4	1 2 3 4	1 2 3 4	1 2 3 4	1 2 3 4	1 2 3 4	1 2 3 4	1 2
7:00 AM		1 2 3 4	1 2 3 4	1 2 3 4	1 2 3 4	1 2 3 4	1 2 3 4	1 2 3 4	1 2
7:30 AM		1 2 3 4	1 2 3 4	1 2 3 4	1 2 3 4	1 2 3 4	1 2 3 4	1 2 3 4	1 2
8:00 AM		1 2 3 4	1 2 3 4	1 2 3 4	1 2 3 4	1 2 3 4	1 2 3 4	1 2 3 4	1 2
8:30 AM		1 2 3 4	1 2 3 4	1 2 3 4	1 2 3 4	1 2 3 4	1 2 3 4	1 2 3 4	1 2
9:00 AM		1 2 3 4	1 2 3 4	1 2 3 4	1 2 3 4	1 2 3 4	1 2 3 4	1 2 3 4	1 2
9:30 AM		1 2 3 4	1 2 3 4	1 2 3 4	1 2 3 4	1 2 3 4	1 2 3 4	1 2 3 4	1 2
10:00 AM		1 2 3 4	1 2 3 4	1 2 3 4	1 2 3 4	1 2 3 4	1 2 3 4	1 2 3 4	1 2
10:30 AM		1 2 3 4	1 2 3 4	1 2 3 4	1 2 3 4	1 2 3 4	1 2 3 4	1 2 3 4	1 2
11:00 AM		1 2 3 4	1 2 3 4	1 2 3 4	1 2 3 4	1 2 3 4	1 2 3 4	1 2 3 4	1 2
11:30 AM		1 2 3 4	1 2 3 4	1 2 3 4	1 2 3 4	1 2 3 4	1 2 3 4	1 2 3 4	1 2
12:00 PM		1 2 3 4	1 2 3 4	1 2 3 4	1 2 3 4	1 2 3 4	1 2 3 4	1 2 3 4	1 2

Department of Rehabilitation Medicine
National Institutes of Health

Activity Record
NIH-2637 (7-87)

☆ GPO : 1987 0 – 190–246

Developed by Gloria Furst, MPH, OTR/L and Lynn Gerber, MD, Occupational Therapy Service, National Institutes of Health. Used with permission. SLACK Incorporated, 6900 Grove Road, Thorofare, NJ 08086-9447.

Activity Record

Name _____ Age _____ Day/Date _____ I.D.# _____

Day 2   Afternoon

Half-Hour Beginning At	Key#	Activity Category	Question 1 — During This Time I Felt Pain — 1 = Not At All, 2 = Very Little, 3 = Some, 4 = A Lot	Question 2 — At The Beginning Of This Half-Hour I Felt Fatigue — 1 = Not At All, 2 = Very Little, 3 = Some, 4 = A Lot	Question 3 — I Think That I Do This — 1 = Very Poorly, 2 = Poorly, 3 = Average, 4 = Well	Question 4 — I Find This Activity To Be — 1 = Very Difficult, 2 = Difficult, 3 = Slightly Difficult, 4 = Not Difficult	Question 5 — For Me This Activity Is — 1 = Not Meaningful, 2 = Slightly Meaningful, 3 = Meaningful, 4 = Very Meaningful	Question 6 — This Activity Causes Fatigue — 1 = Not At All, 2 = Very Little, 3 = Some, 4 = A Lot	Question 7 — I Enjoy This Activity — 1 = Not At All, 2 = Very Little, 3 = Some, 4 = A Lot	Question 8 — I Stopped To Rest During The Activity — 1 = Yes, 2 = No
12:30 PM			1 2 3 4	1 2 3 4	1 2 3 4	1 2 3 4	1 2 3 4	1 2 3 4	1 2 3 4	1 2
1:00 PM			1 2 3 4	1 2 3 4	1 2 3 4	1 2 3 4	1 2 3 4	1 2 3 4	1 2 3 4	1 2
1:30 PM			1 2 3 4	1 2 3 4	1 2 3 4	1 2 3 4	1 2 3 4	1 2 3 4	1 2 3 4	1 2
2:00 PM			1 2 3 4	1 2 3 4	1 2 3 4	1 2 3 4	1 2 3 4	1 2 3 4	1 2 3 4	1 2
2:30 PM			1 2 3 4	1 2 3 4	1 2 3 4	1 2 3 4	1 2 3 4	1 2 3 4	1 2 3 4	1 2
3:00 PM			1 2 3 4	1 2 3 4	1 2 3 4	1 2 3 4	1 2 3 4	1 2 3 4	1 2 3 4	1 2
3:30 PM			1 2 3 4	1 2 3 4	1 2 3 4	1 2 3 4	1 2 3 4	1 2 3 4	1 2 3 4	1 2
4:00 PM			1 2 3 4	1 2 3 4	1 2 3 4	1 2 3 4	1 2 3 4	1 2 3 4	1 2 3 4	1 2
4:30 PM			1 2 3 4	1 2 3 4	1 2 3 4	1 2 3 4	1 2 3 4	1 2 3 4	1 2 3 4	1 2
5:00 PM			1 2 3 4	1 2 3 4	1 2 3 4	1 2 3 4	1 2 3 4	1 2 3 4	1 2 3 4	1 2
5:30 PM			1 2 3 4	1 2 3 4	1 2 3 4	1 2 3 4	1 2 3 4	1 2 3 4	1 2 3 4	1 2
6:00 PM			1 2 3 4	1 2 3 4	1 2 3 4	1 2 3 4	1 2 3 4	1 2 3 4	1 2 3 4	1 2
6:30 PM			1 2 3 4	1 2 3 4	1 2 3 4	1 2 3 4	1 2 3 4	1 2 3 4	1 2 3 4	1 2
7:00 PM			1 2 3 4	1 2 3 4	1 2 3 4	1 2 3 4	1 2 3 4	1 2 3 4	1 2 3 4	1 2
7:30 PM			1 2 3 4	1 2 3 4	1 2 3 4	1 2 3 4	1 2 3 4	1 2 3 4	1 2 3 4	1 2
8:00 PM			1 2 3 4	1 2 3 4	1 2 3 4	1 2 3 4	1 2 3 4	1 2 3 4	1 2 3 4	1 2

Department of Rehabilitation Medicine
National Institutes of Health

Activity Record
NIH-2637 (7-87)

Activity Record

Name _____   **Age** _____   **Day/Date** _____   **I.D. #** _____

Day 2   Evening

Half-Hour Beginning At	Activity (Category)	Question 1 During This Time I Felt Pain 1=Not At All 2=Very Little 3=Some 4=A Lot	Question 2 At The Beginning Of This Half-Hour I Felt Fatigue 1=Not At All 2=Very Little 3=Some 4=A Lot	Question 3 I Think That I Do This 1=Very Poorly 2=Poorly 3=Average 4=Well	Question 4 I Find This Activity To Be 1=Very Difficult 2=Difficult 3=Slightly Difficult 4=Not Difficult	Question 5 For Me This Activity Is 1=Not Meaningful 2=Slightly Meaningful 3=Meaningful 4=Very Meaningful	Question 6 This Activity Causes Fatigue 1=Not At All 2=Very Little 3=Some 4=A Lot	Question 7 I Enjoy This Activity 1=Not At All 2=Very Little 3=Some 4=A Lot	Question 8 I Stopped To Rest During The Activity 1=Yes 2=No
8:30 PM		1 2 3 4	1 2 3 4	1 2 3 4	1 2 3 4	1 2 3 4	1 2 3 4	1 2 3 4	1 2
9:00 PM		1 2 3 4	1 2 3 4	1 2 3 4	1 2 3 4	1 2 3 4	1 2 3 4	1 2 3 4	1 2
9:30 PM		1 2 3 4	1 2 3 4	1 2 3 4	1 2 3 4	1 2 3 4	1 2 3 4	1 2 3 4	1 2
10:00 PM		1 2 3 4	1 2 3 4	1 2 3 4	1 2 3 4	1 2 3 4	1 2 3 4	1 2 3 4	1 2
10:30 PM		1 2 3 4	1 2 3 4	1 2 3 4	1 2 3 4	1 2 3 4	1 2 3 4	1 2 3 4	1 2
11:00 PM		1 2 3 4	1 2 3 4	1 2 3 4	1 2 3 4	1 2 3 4	1 2 3 4	1 2 3 4	1 2
11:30 PM		1 2 3 4	1 2 3 4	1 2 3 4	1 2 3 4	1 2 3 4	1 2 3 4	1 2 3 4	1 2
12:00 AM		1 2 3 4	1 2 3 4	1 2 3 4	1 2 3 4	1 2 3 4	1 2 3 4	1 2 3 4	1 2
12:30 AM		1 2 3 4	1 2 3 4	1 2 3 4	1 2 3 4	1 2 3 4	1 2 3 4	1 2 3 4	1 2
1:00 AM		1 2 3 4	1 2 3 4	1 2 3 4	1 2 3 4	1 2 3 4	1 2 3 4	1 2 3 4	1 2
1:30 AM		1 2 3 4	1 2 3 4	1 2 3 4	1 2 3 4	1 2 3 4	1 2 3 4	1 2 3 4	1 2
2:00 AM		1 2 3 4	1 2 3 4	1 2 3 4	1 2 3 4	1 2 3 4	1 2 3 4	1 2 3 4	1 2
2:30 AM		1 2 3 4	1 2 3 4	1 2 3 4	1 2 3 4	1 2 3 4	1 2 3 4	1 2 3 4	1 2
3:00 AM		1 2 3 4	1 2 3 4	1 2 3 4	1 2 3 4	1 2 3 4	1 2 3 4	1 2 3 4	1 2
3:30 AM		1 2 3 4	1 2 3 4	1 2 3 4	1 2 3 4	1 2 3 4	1 2 3 4	1 2 3 4	1 2
4:00 AM		1 2 3 4	1 2 3 4	1 2 3 4	1 2 3 4	1 2 3 4	1 2 3 4	1 2 3 4	1 2

Key#

Department of Rehabilitation Medicine
National Institutes of Health

Activity Record
NIH-2637 (7-87)

Page 6 of 6

Developed by Gloria Furst, MPH, OTR/L and Lynn Gerber, MD, Occupational Therapy Service, National Institutes of Health. Used with permission. SLACK Incorporated, 6900 Grove Road, Thorofare, NJ 08086-9447.

Instructions for Activity Record

The purpose of this questionnaire is to help you to see your day more clearly. For each of two consecutive days during the week (such as Monday and Tuesday, but not to include a Saturday or Sunday), write in the space provided, the activity **that you feel best describes** what you were doing during that half-hour of the day. If what you were doing takes longer than one half-hour, write it again for as long as you continue to do the activity. Do this for each half-hour of the day and night.

After you have completed listing all your activities, give each half-hour period a number from the key below that best describes the **level of physical activity** that was necessary during that half-hour. Please answer all eight questions for each half-hour time period by putting a circle around the number you feel is the **best** answer to the question. You need not answer the questions for sleep.

Key

1. During this half-hour, I was mostly sitting or lying down.
2. During this half-hour, I was mostly standing, walking, lifting, moving around or sitting and working with my hands.

At the end of the day, use the categories on the back of this page to describe your activities.

Example

| | | Name | | | Age | | Day/Date | | | I.D. # | |

Day 1	Afternoon		Activity	Question 1 During This Time I Felt Pain 1 = Not At All 2 = Very Little 3 = Some 4 = A Lot	Question 2 At The Beginning Of This Half-Hour I Felt Fatigue 1 = Not At All 2 = Very Little 3 = Some 4 = A Lot	Question 3 I Think That I Do This 1 = Very Poorly 2 = Poorly 3 = Average 4 = Well	Question 4 I Find This Activity To Be 1 = Very Difficult 2 = Difficult 3 = Slightly Difficult 4 = Not Difficult	Question 5 For Me This Activity Is 1 = Not Meaningful 2 = Slightly Meaningful 3 = Meaningful 4 = Very Meaningful	Question 6 This Activity Causes Fatigue 1 = Not At All 2 = Very Little 3 = Some 4 = A Lot	Question 7 I Enjoy This Activity 1 = Not At All 2 = Very Little 3 = Some 4 = A Lot	Question 8 I Stopped To Rest During The Activity 1 = Yes 2 = No
Key#	Half-Hour Beginning At	Category									
2	12:30 p.m.	HA	Prepare Lunch	1 2 3 ④	1 2 ③ 4	1 2 ③ 4	1 ② 3 4	1 ② 3 4	1 2 ③ 4	1 2 ③ 4	① 2
1	1:00 p.m.	SC	Eat Lunch	1 2 ③ 4	1 ② 3 4	1 2 ③ 4	1 2 ③ 4	1 2 ③ 4	1 2 ③ 4	1 ② 3 4	1 ②
2	1:30 p.m.	HA	Clean Kitchen	1 2 3 ④	1 ② 3 4	1 2 ③ 4	1 2 ③ 4	1 2 ③ 4	1 2 ③ 4	1 2 ③ 4	1 ②

In question #4 - an activity may be difficult to do for several reasons. For example, it may be difficult physically while you are doing it. Or, it may be difficult because it requires a lot of advance planning or preparation, or because it takes a long time, or is very tiring or painful.

In question #8 - circle 1 **(Yes)** if you stopped to rest for a 5 or 10 minute break **during** the half-hour activity period; or circle 2 **(No)** if you did the activity for the full half-hour without a rest break.

To make remembering easier, it is recommended that you do this for each of the three time periods (morning, afternoon, and evening) rather than the whole day at one time. **It is important to be accurate.**

Department of Rehabilitation Medicine
National Institutes of Health

Activity Record
NIH-2637 (7-87)

Developed by Gloria Furst, MPH, OTR/L and Lynn Gerber, MD, Occupational Therapy Service, National Institutes of Health. Used with permission. SLACK Incorporated, 6900 Grove Road, Thorofare, NJ 08086-9447.

Categories

Rest (RE) - rest periods taking one-half hour or longer

Self-Care (SC) - personal care activities including dressing, grooming, exercises, normal meals, showering, or other similar activities

Preparation or Planning (PP) - time spent preparing to do an activity or planning when and how to do your daily or weekly activities

Household Activities (HA) - cooking, cleaning, mending, shopping for or putting away groceries, gardening, or other similar activities

Work (WK) - paid or volunteer activities in or out of the home, school work, writing papers, attending classes, studying, or other similar activities

Recreation or Leisure (RL) - hobbies, TV, games, reading (unless done during short rest breaks), sports, out-for-meals, movies, adult education classes, shopping, gardening, talking with friends, or other similar activities

Transportation (TR) - traveling to and from activities

Treatment (RX) - doctor or therapy appointments, home exercise, etc.

Sleep (SL) - when you go to bed for the night

Developed by Gloria Furst, MPH, OTR/L and Lynn Gerber, MD, Occupational Therapy Service, National Institutes of Health. Used with permission. SLACK Incorporated, 6900 Grove Road, Thorofare, NJ 08086-9447.

The Level of Interest in Particular Activities

Directions: For each activity listed check (✓) all columns that describe your level of interest in that particular activity.

ACTIVITY	WHAT HAS BEEN YOUR LEVEL OF INTEREST?						Do you currently participate in this activity?		Would you like to pursue this in the future?	
	IN THE PAST TEN YEARS			IN THE PAST YEAR						
	STRONG	SOME	NO	STRONG	SOME	NO	YES	NO	YES	NO
Gardening/Yardwork										
Sewing/Needlework										
Playing cards										
Foreign Languages										
Church activities										
Radio										
Walking										
Car repair										
Writing										
Dancing										
Golf										
Football										
Listening to popular music										
Puzzles										
Holiday activities										
Pets/livestock										
Movies										
Listening to classical music										
Speeches/lectures										
Swimming										
Bowling										
Visiting										
Mending										
Checkers/Chess										
Barbecues										
Reading										
Traveling										
Parties										
Wrestling										
Housecleaning										
Model building										
Television										
Concerts										
Pottery										

Adapted from Matsutsuyu (1967) by Scaffa (1982) Kielhofner & Neville (1983) Occupational Therapy Service, Department of Rehabilitation Medicine, National Institutes of Health. Used with permission. SLACK Incorporated, 6900 Grove Road, Thorofare, NJ 08086-9447.

Directions: For each activity listed check (✓) all columns which describe your level of interest in that particular activity.

ACTIVITY	WHAT HAS BEEN YOUR LEVEL OF INTEREST?						Do you currently participate in this activity?		Would you like to pursue this in the future?	
	IN THE PAST TEN YEARS			IN THE PAST YEAR						
	STRONG	SOME	NO	STRONG	SOME	NO	YES	NO	YES	NO
Camping										
Laundry/Ironing										
Politics										
Table games										
Home decorating										
Clubs/Lodge										
Singing										
Scouting										
Clothes										
Handicrafts										
Hairstyling										
Cycling										
Attending plays										
Bird watching										
Dating										
Auto-racing										
Home repairs										
Exercise										
Hunting										
Woodworking										
Pool										
Driving										
Child Care										
Tennis										
Cooking/Baking										
Basketball										
History										
Collecting										
Fishing										
Science										
Leatherwork										
Shopping										
Photography										
Painting/Drawing										

Adapted from Matsutsuyu (1967) by Scaffa (1982) Kielhofner & Neville (1983) Occupational Therapy Service, Department of Rehabilitation Medicine, National Institutes of Health. Used with permission. SLACK Incorporated, 6900 Grove Road, Thorofare, NJ 08086-9447.

Social Environment Interview

This care giver interview is based on the hospice principle of "treating the family as the unit of care." In our work with people with HIV and AIDS, it is essential that we recognize the need to redefine "family." This new definition includes the lover, spouse, roommate, friend and even community organization working with the person with HIV infection.

It is an often stated health care assumption that when one cares for himself/herself, one can better care for others. This interview helps the therapist to support the care giver in doing that very thing—care for himself/herself so that improved care for the person with HIV can/will occur. It also assists the therapist in helping the care giver and person with HIV develop strategies to work with occupational role loss and transition within this newly defined family system.

NOTE: These questions must be viewed as guiding questions. They must be adapted to the level of understanding of the individual being interviewed.

INTERVIEW QUESTIONS

1. What was your daily routine like before the diagnosis of your family member? After the diagnosis and currently?

2. How do you currently manage your time? Do you feel productive?

3. Are you involved in any leisure activities or hobbies? Do you do things just for fun?

4. Have you altered your activity level since the diagnosis of your family member? How do you feel about this alteration? What would you change, if anything?

5. How has this current situation affected your work? Productivity level? Your relationships? Your daily responsibilities and their performance? Your communication with others?

6. Do you feel competent in caring for your loved one? In what areas, if any, do you feel you need assistance and/or support?

Appendix D

Fatigue Survey

1. Were you ever bothered by fatigue before your diagnosis with HIV-related illness?
   YES   NO

2. Have you been bothered with fatigue since your diagnosis with HIV related illness?
   YES   NO   (If you answered no, you are now finished).

3. Are you experiencing fatigue now?
   YES   NO

4. Is the fatigue you have experienced since your diagnosis different from the fatigue you experienced before?
   YES   NO   If yes, how is it different?
   _____
   _____

5. If you have experienced fatigue since your diagnosis, how long ago did it first begin?
   _____

6. How often does your fatigue occur?
   1-3 times/month   1-3 times/wk   daily   constant   variable

7. How long does your fatigue occur at a time?
   a day   a few days   a week   a few weeks   constantly   variable

8. What time of the day is your fatigue the worst?
   early a.m.   late a.m.   early p.m.   late p.m.

9. If you are taking AZT, was there a change in your fatigue once you started taking the medication?
   a lot better   a little better   no change   a little worse   a lot worse

10. When you experience fatigue, how do you cope with it?
    _____
    _____
    _____

11. Does fatigue interfere with caring for yourself, such as (circle one answer from each line):

eating	a lot	somewhat	none
dressing	a lot	somewhat	none
grooming	a lot	somewhat	none
bathing	a lot	somewhat	none
using the bathroom	a lot	somewhat	none

12. Does your fatigue interfere with the following activities?
(Circle one answer from each line)

getting around in your home	a lot	somewhat	none
getting around outside your home	a lot	somewhat	none
in recreational activities	a lot	somewhat	none
in shopping for food/clothes	a lot	somewhat	none
in housework	a lot	somewhat	none
in meal preparation	a lot	somewhat	none
in sexual relations	a lot	somewhat	none
in using public transportation	a lot	somewhat	none

13. If you are not working, was fatigue a factor in your stopping work?
a major factor   a minor factor   not a factor

14. If you are working, have you had to decrease your activity at work because of fatigue?
a lot   somewhat   not at all

Developed by Micheal O'Dell, MD and John L. Turner, MD at Graduate Hospital, Philadelphia, PA. Used with permission. SLACK Incorporated, 6900 Grove Road, Thorofare, NJ 08086-9447.

Appendix E

A Guide to Assessing the HIV Seropositive Patient

Pain is an indication of pathology, either HIV or opportunistic infection oriented, and its locations and characteristics provide the medical professional with information about the etiology of the problem and the course of treatment. The practitioner, therefore, is encouraged to conduct the clarifying evaluation and, if possible, attempt to eliminate the cause of the pain rather than simply resorting to symptomatic treatment. Determining the structure from which pain is arising is of utmost importance in formulating a treatment plan, as well as in deciding on optimum sites for electrode placement.

I. Observation of Patient
   A. Limp or shuffle — (advancement of Kaposi's sarcoma (KS) lesions, peripheral neuropathy, rheumatologic disorder)
   B. Slow sitting may signify an acute twinging pain
   C. Facial expression

II. History
   This should be as complete as possible. Many times, the problem may become apparent from the history, but this should not take the place of a thorough physical evaluation. Give the patient adequate time to answer your questions so that the responses will be clear. Questions should be developed in relation to the following topics or parameters:
   A. Cause of the pain or condition
      1. Accident, surgery, disease, unknown
      2. Onset: sudden or gradual
      Note: Many conditions can occur without an obvious precipitating event.
   B. Length of time that pain has been present-distinguish between acute vs chronic condition
      1. When pain does occur, consider its duration

   a. Frequent recurrences-mechanical instability
   b. Continuous but fluctuating in intensity-muscular/nerve
   c. Rhythmic pulses — headache (can be indicative of HIV CNS lesion or opportunistic infection)
   d. Long and less rhythmic phases — intestinal colic
   e. Increasing in frequency and severity-(progressive demyelination/peripheral neuropathy)
   f. Occurring every few months — loose disk fragment
   g. Consider family, environmental problems or chronicity of HIV as source of stress or tension that may affect pain intensity

C. Is the condition worsening, remaining the same, or getting better?
   1. A pain that disappears and then is replaced by numbness and weakness is not indicative of improvement
   2. Compare pain at present to that at time of onset

D. Do activities or postures influence the pain?
   1. Sleeping, work, sports
   2. Pain-free position or activities
   3. Painful position or activities
      a. Visceral pain is unrelated to posture
      b. Once a nerve root swells and neuritis sets in, relief will not occur with any posture
      c. If standing on the involved leg causes increased pain, consider possibility of sacroiliac joint involvement

4. What is the effect of rest on the pain? Pain alleviated by rest is not so significant, but pain that increases or is not relieved by rest is important. This could signify a malignancy (KS) or other pathology.
5. AM vs PM
   a. Carpal tunnel and thoracic outlet syndromes produce paresthesia at night
   b. Increased pain at night with peripheral neuropathies

E. Have the patient describe the pain
1. Where did it start?
2. Where is it now?
3. Sharp, superficial pain
4. Dull, sore, achy, deep pain
5. Tiring, suffocating, pushing-signs of chronic problem—Sensory loss vs paresthesia
6. Draw or color in area of pain on a body diagram
   a. Mark the beginning and end of painful area
   b. Darken most intense region
   c. Place an X on very sensitive spots (possible trigger points)
   d. Differentiate between kidney and L-S area, hip and SI area, and anterior vs lateral thigh
7. Bilateral (cord, dura mater), unilateral (sciatic, facet), back only (may be visceral)
8. Hard to localize pains (scieratogenous) may be indicative of visceral or dura mater involvement
9. Does pain originate in the neck or shoulder (lymphoma)?
10. Is there pain referred-where, how far? KS may refer to low back pain
11. Does the pain follow the pathway of a peripheral nerve, dermatome, myotome, sclerotome, or trigger point pattern of referral?
12. Have the patient rate the intensity of the pain on a scale of 1 to 10

F. Severity of pain
1. Neuralgic (radiculitis, neuritis or causalgia) is severe; muscular from fatigue backache is achy, dull and not too unbearable

2. Malignancy may be severe and constant
3. Signs of serious pathology
   a. Vague pain reference
   b. Gradual, progressive, worsening
   c. Onset of fresh symptoms
   d. Pain unaffected by treatment
   e. Constant pain (24 hr/day)

G. Any associated symptoms
1. Weakness (myopathy, polymyositis, wasting syndrome)
2. Bowel or bladder problems—cauda equine, involvement (could be progressive inflammatory polyradiculopathy, or vacuolar myelopathy)
3. Coughing or sneezing increases intracranial pressure, puts pressure on weight-bearing structures (facets, disks), and may also distract the sacroiliac joint causing unilateral buttock pain.

H. Does the patient do anything to the involved area that relieves the pain?
1. They may point to a specific area or give a clue to treatment approach

I. Prior treatment
1. Do not repeat that which already has been unsuccessful

J. Diet
1. In relation to headaches, lymphoma or toxoplasmosis may be ensuing, constant low-grade achiness may be due to dietary deficiencies. (B6, B12)

K. Medication (certain drugs may interfere with actual treatment by increasing awareness to pain)
1. Type and amount may provide information about severity of pain. Is medication taken regularly, even when pain is not present? Is medication helpful and what percentage of pain is relieved by it?

L. Consider other information such as x-rays, general health history, related conditions and prior occurrences

M. Conclude by allowing the patient to mention anything else that he or she may consider to be in any way related

Adapted from Mannheimer & Lampe: Pain evaluation and pain diagram. In Clinical Transcutaneous Electrical Nerve Stimulation. Philadelphia, F.A. Davis Company, 1984-86.

Appendix F

Summary of the Classification of HIV Infection in Children Under 13 Years of Age

CLASS	CLASSIFICATION
P-O	**Indeterminate infection**
P-1	**Asymptomatic infection**
Subclass A	Normal immune function
Subclass B	Abnormal immune function
Subclass C	Immune function not tested
P-2	**Symptomatic Infection**
Subclass A	Nonspecific findings
Subclass B	Progressive neurologic disease
Subclass C	Lymphoid interstitial pneumonitis
Subclass D	Secondary infectious disease
Category D-1	Specific secondary infectious diseases listed in the CDC surveillance definition for AIDS
Category D-2	Recurrent serious bacterial infections
Category D-3	Other specified secondary infectious diseases
Subclass E	**Secondary cancers**
Category E-1	Specified secondary cancers listed in the CDC surveillance definition for AIDS
Category E-2	Other cancers possibly secondary to HIV infection
Subclass F	Other diseases possibly due to HIV infection

Adapted from Centers for Disease Control: (1987). Classification system for human immunodeficiency virus (HIV) infection in children under 13 years of age. MMWR 36:227.

Appendix G

Texas Statute Addressing Confidentiality

V.T.C.A. Health and Safety

81.103. Confidentiality; Criminal Penalty

(a) A test result is confidential. A person that possesses or has knowledge of a test result may not release or disclose the test result or allow the test result to become known except as provided by this section.

(b) A test result may be released to:
   (1) the department under this chapter;
   (2) a local health authority if reporting is required under this chapter;
   (3) the Centers for Disease Control of the United States Public Health Service if reporting is required by federal law or regulation;
   (4) the physician or other person authorized by law who ordered the test;
   (5) physician, nurse, or other health care personnel who have a legitimate need to know the test result in order to provide for their protection and to provide for the patient's health and welfare;
   (6) the person tested or a person legally authorized to consent to the test on the person's behalf;
   (7) the spouse of the person tested if the person tests positive for AIDS or HIV infection, antibodies to HIV, or infection with any other probable causative agent of AIDS and if the physician who ordered the test makes the notification; and
   (8) the victim of an offense listed in Article 21.31, Code of Criminal Procedure, if the person tested allegedly committed the of-

fense and the test was required under that article.

(c) The court shall notify an alleged victim to whom test results are released under Subsection (b)(8) of the requirements of this section.

(d) A person tested or a person legally authorized to consent to the test on the person's behalf may voluntarily release or disclose that person's test results to any other person, and may authorize the release or disclosure of the test results. An authorization under this subsection must be in writing and signed by the person tested or the person legally authorized to consent to the test on the person's behalf. The authorization must state the person or class of persons to whom the test results may be released or disclosed.

(e) A person may release or disclose a test result for statistical summary purposes only without the written consent of the person tested if information that could identify the person is removed from the report.

(f) A blood bank reports positive blood test results indicating the name of a donor with a possible infectious disease to other blood banks. A report under this subsection is not a breach of any confidential relationship.

(g) A blood bank may report blood test results to the hospitals where the blood was transfused, to the physician who transfused the infected blood, and to the recipient of the blood. A blood bank may also report blood test results for statistical purposes. A report under this subsection may not disclose the name of the donor or person tested or any information that could result in the disclosure of the donor's or person's name, including an address, social security number, a designated recipient or replacement information.

(h) A blood bank may provide blood samples to hospitals, laboratories and other blood banks for additional, repetitive or different testing.

(i) An employee of a health care facility whose job requires the employee to deal with permanent medical records may view test results in the performance of the employee's duties under reasonable health care facility practices. The test results viewed are confidential under this chapter.

(j) A person commits an offense if, with criminal negligence and in violation of this section, the person releases or discloses a test result or other information or allows a test result or other information to become known. An offense under this subsection is a Class A misdemeanor.

Appendix H

Abbreviations and Acronyms

Ab	antibodies	CT	computed tomography
ACTH	adrenocorticotropin hormone		
ADC	AIDS dementia complex	DdC	dideoxycytidine
ADL	activities of daily living	DdI	dideoxyinosine
Ag	antigen	DFMO	difluoromethylornithine
AIDS	acquired immunodeficiency syndrome	DHPG	gancidozia
ANOVA	Analysis of Variance	DNA	deoxyribonucleic Acid
ANS	autonomic nervous system	DNR	Do Not Resuscitate
AOTA	American Occupational Therapy Association	DSM-III-R	Diagnostic & Statistical Manual of Mental Disorders, Third Revised Edition
AOTF	American Occupational Therapy Foundation		
APTA	American Physical Therapy Association	DSPN	distal symmetric polyneuropathy
APTF	American Physical Therapy Foundation	DTR	deep tendon reflexes
ARC	AIDS-related complex		
AROM	active range of motion	E	epinephrine
ARV	AIDS-related virus	EEG	electroencephalogram
ASPEN	American Society for Parenteral and Enteral Nutrition	ELISA	enzyme-linked immunosorbent assay
		EMG	electromyography
ATP	adenosine triphosphate	EPA	Environmental Protection Agency
AZT	azidothymidine		
		FAOF	Family Assessment of Occupational Functioning
BEE	basal energy expenditure		
BMR	basic metabolic rate	Fc	fraction/centrifuge
BRM	biologic response modifier	FDA	Food and Drug Administration
		FIM	Functional Independence Measure
CAMP	cyclic adenosine monophosphate	FO	foot orthosis
CAOT	Canadian Association of Occupational Therapy	GDS	Global Deterioration Scale
		GBS	Guillain Barre syndrome
CASA	A Special Hospital in Houston	GI	Gastrointestinal
CPA	Canadian Physiotherapy Association		
CBC	complete blood count	HBV	hepatitus B virus
CDC	Centers for Disease Control	HBsAg	hepatitus B surface antigen
CIDP	chronic inflammatory demyelinating polyneuropathy	HIV	human immunodeficiency virus
		HIV-1	human immunodeficiency virus type 1
CMV	cytomegalovirus	HIV-2	human immunodeficiency virus type 2
CNS	central nervous system	HKAFO	hip-knee-ankle-foot orthosis
CO	carbon monoxide	HPAC	hypothalamic-pituitary adrenocortical system
COG	center of gravity		
CPN	central parenteral nutrition	HR	Heart Rate
CRH	corticotropin-releasing hormone	HRSUB	Submaximal Heart Rate
CSF	cerebrospinal fluid	HSV	herpes simplex virus

HTLV	human T-cell lymphotropic virus
HTLV-III	human T-cell lymphotropic virus type three
HZV	herpes zoster virus
I-ADL	instrumental activities of daily living
IBW	ideal body weight
ICU	intensive care unit
IDP	inflammatory demyelinating neuropathy
IFN	interferon
Ig	immunoglobulin
INH	isoniazid
IPPB	intermittent positive pressure breathing
IQ	intelligence quotient
IV	intravenous
KAFO	knee, ankle, foot orthosis
KS	Kaposi's sarcoma
LAV	lymphadenopathy-associated virus
LIP	lymphocytic interstitial pneumonitis
MA	milliamp
MAC	midarm circumference
MAI	*mycobacterium avium-intracellulare*
MAMC	midarm muscle circumference
MICU	Medical Intensive Care Unit
MMPI	Minnesota Multiphasic Personality Inventory
MMS	Mini-Mental State
MOHO	Model of Human Occupation
MRI	magnetic resonance imaging
NDT	neurodevelopmental treatment
NE	norepinephrine
NG	nasogastric
NIH	National Institutes of Health
NIMH	National Institute of Mental Health
NIOSH	National Institute for Occupational Safety and Health
NK	natural killer
NRS	National Research Council
NSAID	nonsteroidal anti-inflammatory drug
OMD	organic mental disorder
OSHA	Occupational Safety and Health Association
OT	occupational therapy
PADL	personal activities of daily living
PaO$_2$	Arterial Oxygen Tension
PCM	protein calorie malnutrition
PCP	*Pneumocystis Carinii pneumonia*
PDI	Pain Disability Index

PET	positron emission tomography
PHA	phytohemagglutinin
PLWA	person living with AIDS
PML	progressive multifocal leukoencephalopathy
PMHR	predicted maximum heart rate
PMN	polymorphonuclear neutrophil
PNF	proprioceptive neuromuscular facilitation
PNI	psychoneuroimmunology
PNS	peripheral nervous system
POMS	Profile of Mood States
PPN	peripheral parenteral nutrition
PPT	pulmonary physical therapy
PRE	progressive resistance exercise
PROM	passive range of motion
PT	physical therapy
PWA	person with AIDS
RDA	Recommended Daily Allowances
RHR	resting heart rate
RNA	ribonucleic acid
ROM	range of motion
RR	respiratory rate
SAM	sympathoadrenomedullary
SIV	simian immunodeficiency virus
SOB	shortness of breath
SUNY	State University of New York
TB	tuberculosis
TEE	total energy expenditure
TENS	transcutaneous electrical nerve stimulation
TIBC	total iron binding capacity
TMP/SMX	trimethoprim-sulfamethoxazole
TPN	total parenteral nutrition
TSF	triceps skinfold
ua	microamperage
UBW	usual body weight
US	United States
USDH & HS	United State Department of Health and Human Services
USRDA	United States Recommended Daily Allowance
WB	Western Blot
WHO	World Health Organization
WR	Walter Reed (Staging System)
ZDV	azidothymidine

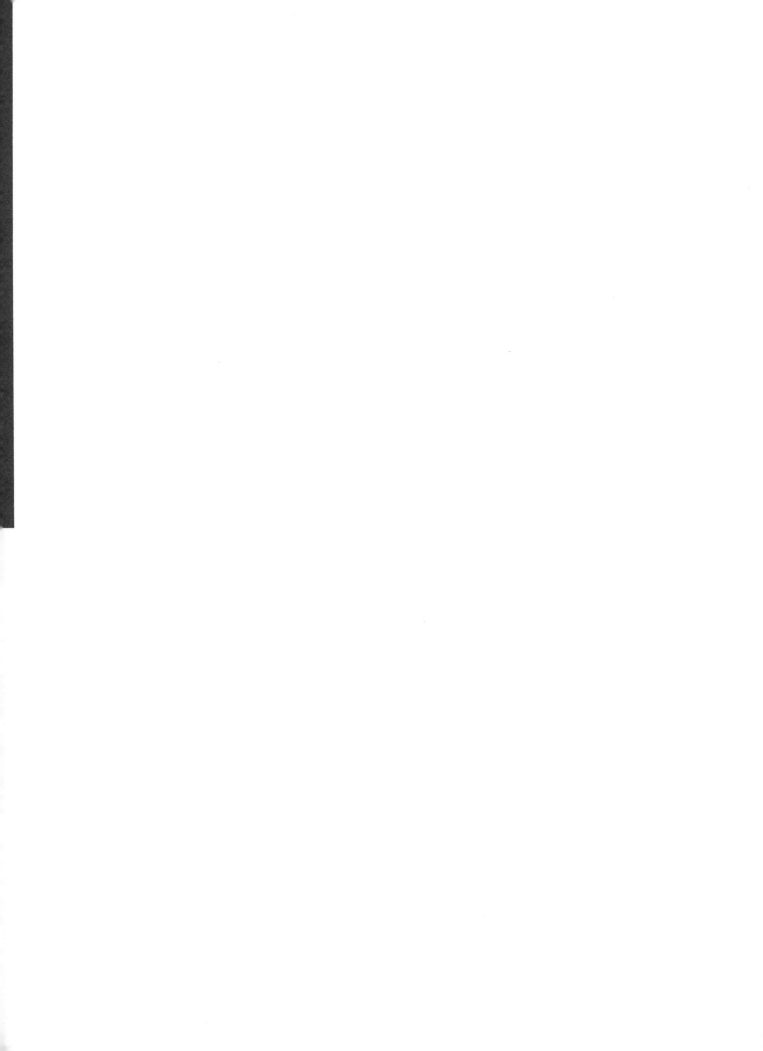

Glossary

ACTH (Adrenocorticotropic Hormone)—hormone secreted by anterior pituitary gland, which stimulates glucocorticoid steroid hormone production by the adrenal cortex.

Aerobic exercise—physical activities performed with oxygen intake which utilizes fat as an energy source.

Afferent phase—the period of the immune response when the leukocyte (white blood cells) move toward the lymphoid tissue.

Agglutination—the clumping of cells, especially red blood cells.

Agranular leukocytes—the type of white blood cells (leukocytes) that do not contain microscopically distinct cytoplasmic granules, namely lymphocytes and monocytes.

Anaphylaxis—the anaphylactic reaction whereby the body is in a state of shock due to the hypersensitivity response to an antigen, eg. allergic response to a bee sting.

Antibody—the immunoglobulin, IgA, IgE, IgG, IgM or IgD, synthesized and released by plasma cells in response to the presence of a specific antigen.

Antigen—the particle in the body recognized as foreign, which evokes an immune response, eg. pollen or bacteria.

Antitoxin—the substance that neutralizes the toxin produced by certain bacteria.

Anxiety—an unpleasant emotional state whose causes may not be easily identified (distinguished from fear which is an emotional and physiologic response to a recognized threat) and which has accompanying symptoms of worry (apprehensive expectation); motor tension or restlessness; fatiguability; shortness of breath; fast heart rate; sweating; dizziness or light headedness; dry mouth, nausea, diarrhea, or other abdominal distress; flushes or chills; frequent urination; difficulty swallowing; feeling on edge; exaggerated startle response; concentration problems; trouble falling or staying asleep; irritability. Other anxiety disorders include phobias, panic states and obsessive-compulsive disturbances.

Anxiolytic—a chemical compound that reduces or dispels anxiety. Most common are the benzodiazepines, such as diazepam (Valium), alprazolam (Xanax), lorazepam (Ativan), oxazepam (Serax), temazepam (Restoril), chloretiazepoxide (Librium), and clorazepate (Tranxene). Buspirone (Buspar) is a nonbenzodiazepine anxiolytic that achieves its effect after multiple doses, but without sedation, motor slowing or potentiation by other depressants such as alcohol.

Autonomic nervous system—the part of the nervous system concerned with control of involuntary bodily functions. It controls function of glands, smooth muscle tissue and the heart.

Autonomy—a term derived from the Greek *autos* (self) and *nomos* (rule, governance, or law) and was first used to refer to self-rule of self-governance in Greek city-states. The most general idea of personal autonomy is still that of self-governance: being one's own person, without constraints either by another's action or by psychological or physical limitations.

B-cells—abbreviated name for the B-lymphocytes derived from the bursa of Fabricius. It is the major cell involved in the humoral immune response.

B-lymphocytes—one of two distinct types of lymphocytes, namely B-lymphocytes and T-lymphocytes. It is also known as a B-cell.

Basophils—a type of granular leukocyte containing large, bluish-black, cytoplasmic granules visible with a light microscope.

Beck depression scale—a 20-item scale designed to tap clinical levels of depression.

Beneficence—the duty to help others further their important and legitimate interests. The duty to confer benefits and actively to prevent and remove harms.

Beta adrenergic receptor—a site in autonomic nerve

pathways wherein inhibitory responses occur when adrenergic agents such as norepinephrine and epinephrine are released.

Bursa cells—the B-cells derived from the bursa of Fabricius.

Bursa of Fabricius—the area of the cloaca of the chicken responsible for the production of B-cells. The corresponding part in humans is located in the gut.

C3B receptor—in the complement system, the third complement protein whose receptor side can be activated to enhance the immune response.

Cardiovascular endurance—low muscle forces in human movement during maximum performance; may be subdivided into aerobic or anaerobic-aerobic endurance.

Cardiovascular fitness—can be compared by the response of heart rate to a given amount of work.

CD4 (T-helper/inducer cell)—the regulatory functions carried out by T-helper lymphocytes are essential to B-cell differentiation and proliferation into antibody-producing plasma cells. CD4 cells help is both indirect, ie. mediated by T-cell products, such as interleukin-2, and direct.

CD45RA+CD4+—a subset of CD4 cells, which induce the production of T-suppressor cells clones, which inhibit B-cell maturation.

Cell-fixing—when freshly gathered live cells are immersed in a solution that preserves or "fixes" cell organelles such as mitochondrial and the golgi apparatus, eg. ethanol.

Cell-mediated immune response—one of the immune responses involving T-lymphocytes and their production of lymphokines to combat intracellular antigens primarily.

Cellular immunity—the reaction to antigenic material of specific defensive cells (macrophages) rather than antibodies. This reaction is thought to break down in AIDS.

Clinical trial—studies with human subjects.

Clone—cells derived from the same cell line.

Complement system—nine interacting proteins, C1-C9, circulate in the blood in inactive form. Complement-fixing antibodies, IgG and IgM, can activate the various complement proteins by binding to C1, which causes a cascade reaction resulting in the enhancement of the immune response.

Confidentiality—the duty to keep secret all information about a patient gained in the course of professional-client relationship unless given permission to disclose by the patient or if there is threat of harm by keeping the information secret.

Corticosteroids—a steroid substance obtained from the cortex of the adrenal gland.

Corticotropin-releasing hormone (CRH)—a neurohormone, produced in the paraventricular nucleus of the hypothalamus, which regulates the release of adrenocorticotropic hormone (ACTH) from the pituitary gland and is itself regulated by inhibitory feedback of ACTH and its hormonal products, cortisol and corticosterone.

Cortisol—a glucocorticoid hormone secreted by the adrenal cortex. Cortisol regulates carbohydrate, protein, and lipid metabolism, and also acts as an anti-inflammatory.

Cyclic AMP (cyclic adenosine monophosphate [cAMP])—a ubiquitous nucleotide, cyclic AMP acts as a "second messenger" within the cytoplasm of the cell, mediating the effects of a first messenger (hormone, or neurotransmitter) upon the distinctive functional properties of the cell. This complex chain of events, which includes the phosphorylation of proteins by cAMP-dependent kinase enzymes, is initiated by the coupling of a first messenger molecule (ligand) with a specific receptor at the cell membrane.

Cytotoxicity—the process by which a cell (T-lymphocyte, natural killer cell) attacks and kills a viral-infected cell.

Dementia—acquired deterioration of cognitive functions from a previous level, including loss of memory, abstract thinking, linguistic functions and personality change. There is no clouding of consciousness. "Subcortical" dementia may appear as cognitive forgetfulness with awareness and motoric disruption; whereas dementia may involve aphasia, amnesia without awareness or visuospatial disturbances.

Depression—a disorder of affect that includes pervasive depressed mood, loss of interest or pleasure in activities, significant weight loss or gain, insomnia or increased sleep, psychomotoric slowing or agitation, inappropriate loss of energy or fatigue, feelings of worthlessness or guilt, difficulty with concentration or decision making and recurrent thoughts of death or suicide. Depression is sadness over a situational stressor or grief and bereavement over a real or anticipated loss.

EEG (electroencephalogram)—the recording of the brain's spontaneous bioelectrical activity from electrodes placed on the scalp. An array is usually used to survey the entire surface of the brain. However, the recording reflects the summation of electrical potentials under the electrode and is the record of functioning of millions of cells. Certain rhythms and wave forms are indicative of different states of alertness and mental activity, as well as electrical dysfunctions, such as seizures. Some patterns are correlated with brain metabolism dysfunction and destructive lesions, such as tumors or infections.

Endogenous opiates—a group of polypeptides that can act both as a neuromodulator and hormone. The endorphins derived from the prohormone beta-lipotropin mediate analgesia, and play a role in adaptive behavior and affective disorders. Also includes methionine [MET]- and leucine [LEU]-enkephalin.

Eosinophils—one of the three types of granular leukocytes: eosinophils, basophils and neutrophils. Its cytoplasm contains large, reddish-pink granules visible with a light microscope. It is primarily involved in allergic and parasitic reactions.

Epidemiology—study of the relationships of the various factors determining the frequency and distribution of diseases in a human environment.

Epinephrine—one of the two active hormones produced by the adrenal medulla. Its effects are similar to those brought by stimulation of the sympathetic division of the autonomic nervous system.

Etiology—study of the factors that cause disease.

Evoked potentials—neural electrical responses to various kinds of stimulation, sensed by electronic amplification of those responses picked up through externally applied electrodes (usually to the scalp overlying brain regions that sense these stimuli). Auditory evoked potentials are usually averaged responses to clicks; visual evoked responses are responses to light flashes or changing visual pattern presented to the eyes; somatosensory evoked potential are responses to electrical stimulation of peripheral muscles and nerves.

Fox equation—a method of estimating VO^2max.

Glucocorticoid—a general classification of adrenal cortical hormones that are primarily active in protecting against stress and in affecting protein and carbohydrate metabolism.

Heuristic—a device that organizes principles and theories for the purpose of guiding future research.

HIV testing (ELISA)—programs to provide a confirmatory test, principally the Western Blot, to individuals who have positive ELISA results.

HPAC—hypothalamic pituitary adrenocortical system.

Humoral immunity—an immune response involving B-lymphocytes and their production of antibodies to combat extracellular antigens primarily.

Hydraulic resistance—the opposition to the force created when a piston-like device is set in motion against a fluid-filled chamber.

Informed consent—the giving of consent for diagnostic, therapeutic or experimental medical procedures after a thorough explanation of the risks and benefits of the procedure.

Interleukin-1 (IL-1)—a polypeptide compound (monokine) derived from activated macrophages, which promotes T-lymphoblast differentiation to the T-helper (CD4) cell subclass.

Interleukin-2 (IL-2)—a mediator substance (lymphokine) released by T-helper (CD4) cells, which affects the proliferation and differentiation of B-lymphocytes, T-suppressor (CD8) cells, and cytotoxic T-lymphocytes.

Justice—the distribution of health resources based on some formulation of the concept of fairness.

Kaposi's sarcoma (KS)—a rare form of skin cancer, characterized by raised, nontender, purplish lesions. These lesions may occur on any part of the body, notably the upper body and extremities.

Kuppfer cells—Scavenger macrophages confined to the liver.

Lentiviruses—the subfamily of retroviruses including HIV. These viruses have long incubation periods and severely impair immune system functions.

Lymphocytes—a type of agranular leukocyte primarily responsible for humoral immunity (B-cells) and cell-mediated immunity (T-cells).

Lymphoid—the tissue that contain aggregates of B- and T-cells, eg. tonsils, spleen, lymph nodes and lymph nodules.

Lymphokines—chemical produced by T-cells to destroy intracellular parasites such as the tubercle bacillus (TB) and the AIDS virus (HIV).

Macrophages—a type of phagocytic cell primarily responsible for phagocytosis.

Mania—or manic episode, is a state of persistently elevated, expansive or irritable mood; inflated self-esteem or grandiosity; decreased need for sleep and increased talkativeness; flight of ideas or feeling that thoughts are racing; distractibility; increase in goal-oriented activities or agitations; and excessive involvement in pleasurable activities that have a great potential for painful consequences that the individual seems unable to recognize (eg. spending lots of money, sexual sprees).

Mast cells—connective tissue cells that synthesize and release histamines and heparin in the early inflammatory response and in the immune response.

Maximum oxygen consumption (VO^2max)—an indicator of aerobic fitness level.

Memory cells—in the humoral response, when an antigen stimulates an immature lymphocyte, it causes the cell to divide. One of the two cells formed proliferates and matures to form a specific antibody-producing plasma cell, and the other proliferates to become a memory cell. The memory cell remains dormant until the next encounter with the same specific antigen months or years later. The memory cell then becomes activated to proliferate and differentiate into mature plasma cells, the end line of B-cell differentiation.

Monocyte—one of the two types of agranular leukocytes, lymphocyte and monocyte. It is the stem cell of the macrophage derived from the bone marrow promonocyte. After differentiation, it forms the monocyte found in the blood. Due to its ameboid action, the monocyte meanders to the outside of the blood vessel to become the mature macrophage whose function is phagocytosis.

Morbidity—frequency of disease occurrence in proportion to the population.

Mortality—frequency of number of deaths in proportion to population.

MRI (magnetic resonance imaging)—a technique for deriving an image of body structures in which the body is put into an intense magnetic field to align all atoms, usually hydrogen, in a certain direction. The field is then released and sensors detect the configuration of the atoms as compared to their prealigned state and an image is formed. The T2-weighted isotope is especially helpful in imaging subtle distinctions of the white matter of the brain.

Neurobehavioral—the consideration of behavior, cognitive and emotion based on the brain structures and functions that subserve these activities.

Neuroendocrine—pertaining to the nervous and endocrine systems as an integrated functioning mechanism.

Neuropeptide—peptide hormone produced by neurons and neurosecretory cells, which demonstrates neurotransmitter like activity. Hypothalamic releasing hormones, adenohypophyseal and neurohypophyseal hormones secreted by the pituitary gland, and the endogenous opioids are all neuropeptides.

Neutrophils—the smallest of the three granular leukocytes, it is one of the major phagocytic cells, along with the macrophage. The neutrophil is predominantly found in blood except during an acute inflammatory response, when it is summoned to the inflammatory side. The neutrophil and macrophage are the major phagocytic cells of the body.

Nonmaleficence—the duty not to injure or to avoid harming a patient.

Norepinephrine (NE)—a widely distributed neurotransmitter in the central nervous system, norepinephrine is also an agent of sympathetic nervous system activity, as well as a hormone released in the general circulation from the chromaffin tissue of the adrenal medulla.

Norepinephrine is important in blood pressure control, muscular coordination, defensive reactions, and in the mediation of mood.

OKT3 and OKT4—Ortho Corporation markers for total T-lymphocytes and CD4+ subset.

Opsonizing—when antibodies attach themselves to the surface of bacteria, enhancing phagocytosis.

Paternalism—the principle and practice of paternal administration; government as by a father; the claim or attempt to supply the needs or to regulate the life a patient in the same way a father does those of his children. Often places autonomy in conflict with beneficence.

PHA—mitogen phytohemagglutinin.

Phagocytosis—the process whereby scavenger cells, namely macrocytes and polys, engulf foreign matter and cellular debris.

Phagosome—when the macrophage has engulfed the antigen, it form a food vacuole known as a phagosome.

Plasma cell—the most highly differentiated cell of the B-lymphocyte line responsible for the production of antibodies.

Polymorphonuclear leukocytes—another name for neutrophils, sometimes also referred to as polymorphonuclear neutrophils (PMNs) or polys.

POMS—profile of mood states.

Positron-emission tomography (PET) scan—technology whereby functioning of a tissue (eg. the brain) is imaged by the utilization of glucose tagged with a radioactive element (radioactive fluorine). The gradations of amount of glucose sensed by multiple external sensors is portrayed as an image of the working of the tissue.

Positive HIV test—a sample of blood that is reactive on an initial ELISA test, repeatedly reactive on a second ELISA run of the same specimen and reactive on Western Blot, if available.

Post-test counseling—programs that provide individual counseling after HIV testing and that include the results, whether positive or negative, the implications of an individual's HIV status and any necessary referrals for additional counseling or medical assessment.

Predictive of AIDS—indicating presence of HIV infection.

Predictive value positive (PVP)—the probability that a person with a reactive test has the disease and is not falsely reactive.

Pre-test counseling—programs to provide individual counseling before HIV testing that detail the reasons for, possible risks of and implications of possible results of HIV testing.

Prevalence—the total number of persons with a disease in a given population at a given time. Prevalence is usually expressed as the percentage of the population that has the disease.

Primary immune response—the first response of the immune system to an antigen (humoral response). Upon infection, there is a latency period usually of several days before significant amounts of antibody accumulate in the body. In this primary response, antibody levels slowly rise and then gradually diminish; however, memory cells are retained.

Psychoneuroimmunology (PNI)—a growing area of behavioral medicine research that studies the interaction of biobehavioral, cognitive/affective, psychosocial, neuroendocrine/neuropeptide and immunologic phenomena. It establishes an area of scientific research that demonstrates an interrelationship between the brain and altering immune responses.

Retrovirus—viruses whose genetic information is encoded in ribonucleic acid (RNA) instead of the common desoxyribonucleic acid (DNA). Therefore, the expression of 15 the viral RNA can take place only after its conversion to DNA.

Reverse transcriptase—the enzyme that transcribes in a reverse order, converting an RNA genome to a complementary strand of DNA. HIV is a retrovirus whose genetic information is transcribed through the use of this enzyme during replication.

SAM—sympathoadrenomedullary system.

Secondary immune response—when antigen is presented the second time, after the primary immune response. Immunoglobulins appear after a short latency period in higher concentration and at a faster rate.

Sensitivity—the probability that a test will be positive when infection is present.

Seroconversion—the point at which an individual exposed to the Human Immunodeficiency Virus becomes serologically positive.

Serologic—pertaining to blood serum.

Seropositive—condition in which antibodies to a specific antigen are found in blood.

Seroprevalence—prevalence based on blood serum tests.

Serotonin—in an allergic reaction, Ig E attaches itself to the surface of most cells and basophils. Then, when a specific antigen subsequently reacts with the specific antibody, exceedingly large quantities of histamine, heparin, bradykinin and serotonin are released, resulting in severe local vascular and tissue responses. It is also a well established neurotransmitter synthesized from tryptophan.

Stem cell—the undifferentiated pluripotential baseline cell, which upon stimulation, develops into a highly organized, well-differentiated cell.

Suppressor T-cells—there are two basic types of T-cells: T-suppressor cells and T-helper cells. T-suppressor cells depress the function of T-helper cells.

Surveillance—process of monitoring public health conditions such as epidemics. Passive surveillance monitors conditions through the receipt of reports; active surveillance uses investigative techniques.

T-cell rosetting—a formation of a cluster (rosette) of cells consisting of sheep erythrocytes and human T-lymphocytes.

T-cells—abbreviated name for T-lymphocytes derived from the thymus. It is the major cell involved in the cell-mediated immune response.

Thymus—the gland that provides the immune system with T-lymphocytes, otherwise known as T-cells.

Thymus cell—the cells of the thymus gland that are progenitor cells of the T-lymphocytes.

T-lymphocyte—one of two types of lymphocytes. It is the major cell involved in the cell-mediated immune response.

Western blot—blood test that involves the identification of antibodies against specific protein molecules. This test is more specific than the ELISA test in detecting antibodies to HIV in blood samples. It is used to confirm a positive ELISA test. The Western blot requires more sophisticated lab technique than the ELISA and is more expensive.

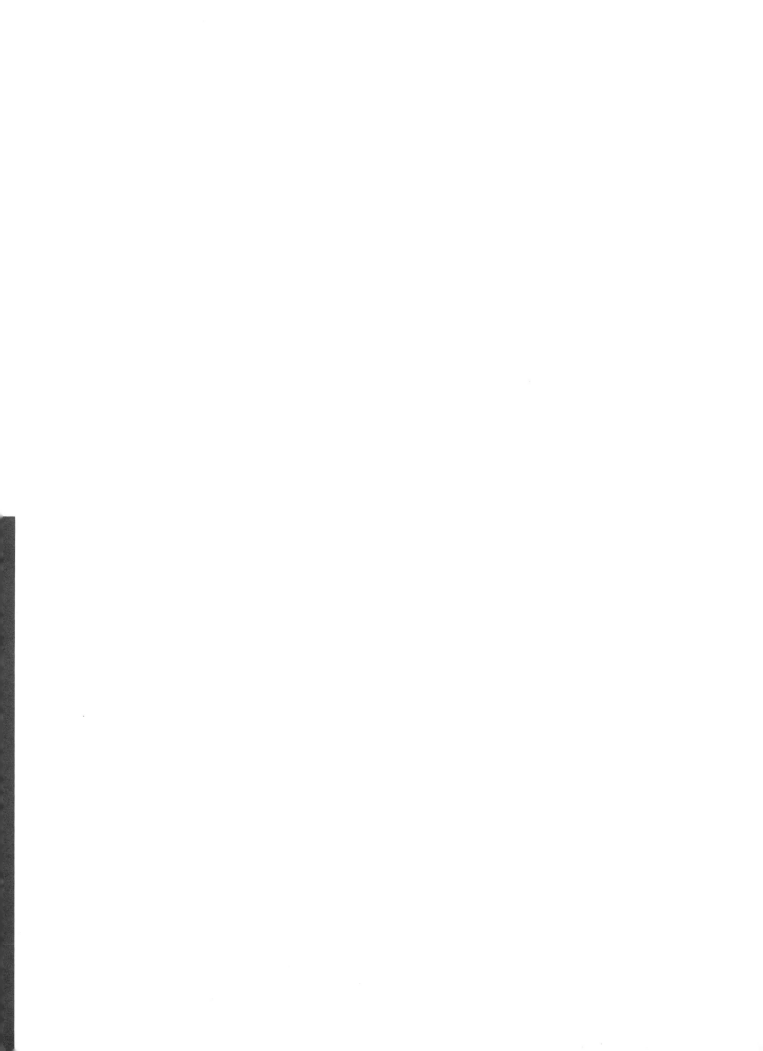

Index